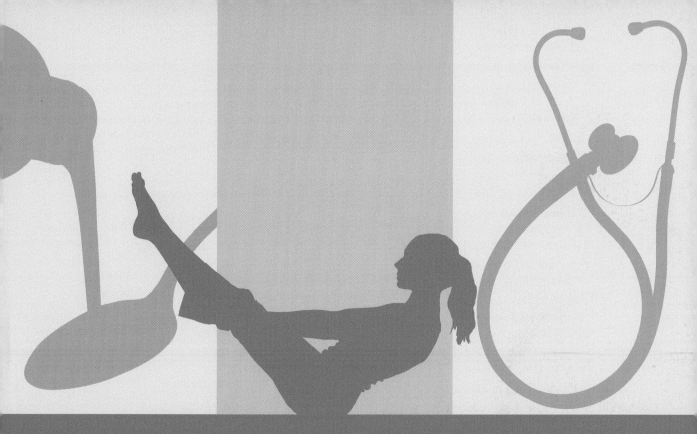

what works
what doesn't

THE BOTTOM LINE ON
EVERYTHING HEALTH

Reader's Digest

The Reader's Digest Association, Inc.
Pleasantville, New York | Montreal

Project Staff

Editor
Marianne Wait

Designer
Rich Kershner

Layout/Production
Erick Swindell

Writers
Ron Geraci, Debra Gordon,
Timothy Gower, Sarí Harrar,
Amy Paturel

Copy Editor/Proofreader
Jane Sherman

Indexer
Cohen Carruth Indexes

RDA Content Creation Studio

VP, Editor in Chief
Neil Wertheimer

Creative Director
Michele Laseau

Executive Managing Editor
Donna Ruvituso

Associate Director, North America Prepress
Douglas A. Croll

Manufacturing Manager
John L. Cassidy

Marketing Director
Dawn Nelson

The Reader's Digest Association, Inc.

President and Chief Executive Officer
Mary G. Berner

President, Emerging Businesses
Alyce C. Alston

SVP, Chief Marketing Officer President & CEO, Direct Holdings
Amy J. Radin

Library of Congress Cataloging-in-Publication Data
What works what doesn't : the bottom line on everything health.
    p. cm.
 ISBN 978-0-7621-0558-8
 1.   Medicine, Popular—Encyclopedias.
 RC81.A2W53 2008
 616.003—dc22
                                    2008018006

Address any comments about *What Works, What Doesn't* to:
The Reader's Digest Association, Inc.
Editor in Chief, Books
Reader's Digest Road
Pleasantville, NY 10570-7000

To order copies of *What Works, What Doesn't*,
call 1-800-846-2100.

Visit our online store at **rdstore**.com

Printed in the United States of America

7 9 10 8 6

US 6003/IC

Note to Readers
The information in this book should not be substituted for, or used to alter, medical therapy without your doctor's advice. For a specific health problem, consult your physician for guidance. The mention of any products, retail businesses, or Web sites in this book does not imply or constitute an endorsement by the authors or by the Reader's Digest Association, Inc.

Among the scores of top experts we consulted are ...

M. Christie Ballantyne, MD, FACC
Director, Center for Cardiovascular
Disease Prevention
Baylor College of Medicine

Joan Salge Blake, MS, RD, LDN
Clinical Assistant Professor
of Nutrition
Boston University

Ian Blumer, MD

Shanthy Bowman, PhD
Nutrient Data Laboratory
US Department of Agriculture

Tod Cooperman, MD
President
ConsumerLab.com

Felicia Cosman, MD
Clinical Director
National Osteoporosis Foundation

Joseph Dello Russo, MD
Lasik surgeon

Karl Doghramji, MD
Director, Sleep Disorders Center
Thomas Jefferson University

Joann G. Elmore, MD, MPH
Professor of Medicine
Adjunct Professor of Epidemiology
University of Washington School
of Medicine

Mary B. Engler, PhD, RN, MS
Director, Cardiovascular and
Genomics Graduate Program
University of California,
San Francisco

Edzard Ernst, MD, PhD
Laing Chair In Complementary
Medicine
Peninsula Medical School

Joshua J. Fenton, MD, MPH
Assistant Professor
Department of Family and
Community Medicine
University of California, Davis

Matthew Freeman, CNP, MPH

Keri M. Gans, RD, MS, CDN
President, New York State
Dietetic Association
Spokesperson, American
Dietetic Association

Jeannie Gazzaniga-Moloo, PhD, RD
Spokesperson, American
Dietetic Association

Chuck Gerba, PhD
Professor of Microbiology
University of Arizona

Christine Gerbstadt, MD, RD

Hayes Gladstone, MD
Director of Dermatologic Surgery
Stanford University School
of Medicine

Elizabeth A. Gollub, PhD, MPH, RD
Nutrition Consultant

William S. Harris, PhD
Research Professor of Medicine
Sanford School of Medicine
University of South Dakota

Randy C. Hatton, PharmD
Co-Director, Drug Information
and Pharmacy Resource Center
Clinical Professor
University of Florida College
of Pharmacy

Katherine Hillblom, PharmD
American Pharmacists Association

Robert H. Hopkins, MD, FACP, FAAP
Associate Professor of Internal
Medicine and Pediatrics
University of Arkansas
for Medical Sciences

Mady Hornig, MA, MD
Associate Professor
of Epidemiology
Mailman School of Public Health
Columbia University

Carolyn Jacob, MD
Dermatologist

Ed Kang
Spokesperson, Consumer Product
Safety Commission

Bruce Katz, MD
Clinical Professor of Dermatology
Mt. Sinai School of Medicine

D'anne M. Kleinsmith, MD
Dermatologist

Robert Kotler, MD, FACS
Clinical Instructor
University of California, Los Angeles

Sarah Krein, PhD, RN
Research Investigator
University of Michigan
Health System

Kelly McGonigal, PhD
Editor in Chief, *International
Journal of Yoga Therapy*

Robert Pallay, MD
Program Director, Family Medicine
Memorial University Medical Center

Laurie Polis, MD
Cosmetic Dermatologist

Vicki Rackner, MD

Sandra Read, MD
Dermatologist

Leif Rogers, MD
Plastic and Reconstructive Surgeon

Jonathan Scher, MD
Assistant Clinical Professor of
Obstetrics, Gynecology
and Reproductive Science
Mt. Sinai Medical Center

Peter S. Sebel, MD, PhD
Professor of Anesthesiology
Emory University

Michael Shannon, MD
Professor and Chair of
Emergency Medicine
Children's Hospital Boston

Robert H. Shmerling, MD
Clinical Chief, Division of
Rheumatology
Beth Israel Deaconess
Medical Center

Lauren Streicher, MD
Clinical Assistant Professor
Department of Obstetrics
and Gynecology
Northwestern University
Feinberg School of Medicine

Anne Thurn
NIH Office of Dietary Supplements

Peter Wyer, MD
Associate Clinical Professor
of Medicine
Columbia University College
of Physicians & Surgeons

Ann Yelmokas McDermott, PhD, MS, LN
Director, Center for Obesity
Prevention and Education
California Polytechnic
State University

contents

What This Book Can Do for You/9

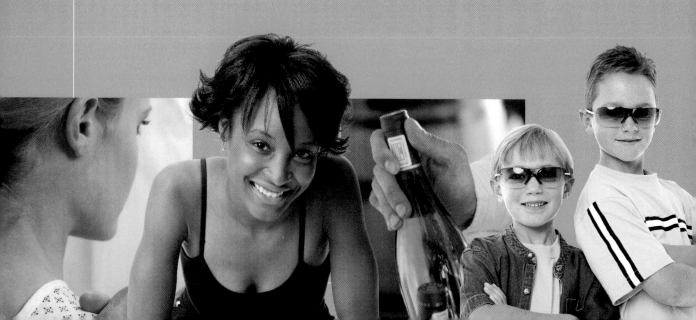

PART 3
treating what ails you

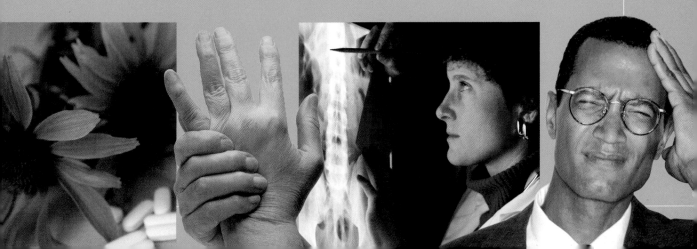

PART 4
is it safe or dangerous?

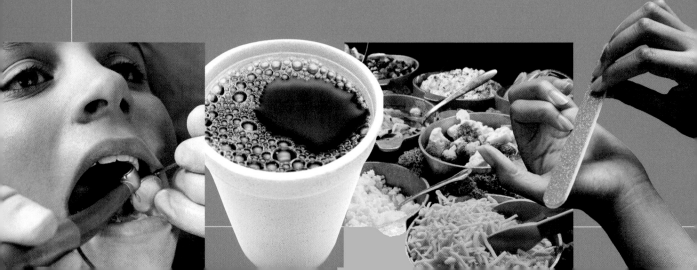

what this book can do for you

Why do people take cough syrup? To stop coughs! But what if we told you that a review of 15 studies, published in the prestigious *British Medical Journal*, cast serious doubt on whether these vile-tasting elixirs work? And that a group of chest physicians now discourages their use because there's simply no evidence that they do anything? You might stop pouring money down your throat and fire up an old-fashioned vaporizer instead.

Before you take a medicine, start a new diet or exercise regimen, get a medical test, or swallow a supplement, why not find out first if it's worth the effort—and whether something else might work better? It's easy to do with *What Works, What Doesn't*. To create this book, we pored over hundreds of the best quality, most definitive studies ever conducted and talked to scores of leading doctors and health specialists about everything from weight-loss pills to water filters to figure out—you guessed it—what works and what doesn't when it comes to improving your health.

Some of the answers surprised us. A simple salt-water rinse for allergies? It works! Botox for killer head pain? Worth trying. Beta-blockers for high blood pressure? Despite the widespread use of these drugs, according to the hard evidence, they aren't your best choice. Cutting calories? Shockingly, not the best way to lose weight.

Whether it's something you eat, take, do, or use around the house, if it has to do with your health, we investigated it. Of course, we paid special attention to the treatments we use to cure what ails us, from vitamin C for the common cold (thumbs down) to fiber supplements for constipation (you may not be happy with the results) to angioplasty for blocked arteries. While we were at it, we looked into the safety of some common products and practices, putting everything from artificial sweeteners to acupuncture under the microscope. Does MSG really cause headaches? Can vaccinations trigger autism? You'll find some unexpected answers—for instance, hormone replacement therapy may be considerably safer than you think, while generic drugs aren't always the foolproof substitutes they're made out to be.

This book provides the most comprehensive, most reliable advice on what's worth spending your time, money, and energy on and what you should simply walk away from. We based the information on the best available scientific evidence, but keep in mind a couple of points. Sometimes there simply aren't enough good studies to allow a firm conclusion to be drawn. And even the best studies don't always tell the whole story. Every person and every case is different. There is no guarantee that something that "works" will work for you—or that something that "doesn't" won't. It's important that you team up with your doctor to determine the right course of action. But do your research first. We've done a lot of it for you, and you can do more at any time by using the tips in the chapter "How to Be a Smart Medical Consumer." The more you know the better you'll feel, in so many ways.

—**Marianne Wait**
Associate Editorial Director,
Reader's Digest Health Books

PART 1

getting to
the truth

how to be a smart
medical
consumer

Will eating more fish stave off a heart attack—or make us sick from toxins? Does sunblock prevent skin cancer? Do cell phones *cause* cancer? These questions, and countless others like them, aren't just interesting research topics for curious scientists. The fact is, we all want and need the answers because our health depends on them.

In the past, when people wondered whether eating sugar caused diabetes or if taking vitamins was a waste of money, they asked their doctors. After all, the men and women in white coats were the gatekeepers of all medical knowledge. No more. The gates have been overwhelmed by a torrent of scientific research. Hardly a week passes without a new discovery—often one that purports to turn an old one on its head. How can a doctor who's racing from one exam room to the next to keep up with his patient load also keep up with every last development? It's simple: He can't.

The rise of the Internet has created another kind of deluge: the flood of medical information that spills onto a computer screen with just a few keystrokes—some of it valuable, some scary, and some just plain wrong. Anyone with a laptop and a Web browser can find their way to both groundbreaking studies published in respected journals and medical quackery masquerading as science.

News stories about health aren't wholly reliable either. They bombard the eye and ear, aimed at an aging population suddenly worried about becoming sick. But the headlines are often misleading, and the messages seem to change faster than the seasons, partly because they weren't always right to begin with. If today's paper brings news that your favorite food causes cancer, don't panic; next month you're just as likely to read that it's harmless.

The real truth often lies buried, and you may have to do some digging to find it. It's worth the effort: There's no doubt that the smartest, best-informed medical consumers get superior care—and ultimately enjoy longer, healthier lives. To get the best that modern healthcare has to offer you and your family, you must learn how to make sense of the bewildering variety of choices and information available to you.

In this chapter, we'll arm you with the tools you'll need. We've also done our own digging—you might call it a major excavation, in fact—in the quest for solid, objective answers to your most pressing health questions, and you'll find the results throughout the rest of this book. How often should you have a physical exam? What really works for headaches? Is it safe to eat barbecued meat? We've put these and many, many other questions to the test by poring over the latest, best-quality research and calling upon key experts to deliver the truth. Some of the answers will surprise you; you'll see that many deeply entrenched ideas about medicine are based on flimsy research or none at all. The next time you confront a health conundrum—Is surgery the best option for my aching back? Is organic food worth the price?—you can look up the answers here.

Getting the Best Healthcare

It always pays to be a smart medical consumer, but never more than when you're sick. Gone are the days when there was one approach to getting you well, and you accepted it without question. Today, smart patients search for the right treatment or surgeon the way they shop for a new car or dishwasher. They do research. They arm themselves with healthy skepticism. They ask a lot of questions. In a world where medical treatment is expensive and options abound, more and more patients want to know: Am I getting the best bang for my healthcare buck? Is this really the best medical treatment for my condition? How do you know?

When Stephen H. Schneider learned he had a rare form of non-Hodgkin's lymphoma, a type of cancer, he realized he had two options. He could become an average patient, doing everything his doctors told him and hoping for the best, or he could learn everything he could about his disease and put his knowledge to use. He took the latter course, reading up on all the treatment approaches available, both standard and experimental. And he questioned his doctors every step of the way.

Not that he kicked and screamed. Schneider simply asked his doctors to let him participate in making decisions about his treatment. They were reluctant at first but eventually saw that he truly understood his disease, and then they took his input seriously. In several instances, he persuaded them to bend the rules and try nonstandard therapies—which may be one reason he lived to write about his experience in *The Patient from Hell.*

Schneider had an advantage over most patients in terms of understanding the nuances of medical research, since he's a noted scientist who studies global warming at Stanford University. But an advanced degree isn't required to become a better medical consumer. All you need is persistence, a willingness to ask questions, and a perception of yourself as a key player in your care instead of a victim.

"Becoming a participant in your treatment tells your doctors you are a savvy patient and that they had better stay on their toes," says Schneider. "It can make a big difference in getting the best—not just average—care."

You can gain a greater sense of control over your health and healthcare by applying the same philosophy to all the quandaries you confront that affect your wellbeing, both large and small. Here, in Part 1 of this book, we'll show you how to:

- Work with doctors in a way that improves your chances of getting top-quality treatment.

Smart patients search for the right treatment or surgeon the way they shop for a car or dishwasher:

They do research.

- Make sense of medical news by knowing when to heed alarming headlines and when to ignore them.
- Find accurate, unbiased information about medical conditions, which will help you make better healthcare decisions.

Understanding Doctors

A century ago, a famous doctor named William Osler, MD, told a group of students, "The practice of medicine is an art, not a trade; a calling, not a business … "

Try telling that to an increasingly common breed of medical consumer, who might respond: "If medicine isn't a business, then why does my orthopedist accept Visa and MasterCard? Furthermore, if my doctor can't fix what's wrong with me, I'll drop him like that mechanic who messed up my muffler."

Medicine may indeed be a calling, like religious ministry, but if doctors were once viewed as god-like, they are now mortals providing a service for which you pay. Remembering that fact can help you get better medical care.

Remember That Doctors Are Fallible

If you cling to the idea that doctors are infallible, you must not watch much television. In the past, fictional doctors were portrayed as twinkle-eyed father figures or dashing heroic types. Today's warts-and-all TV docs wear their flaws and failings—bad marriages, addictions, sour attitudes—on the sleeves of their white coats. The message amid the melodrama is an important one: Doctors are human.

More important, studies show that doctors can—there's no nice way to put it—screw up. The alarming frequency with which mistakes happen in medicine came to light in 1999, when the Institute of Medicine published a report titled "To Err Is Human." The institute, which advises the US government on health issues, estimated that as many as 98,000 people die each year in the United States alone due to medical errors. That means medical errors kill more people than breast cancer and motor vehicle accidents *combined*.

A more recent estimate that appeared in the *Journal of the American Medical Association* places the number of deaths from unnecessary surgery, errors and infections in hospitals, and adverse effects from medications at approximately 225,000 per year. That still makes dying from medical treatment the third leading cause of death in the United States.

Doctors aren't the only people in the healthcare system who can make mistakes that affect the welfare of patients; nurses, pharmacists, and others can err, too. However, Jerome Groopman, MD, of Harvard Medical School and Boston's Beth Israel Deaconess Medical Center, offered an insider's view of why doctors sometimes misdiagnose diseases and recommend the wrong therapies in his book *How Doctors Think*. Simply put, they're just like you and me: Sometimes doctors allow personal biases and feelings to get in the way of dispensing good medicine. Here are three reasons a doctor may give you the wrong diagnosis or miss what's ailing you altogether.

Appearances are deceiving. Dr. Groopman tells the story of an anxious-seeming young woman who was losing weight even though her doctor had advised her to eat a high-calorie diet. The doctor suspected the woman had an eating disorder, such as anorexia. In fact, she had celiac disease, which interferes with the body's ability to absorb nutrients from food.

Everyone makes assumptions. A doctor who's treated a dozen flu patients in a row at the height of an epidemic might unwittingly assume that the next person to enter the exam room with a fever and trouble breathing has the flu, too. However, fever and respiratory problems are also symptoms of many other conditions. In one case Dr. Groopman describes, a woman who had several of the classic signs of the flu mentioned that she had taken "a few aspirin," a remark her doctor dismissed. Doctors later discovered that the woman had actually popped dozens of the white pills. Instead of having the flu, she was in the throes of an aspirin overdose.

Doctors have feelings, too. For their patients, that is. The best doctors are caring and compassionate, of course. But Dr. Groopman points out that caring too much for patients may cause doctors to miss a problem or make the wrong diagnosis. Once he was checking in on a man with cancer who had become his favorite patient on the ward; they shared a love of running and literature, and they talked often. While examining the man's skin, Dr. Groopman became concerned that the patient felt uncomfortable, so he stopped. As a result, he failed to notice an abscess that became infected and could have killed the patient. (Fortunately, he survived.) On the other hand, Dr. Groopman cautions, if you get the strong impression that your doctor does *not* like you, it's time to find a new doctor.

Gut Instincts Can Be Wrong

Even if your doctor gets the diagnosis right, he also needs to get the treatment approach right. It's not usually a guessing game; in most cases, there are clear treatment guidelines published in medical journals and textbooks. These guidelines represent the collective wisdom of scientists who have studied a disease and how best to cure it. They aren't guaranteed to work, but according to scientific studies, they are your best shot at getting better.

Nevertheless, a surprising number of doctors ignore them. For example, researchers at the RAND Corporation, a nonprofit think tank, analyzed the medical records of several thousand patients with a variety of medical conditions in a dozen US cities. The survey determined that patients received the standard recommended preventive care and treatment for their conditions just 55 percent of the time. In some cases, the lapses could have had fatal consequences. For instance, only 45 percent of patients who had suffered heart attacks received prescriptions for beta-blockers, even though these drugs are known to lower the risk of death in this population. What's most shocking about this particular finding is that well-publicized studies confirmed the benefits of beta-blockers for heart attack patients *more than 25 years ago.*

What's going on? Many doctors practicing today continue to base their treatment decisions on the opinions of respected experts within their medical specialty or simply go with their gut

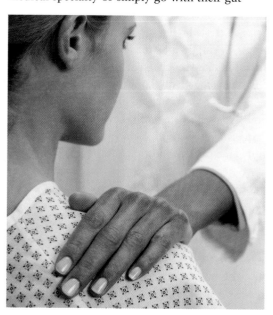

instincts, even when those decisions are at odds with the current medical science, says Peter Wyer, MD, of Columbia University College of Physicians and Surgeons. Dr. Wyer heads a program designed to help doctors understand—and use—clinical research. While he feels there is still a place for doctors to use their intuition and experience when making diagnoses and prescribing treatments, he and many other physicians believe their fellow doctors should use the vast body of scientific data, or evidence, that's available, too. "We want doctors to be evidence-literate," says Dr. Wyer.

How to Be a Better Patient

If you just have a cold, you probably don't need to read this section now. But if you have something more serious, whether it's high blood pressure or cancer, you'll want to learn how to be the best patient you can be in order to make sure you get the best possible medical care. In short, be polite but not a pushover. Be assertive but not bossy. Be informed but not a know-it-all. Taking the following steps will help you build a healthy, balanced relationship with your doctor and get the right care for you, with risks and benefits you're comfortable with.

Understand Your Condition

If you are diagnosed with a disease or disorder, learn all you can about it. You don't need to become an authority—and without going to medical school, you won't become the expert your doctor is—but understanding the basic facts can relieve anxiety by making your condition seem less scary, and it may even improve your odds of getting better. Most important, try to find out what treatment options are available for your condition. If your doctor doesn't offer you one form of therapy, ask why.

If you're not comfortable surfing the Internet for medical information (we'll show you how to do that effectively later on), ask a computer-literate friend or relative to work with you. Furthermore, your local hospital probably has a medical library; call and ask a librarian for help. You can hire a professional service to search for medical literature related to your condition, too. Some employers offer access to services such as Consumer's Medical Resource (www.medicaldecisionsupport.com) as part of employee health plans; ask your human resources representative.

It's also important to understand what your doctor tells you about your condition and your treatment options. Too often, people walk away from an office visit more confused than when they walked in. To ensure that you come away with all the pertinent facts, take the following steps.

- Take along a friend or relative, preferably someone who is a good listener and won't be afraid to speak up on your behalf.
- Carry a pen and notepad and write down important information. If you don't think you can capture the information and listen at the same time, you may want to use a tape recorder.
- Ask your doctor to explain and spell any unfamiliar terms.

Ask Questions

If you get sick enough to need a doctor's care, you may be consumed by a big question: Why me? That's understandable, but moving beyond life's imponderable matters and asking some practical questions can help you feel more at ease and maybe even heal faster. Be sure to ask your doctor to explain anything that you don't understand or that worries you. Here's a short list of questions to get you started.

IF YOU RECEIVE A PRESCRIPTION

- ☐ What is the name of the medicine? How do you spell it?
- ☐ What is it for?
- ☐ How should I take it?
- ☐ What side effects can it cause?

- ☐ Will it interact with other drugs or supplements I take?

IF YOUR DOCTOR ORDERS A DIAGNOSTIC TEST

- ☐ What will this test tell you?
- ☐ How is it performed? Is it painful?
- ☐ How accurate is it?
- ☐ How will you use the results?

IF YOU RECEIVE A DIAGNOSIS

- ☐ What is the technical name of this disease?
- ☐ What is my outlook? What can I expect to happen?
- ☐ What treatment do you recommend?

IF YOUR DOCTOR PRESCRIBES A TREATMENT PLAN

- ☐ What are the risks and benefits?
- ☐ How effective is it?
- ☐ How long before we know whether it's working?
- ☐ What other options do I have?

Understand the Risks of Treatment

If your doctor prescribes a drug, recommends surgery, or suggests any other form of treatment, you will naturally want to know the answers to a few specific questions, such as how well it works and whether the cure is worse than the disease. Your doctor should be able to offer you a clear idea of a treatment's potential benefits as well as its risk of side effects, preferably in the form of statistics from studies of patients who received the therapy. But those numbers can be tricky to interpret.

When a doctor tells you that a drug or procedure will reduce the risk that something bad will occur as a result of your condition, he may describe the drop in *relative risk*, that is, how much the risk will be reduced in someone who receives the therapy as compared to someone who does nothing. For example, studies have shown that widely prescribed cholesterol-lowering drugs called statins reduce the risk of heart attacks by 24 to 37 percent. That sounds pretty impressive, but keep in mind that the likelihood of the average person having a heart attack in a given year is low. Even someone with high cholesterol and other risk factors for heart disease may have only about a 5 percent chance of having a heart attack. Reducing a 5 percent risk by 24 percent brings the risk down to about 3.75 percent. When millions of people take a drug, small benefits like those add up, but that doesn't mean that you personally will see a benefit.

That means doctors end up prescribing statins to many patients who probably never would have developed serious heart trouble. In fact, some studies suggest that at least 63 people need to take a statin for a year in order to prevent a single heart attack. Among patients whose actual heart attack risk is relatively low, studies suggest that the number of patients who must be treated for one year in order to prevent one heart attack in one person is even higher.

If drugs were free and completely safe, none of this would matter much. But medications can be expensive and can cause serious side effects (such as liver and muscle damage in the case of statins). That's why it's important to have a serious discussion with your doctor about whether the benefit of a drug or procedure outweighs the risks.

You don't have to be a math whiz to talk statistics with your doctor. Simply ask what

Talk with your doctor about whether the **benefit of a drug or procedure** outweighs the risks.

Stephen Schneider calls the "100 patients like me" question. For instance, "Out of 100 patients who have my condition, how many will recover if they take treatment A, treatment B, or receive no treatment at all?" or "Of 100 patients who take the medication you're prescribing, how many will develop side effects?"

If your doctor can't give you estimates, ask for her best informed opinion about how well the therapy works, then crosscheck it with another doctor or another source, such as a trusted Web site (you'll get advice on how to find one later in this chapter).

Don't Let the Doctor Rush You

Have you had a long talk with a family doctor recently? If you have, chances are it was on an airplane or at a cocktail party—anywhere but the exam room. The drive-by office visit has become the norm in many clinics. Doctors rush from one appointment to the next, keeping one eye on a patient's chart and the other on the clock.

It's not necessarily their fault. Primary care doctors are unlike auto mechanics and plumbers in one key respect: They get paid per appointment, not for how much time they spend with a patient. Some general practitioners have publicly complained that insurers require them to spend no more than seven minutes with a patient on average.

There is evidence that when doctors rush, good medicine suffers. For example, a 2006 study found that gastroenterologists in one practice who spent more than six minutes performing the critical withdrawal phase of a colonoscopy detected polyps (potentially cancerous growths) in 28 percent of patients. Meanwhile, doctors who spent less than six minutes withdrawing the scope detected polyps in just 12 percent of patients. Even more worrisome: The go-go doctors who raced through colonoscopies detected full-blown colon cancer less than half as often as their more methodical colleagues.

If you feel your doctor is rushing through your office visits, "find another doctor" says Arthur

Levin, director of the Center for Medical Consumers, a nonprofit advocacy organization based in New York City. "There are practices out there that are organized very efficiently," he says, allowing doctors to take more time with patients and still turn a profit.

Take Your Medicine

Drugs don't work if you don't take them. It sounds awfully obvious, yet there are plenty of patients who fail to take their medications as prescribed or quit taking them altogether. Some studies have found that as few as 43 percent of patients with chronic conditions take all of their needed medication. While drugs can cause serious side effects, more than two-thirds of medication-related hospitalizations occur because patients didn't take the drugs prescribed for them.

There are many reasons why people stop taking prescription drugs or miss doses. Some patients who lack insurance can't afford them. Others stop taking needed medications because they misunderstand a doctor's instructions, they fear side effects, they simply forget, or they don't think the drug is working.

If you're having a problem with a drug you've been prescribed, tell your doctor. Taking your meds the way you're supposed to could mean the difference between life and death. One 2006 study of 1,500 heart attack patients found that about one-third quit taking all or some of the medications their doctors prescribed within one month. A year later, patients who had stopped taking all of their prescribed medications were nearly four times more likely to have died than those who continued their medications.

Don't Hesitate to Get a Second Opinion

If this is the oldest advice in the book, why do so many people ignore it? According to a 2005 poll, just 3 percent of people who receive a medical diagnosis always seek second opinions. About half of the 5,000 adults surveyed said they never ask for second opinions. Yet people who do seek them end up changing their course

GET THE RIGHT DRUG AT THE RIGHT DOSE

Each year, 1.5 million people in the United States alone become ill because they receive the wrong drugs or incorrect doses due to errors in writing or filling prescriptions. Following a few simple rules can help you avoid this fate.

Find a good pharmacy—and stick with it. Always buying your medications from the same pharmacy will reduce the risk of receiving the wrong drug. Also, a pharmacist will be better able to spot a potential drug interaction if she has your complete pharmaceutical records.

Make sure you understand the medicine label. Instructions for taking a medication can be confusing; ask the pharmacist to explain anything that isn't clear.

Look inside the bag. Be sure the drug you've been handed is the one your doctor prescribed. When you go to the pharmacy, take along the name of the medication— which you wrote on a pad before leaving your doctor's office, of course.

If you receive a liquid medication, ask your pharmacist for the best way to measure a dose. Getting a precise amount of medicine is important, but research shows that many people make mistakes when measuring doses. For example, if you need one teaspoon of a medication, don't measure it with a spoon from your kitchen drawer; most household teaspoons don't hold a true teaspoon.

of treatment more often than you might think. For instance, in a 2006 study conducted at the University of Michigan, 52 percent of breast cancer patients who sought second opinions about their mammograms and biopsy results changed their treatment plans.

Overall, studies show that second opinions confirm the original diagnosis far more often than not. However, hearing another doctor say that your original diagnosis was accurate can provide peace of mind. What's the right way to go about seeking a second opinion?

Decide whether you really need one. If you have a headache, and your doctor tells you to take two aspirin, you probably don't need to ask the top neurologist in your area to take another look. If you receive any kind of serious diagnosis, however, obtaining a second opinion is appropriate. Experts agree that getting another viewpoint always makes sense if:

- Your doctor recommends major surgery or any other invasive procedure.
- Your doctor diagnoses a rare or life-threatening disease.
- Your doctor is not experienced in treating your condition.
- You are unhappy with your current treatment.
- You have doubts about a diagnosis or believe you haven't been offered all available treatment options.

Do some research first. Reading up on your condition may tell you all you need to know. "If you're willing to do your own research, you will get second, third, and fourth opinions in the literature—other than the one you got from this one doc," says Levin.

Go to another hospital. You can ask the doctor who's treating you to refer you to another doctor for a second opinion. In most cases, your doc won't be offended, since insurance providers often require you to obtain a second opinion before they will pay for certain procedures. (In some cases, health plans cover the cost of seeking a second opinion even if they don't require you to do so.) If your doctor refers you to a colleague down the hall, however, keep in mind that you may find yourself seated across the desk from his racquetball partner, or the two

doctors may eat lunch together every day. That doesn't mean the second doctor will automatically agree with the first, but even if the two aren't best pals, a sense of what Levin calls collegiality may prevent the second doctor from being completely candid—for instance, failing to mention that he thinks your doctor is a dangerous quack.

Talk to a top doctor. There's no sense in getting a second opinion from a doctor who has less experience and expertise than the one you've been seeing. Ask your family doctor for the names of leading specialists or call a major medical center with a reputation for treating your condition. (Some hospitals now offer second opinions via the Internet.) You can also contact local medical societies or medical schools and ask for the names of the best doctors in your area of concern.

Check with a different type of specialist. A spine surgeon tells you that the best treatment option for your chronic back pain is to surgically remove a disk. What do you suppose you'll hear if you seek a second opinion from another spine surgeon? "Chances are, unless the first surgeon is off the wall, the second one will probably agree," says Levin. Yet the medical literature shows that there is no clear winner among the various approaches to managing back pain, and you probably won't hear a full discussion of the potential role of chiropractic, physical therapy, exercise, and other nonsurgical treatments if you talk to only surgeons. The same holds true for virtually any other medical condition. Explore your options by speaking to one or more doctors or other practitioners from different disciplines.

Most experts agree that if the second opinion confirms the original diagnosis, there's no reason to seek more viewpoints. But what do you do when two doctors disagree on what's best for you?

First, compare success rates for the different treatment approaches that have been

GETTING A SECOND OPINION SAVED HER VISION

The doctor's words were blunt and devoid of hope. "I really can't do anything more for you," he told Jenny Nash. "You are going to go blind."

Nash had known for much of her life that she might one day hear this news. Diagnosed with type 1 diabetes at age 15, she was aware that many people with the disease eventually develop diabetic retinopathy, one of the most common causes of blindness. Yet, instead of grief and despair, Nash felt a sense of relief. She had never felt comfortable with the doctor, even though he was a specialist at a major hospital in New York City. "Okay," she thought, "now I'm free to go check with another doctor."

That was in 1985. Nash, then 27, happened to be dating a medical student, who gave her the name of another eye specialist. When Nash consulted him, he brought up something her former doctor had failed to mention: Several eye surgeons in the United States were performing a new procedure that might help her condition.

She met with one of the surgeons, who was based in her home state of Tennessee. He agreed to treat her, and the procedure preserved most of the vision in her right eye. She eventually lost sight in her left eye, so she can't drive a car, and depth perception can be

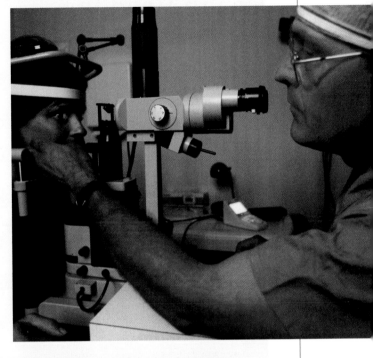

a problem. Two decades after her treatment, however, the "black clouds" that once obscured the view in her right eye are still gone, and she can read, write, and clearly see the faces of her husband and daughter, with whom she lives in Knoxville, Tennessee. "The whole experience," she says, "taught me to trust my gut with doctors."

---

recommended, if they're available. Keep in mind, however, that in the case of surgery and other interventions, these figures represent averages for all procedures performed. A surgeon who specializes in treating a given condition will probably have a better-than-average success rate.

Next, compare the potential side effects and other related factors, such as recovery time from surgery, that accompany each treatment. You may decide that you can't tolerate the risks and requirements of a particular approach.

Finally, seek a third opinion, preferably from an impartial doctor. This may be particularly helpful if doctors from different medical fields have recommended their own unique treatment approaches as the best choice. For example, a urologist may recommend surgery for prostate cancer, while a radiation oncologist is likely to suggest radiation therapy. Some large medical centers now have a medical oncologist on staff who oversees all cancer care and can help patients choose among different treatments.

Looking Beyond the Health Headlines

Why do common foods that once seemed like bit players in your cupboard suddenly become elevated to the status of nutritional saviors, only to have their wondrous health qualities fall into doubt six months later? Why do some drugs that were once touted as "miracle" pills and given the seal of approval by regulatory authorities end up being banned because they're deemed unsafe? In short, why do medical researchers always seem to be contradicting themselves? Why can't they get their stories straight?

It's a major conundrum for average folks interested in protecting their health: How can you trust the results of a new study you heard about on the news when some other study is almost sure to come along next year and prove it wrong?

Why the Story Never Stays the Same

Understanding why the message changes so often will help you maintain a cool head when you hear scary medical news—and use caution when you hear news that sounds too good to be true. There is no single explanation for why medical news seems to shift with the wind, but here are two important reasons.

The media mangles the message. Keeping up with medical news by watching television and reading the newspaper is like watching the trailer for a new movie: You get bits and pieces of the story, but you don't see the whole picture.

Bad or incomplete reporting is one part of the problem. One Canadian study found that three-quarters of the health advice columns published in newspapers omitted critical information, and more than half offered potentially dangerous

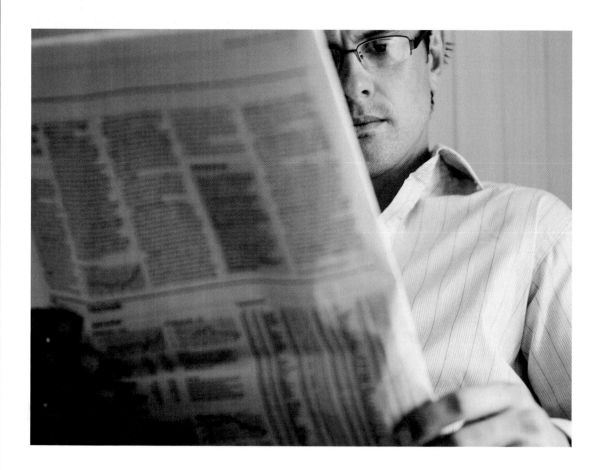

advice. The MTV-style presentation on television doesn't help much either. An Indiana University study found that the typical segment covering health or medicine on local newscasts lasted less than one minute. That's less time than most stations devote to the weather or identifying the latest celebrity to enter rehab.

An even bigger problem occurs when the media misinterpret and overstate the findings of scientific studies. This often happens with observational studies, the kind in which scientists look at a large number of people with similar qualities and track how various aspects of their health change—or don't change—over a given time period, usually at least a few years. In one major ongoing observational study, researchers at the Harvard School of Public Health are following more than 100,000 female nurses. In another, researchers are tracking the health fates of over 50,000 male dentists, optometrists, veterinarians, and other health professionals.

The results of observational studies often produce a big buzz in the media. For example, spaghetti sauce, tomato juice, and even lowly ketchup were hailed in the press during the 1990s as health foods thanks to observational studies showing that men who consumed plenty of foods made from cooked tomatoes had low rates of prostate cancer. Cooked tomatoes have high levels of an antioxidant called lycopene, which researchers believed conferred their cancer-fighting benefit. But in 2007, a major review of the research—one that garnered decidedly smaller headlines—found no evidence that lycopene prevents prostate cancer and "very limited" evidence that cooked tomatoes help.

How could that happen? The problem is that observational studies show only that two things occurred at the same time. In this case, men who ate plenty of cooked tomatoes had low rates of prostate cancer. But does that prove that tomatoes protect the prostate? Nope. It's possible that tomato-loving men tend to have some other habit or quality that protects their prostates.

Bottom line: Observational studies can raise interesting theories, but they don't prove cause

> Bad or incomplete reporting is one part of the problem. The MTV-style presentation on television doesn't help much either.

and effect. Be skeptical the next time a newscaster reports that a food or habit fights or causes some dreaded disease. (To learn more about what to look for in news about medical research, see "How to Interpret a Study" on page 24.)

The rapid rise and fall of new therapies. Why do so many prescription drugs seem to undergo a head-spinning reversal of fortune—panacea one day, poison the next?

For starters, anyone who watches TV or reads consumer magazines knows that the pharmaceutical industry aggressively markets drugs today. Because prescription medications can be patented for only a limited number of years, pharmaceutical companies try to garner as much profit as possible from a new medication before other companies can use the formula and produce copycat drugs. When these imitators reach the market, they may be heavily hyped, too. Some critics charge that marketing drugs directly to consumers through advertising creates a huge demand for these medications that surpasses the actual need.

Again, though, there's an even bigger problem, one that begins before a drug ever hits the market. When a pharmaceutical company wants to sell a new drug, it must show that the drug is effective and safe by conducting experiments known as clinical trials. In these trials, people in one group take the real drug, while volunteers in a comparison group take placebos. The trials reveal how well the drug works and how often it produces unwanted side effects, and we'd be in big trouble without them. They certainly weed out drugs that don't work or cause serious side effects in a lot of people. But they aren't perfect.

The trials used to gain approval for a new drug usually include no more than a few thousand people and last several months or years. Often, patients chosen to participate in these trials have uncomplicated cases of the condition being treated. Once a drug gains approval, however, millions of people may begin taking it, many of them sicker than the people in the trials and battling more than one medical condition—and that's when problems with the drug may become apparent.

Researchers at Harvard Medical School and Cambridge (Massachusetts) Hospital examined the safety record of the 548 new drugs approved by the FDA between 1975 and 1999. One out of 10 of these drugs was eventually taken off the market due to safety concerns or was branded with a "black box" warning—a caution printed in a black box on the drug information sheet and stating that the drug may cause serious or life-threatening side effects. These included heart attacks, liver and kidney failure, a weakened immune system, and the ultimate side effect, death.

In some cases, drugs discovered to carry serious risks are quietly removed from the market. In other cases, the story leads the evening news for weeks. In one of the most infamous examples of this problem, research showed that the heavily advertised and widely used arthritis drug Vioxx increased the risk of heart attack.

To make matters even more confusing, Dr. Wyer says that many drugs that have been pulled off the market actually had very small odds of causing serious side effects. For instance, taking Vioxx increased the risk of having a heart attack by only 1 in 10,000.

"There is as much hype around the adverse effects of high-profile drugs as there is exaggerating their benefits," says Dr. Wyer. "Who gets lost in the middle? The patient."

To protect yourself, always read the information sheet that comes with the medication your doctor prescribes, and ask about the drug's risks and benefits.

How to Interpret a Study

When you hear about a new medical research finding on the news, should you sit up and take notice or turn off the set? We can help you decide. Next time you hear or read about a new study, ask the following questions.

What kind of study was it? There are many different ways to study a scientific question, but the two you hear about most often on the news are observational studies and randomized controlled trials. You've already read about observational studies (see page 23) and why the results of a single such study don't prove much. When many of these studies produce similar results, however, their collective findings can influence how doctors advise and treat patients.

The real "gold standard" of research—as good as research gets—is the randomized controlled trial, or RCT. In a typical RCT, researchers assign people randomly to receive either a treatment or a placebo (the placebo group is the "control" group). Changes that occur or don't occur in the treatment group offer powerful evidence about whether a therapy works. The results of a single RCT must be reproduced by other scientists before they can be trusted, but RCTs are the most reliable way to test a new medical therapy.

Keep in mind, though, that RCTs are expensive to conduct and may not be feasible in some cases due to ethical concerns. For example, you will never see scientists test the cardiovascular benefits of alcohol consumption by asking a group of nondrinkers to start sipping martinis every night.

Who was studied? A study showing that a new drug lowers blood glucose in diabetic lab rats is great news—but only for diabetic rats. What's good for a rat doesn't always turn out to benefit humans. Even when a drug is tested in humans, scientists know that age, sex, race, income bracket, education level, and other factors all influence the outcome of studies. In other words, if you're a 45-year-old woman, the results of a study that included only men over 70 may not apply to you.

How large was the study? Imagine you flipped a coin 10 times, and it came up heads on 8 occasions and tails the other 2. Would you assume that a coin tossed in the air has an 80 percent chance of landing heads up? Of course not. As every schoolchild learns, this result occurred by chance. If you flipped the coin 1,000 times, you'd probably find that it turned up heads roughly half the time. The same thing is true in scientific research. A study involving hundreds or thousands of patients is more likely to produce a reliable result than an experiment that includes a dozen subjects.

Who paid for the study? In the case of many drug studies, it's the pharmaceutical industry. That doesn't mean the study is worthless, but you may want to view results with some skepticism. "There is a correlation between who is funding the study and the results you get," says Paul Brown, a consumer health advocate with the US Public Interest Research Group. For instance, a 2007 review found that studies paid for by drug companies produced positive results 84 percent of the time. By comparison, just 62 percent of independently funded studies turned out positive. The same research paper reported that studies sponsored by the drug industry were more likely to be small and lack control groups.

Finding Reliable Information on the Web

A generation ago, a patient desperate to learn more about a disease or treatment plan had few options outside the doctor's office. If you wanted

FIVE TRUSTWORTHY MEDICAL WEB SITES

The following Web sites aimed at medical consumers were rated either excellent or very good by Consumer Reports Web-Watch, a group created by the famous watchdog magazine to monitor the quality of Internet sites.

1. www.intelihealth.com
Features a broad range of consumer health information provided by Harvard Medical School.

2. www.mayoclinic.com
Draws upon the knowledge of more than 2,500 doctors and scientists from the world-renowned Mayo Clinic.

3. www.medicinenet.com
Offers hundreds of consumer-friendly articles about medicine by practicing doctors, plus a searchable medical dictionary.

4. www.nih.gov
The official Web site of the National Institutes of Health, one of the largest medical research facilities in the world.

5. www.webmd.com
Features a wide variety of medical information, including sections on women's, men's, and children's health.

Another excellent site to know about and use:

www.pubmed.gov
The US National Library of Medicine maintains this massive, up-to-date database, which compiles abstracts of every scientific study published in more than 5,000 medical journals. In some cases, you can link directly to the complete study.

to get more detailed information than you might find at your local bookstore, you could go to the library, blow the dust off a 20-year-old medical reference book, and hope the information you found wasn't hopelessly out of date or incomplete—which it probably was.

Today, gaining access to a vast world of medical information is as simple as flipping open your laptop or kicking your teenager off the family computer. "In the past, the doctor was the portal to medical information," says Vicki Rackner, MD, a Seattle-based surgeon who writes and lectures about the doctor-patient relationship. "But consumers have been given the keys."

To be sure, the Internet is awash in medical information. Knowledge is power, as the old saying goes, but it can also bewilder you or scare the living daylights out of you if you don't know how to use it. Here's how to find accurate medical information online and apply it wisely.

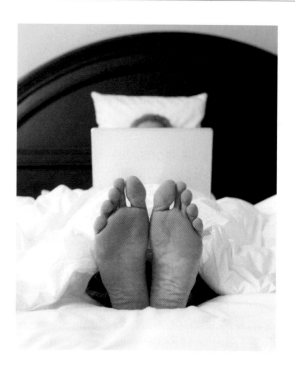

Find Web Sites You Can Trust

The very thing that makes the World Wide Web so democratic—the fact that anyone with a computer, Internet access, and an idea can create a site—also makes navigating cyberspace a challenge. Type the name of a disease or condition into a search engine, and you will undoubtedly find sites promoting questionable treatments and screwball theories about its cause. Amateurish graphics and text riddled with typos are often sure signs that you've come upon a Web page created by someone whose zeal exceeds their medical background. But more polish doesn't necessarily mean a page provides accurate, balanced, or complete information.

Gunther Eysenbach, MD, of Toronto General Hospital, has devised and tested a system patients can use to evaluate facts they find online and the overall credibility of medical Web sites.

Step 1: **Crosscheck the facts.**

Journalists validate facts they pick up from one source by crosschecking them with other sources. Do the same with facts you glean from Web sites. If you learn something critical about your condition on one site, check several others to see if they agree.

Step 2: **Check reliability.**

Evaluate a site by using the acronym CREDIBLE.

CURRENCY

☐ Does the information seem fresh or dated? On some sites, you can check to see when the page was last updated. If the site mentions medical studies, check to see when they were published. If they're years old, more recent studies may have debunked their findings.

REFERENCES

☐ Does the site include citations from medical journals to support its claims? If so, are they from peer-reviewed journals, which publish only studies that have been reviewed for accuracy by panels of experts? You can usually check by going to the journal's Web site.

EXPLICIT PURPOSE

☐ Can you easily determine the intentions of the site's creator? Web sites that are trying to sell products may be less reliable than those designed simply to present information.

DISCLOSURE OF SPONSORS

☐ Can you tell who paid to develop and host the site? Often, sites include a page labeled "Who We Are" or "About Us." These pages identify the people behind the site. If a site doesn't provide this information, be skeptical.

INTERESTS

☐ Could any conflicts of interest interfere with the site's objectivity? For example, does the site tout a miracle cure—and offer to sell it to you?

BALANCE

☐ Does the site's content seem evenhanded? Does it describe both advantages and disadvantages of treatments, for example?

LEVEL OF EVIDENCE

☐ How strong is the scientific evidence cited? For example, are medical claims backed by references to randomized controlled trials?

Step 3: **See what others are saying.**
Put the name of the site into Google or another search engine to see if others have praised the site or challenged its integrity.

Don't Play Doctor

Once you find reliable medical Web sites, don't make the mistake of trying to self-diagnose what ails you. "You're going to find out quickly that it's not an easy thing to do," says Dr. Rackner. For instance, let's say you develop a fever and decide to go online to figure out why. You'll soon learn that it could be because you have the flu. Or an ear infection. Or measles, meningitis, malaria, or any of more than 600 other medical conditions. "It's dangerous to become your own diagnostician," she says. Leave that judgment to your doctor.

Instead, keep a file of your research, take it with you to office visits, and ask your doctor to explain any key point you don't understand. Surveys suggest that the majority of doctors today are comfortable with patients doing their own research online and bringing information to appointments. In a 2007 survey, about two-thirds of doctors called this trend positive.

Finally, don't feel you have to spend hours trawling the Internet. Some people feel that they're bad patients if they *don't* rush home and plug the name of their condition into Google, says Dr. Rackner. If you accept your doctor's diagnosis and feel comfortable with the treatment prescribed—and you want to leave it at that—that's okay, too. Forcing yourself to seek more details or data will probably only increase your anxiety. "You need to know what dose of this information is optimal for you," she says.

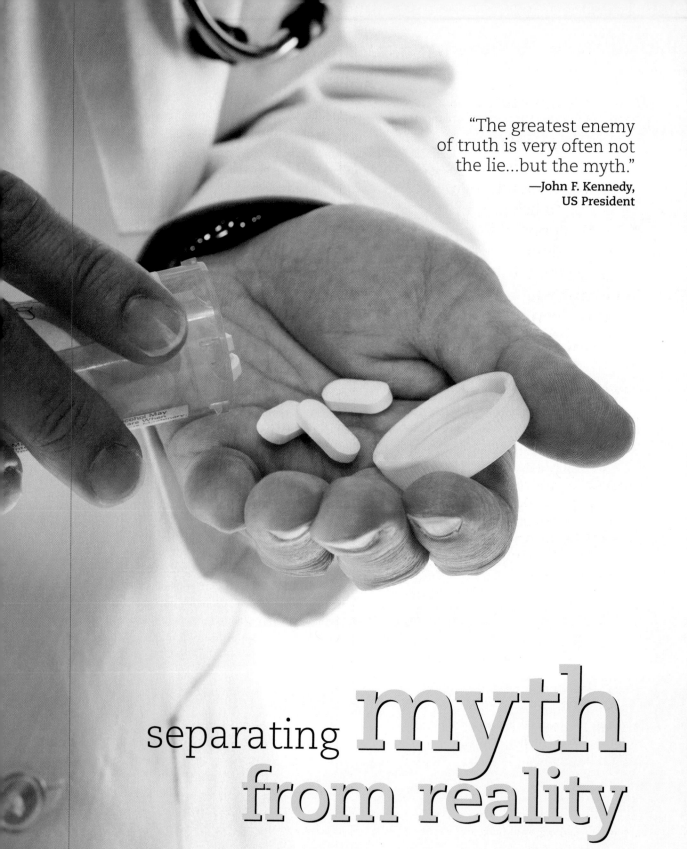

"The greatest enemy
of truth is very often not
the lie...but the myth."
—John F. Kennedy,
US President

separating myth
from reality

You heard this caution as a child and may even have repeated it to your own kids: "Don't sit too close to the television, or you'll go blind!" It sounds logical, yet there is not a lick of scientific evidence to support this advice. A more apt admonition might be "Don't watch too much TV, or you'll raise your risk of obesity and attention problems."

Medical myths and misconceptions are passed along and become accepted as fact over time. Many are relatively trivial and harmless, such as "Don't go swimming for one hour after eating, or you'll get cramps and drown" and "Don't go outside with wet hair on a cold day, or you'll catch a cold." However, some old or misguided ideas can affect your health, such as believing that you can have "just a touch" of diabetes, that vaccines may cause the illness they're meant to prevent, that heart disease is a man's disease, or that your genes are more important to your health than what you eat and how much you exercise.

Why do we continue to believe in medical misconceptions? Sometimes these myths are convenient to us because they justify behavior that in reality isn't so smart. For instance, ardent smokers may choose to believe, despite the evidence to the contrary, that low-tar cigarettes are less dangerous than other cigarettes because it gives them license to smoke. And there are plenty of other reasons, including these, according to Robert H. Shmerling, MD, of Boston's Beth Israel Deaconess Medical Center, who writes about myths in medicine.

Your mother—or father, teacher, or big brother—said it was true. "If a person you respect or fear tells you something, you're likely to believe it without question," says Dr. Shmerling. Sometimes we go on believing "facts" learned from authority figures despite evidence to the contrary.

It just makes sense. "Intuition is powerful," says Dr. Shmerling. If you sit one foot away from a TV and stare at the screen for an hour, your eye muscles may tire from having to alter their normal focus. While that won't cause blindness, your instincts may tell you that the feeling of eyestrain is evidence that you have wrecked your retinas.

It has never been proven false. It takes time and lots of money to formally test a medical question. Who's going to spend thousands of dollars or more to find out whether it's safe to swim after lunch? If no one ever challenges an established belief, it's likely to live on.

Finally, it can take years to get a message across when new research overturns an old idea. And doctors are hardly immune to this phenomenon. For instance, years after scientists had discovered the true cause of most stomach ulcers—the bacterium *Helicobacter pylori*—some physicians continued to prescribe vacations and bland diets to patients with this burning belly pain in the mistaken belief that it was caused by stress and spicy food.

Becoming a smarter medical consumer requires more than seeking out new information and fresh ideas. It means challenging old assumptions, too, by checking their validity with your doctor or other trusted sources (such as the Web sites listed on page 25).

Top Medical Misconceptions

You'll read about medical misconceptions throughout this book. In Part 2, we'll set the record straight about foods, diet strategies, over-the-counter drugs, and more. In Part 3, we'll tell you which treatments work and which don't for dozens of different health conditions, based on evidence and without regard to common wisdom. In Part 4, you'll find out whether common fears—for instance, that cell phones cause brain cancer—represent real risks or senseless worry.

The truth is, an amazing number of our ideas about health are misconceived or simply wrong. Here's a handful that have turned out to be off the mark.

MYTH #1: "Overweight" Means "Unhealthy"

A debate has raged in medicine for years: Can you be fat *and* fit?

To a degree, this debate boils down to a numbers game. Many doctors use body mass index (BMI) to determine whether a patient's weight is healthy or unhealthy. The BMI is a number that describes the ratio of your weight to your height. According to the Centers for Disease Control and Prevention, having a BMI under 25 means your weight is normal, 25 to 25.9 means you are overweight, and 30 or higher means you are obese. It's clear, however, that this breakdown is oversimplified and in some cases inaccurate. For starters,

many buff athletes with chiseled pecs and bulging biceps have high BMIs, since muscle weighs a lot.

More important, research has shown that a person's weight isn't necessarily the best measure of overall health. One study of thousands of men by researchers at the Cooper Institute in Dallas underscored this fact. Researcher Steven N. Blair, PED (who once told the *New York Times*, "I may be short, fat, and bald, but I'm fit."), led a team that tracked more than 25,000 men over 23 years. They recorded who got sick and who died and who didn't.

In the end, Dr. Blair and his colleagues surprised the world by showing that men who were overweight or obese but exercised regularly had half the death rate of normal-weight men who were out of shape. In fact, Dr. Blair's study found that being in poor physical condition was far more dangerous than simply being overweight, increasing the risk of premature death as much as having type 2 diabetes, high blood pressure or cholesterol, or smoking cigarettes does.

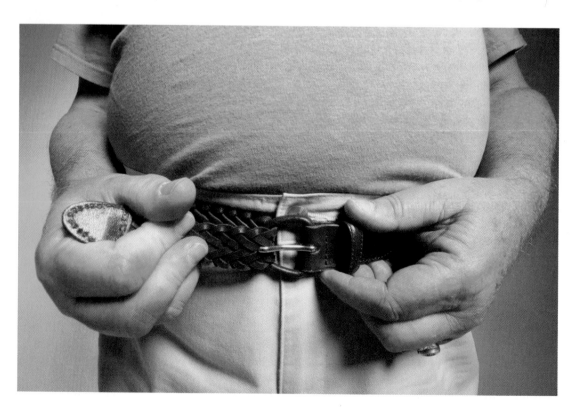

While this study suggests that heavyweights can be healthy people, it's important to keep in mind that lugging around a lot of abdominal fat does appear to be unhealthy. In fact, having a big belly increases the risk of heart disease and type 2 diabetes. (What's big? For men, 40 inches or more; for women, 35 inches or more. To measure your waist, wrap a tape measure around your bare abdomen just above the hipbones so it's snug but not tight. Inhale, exhale, and measure.) Fortunately, exercise burns belly flab, which is all the more reason to keep hitting the treadmill if you're overweight.

MYTH #2: Your Fate Is Already Sealed

You often hear this kind of fatalistic remark from people whose parents died young of heart attacks or cancer: "What's the point of jogging and eating broccoli if my lousy genes are going to kill me anyway?" Furthermore, each passing week seems to bring news that scientists have discovered yet another "disease gene." If our health destinies are preprogrammed, does it really matter whether we take care of our bodies?

In short, yes. The so-called breast cancer gene, BRCA1, offers a good example. There's no doubt the gene is powerful: Some 60 to 80 percent of women who have a mutation of this gene will develop breast cancer as compared to 13 percent of women who don't have the mutation. But that means that as many as 40 percent of women who inherit a BRCA1 mutation never develop breast cancer, suggesting that perhaps their lifestyle choices give them some protection.

What's more, scientists believe that the majority of cancer cases are *not* caused by inherited bad genes. Swedish researchers looked at the incidence of various cancers among nearly 45,000 sets of twins and concluded that "genetic factors make a minor contribution to susceptibility" to most forms of the disease. The evidence clearly shows, they stated, that

If your doctor recommends that you replace your current drug with **a brand new drug,** ask why.

the environment a person lives in has by far the greater influence on cancer risk.

The same scenario seems to hold true for other diseases that can rob you of years. Imagine a pie chart representing all the factors that influence how long you will live. Many studies suggest that the genes you inherited from your parents make up only about one-third of the pie, and maybe less. The other items in the pie include diet, physical activity level, and personal habits, such as tobacco use and alcohol consumption. In other words, you can't change your DNA, but what makes up the rest of the pie is largely up to you.

MYTH #3: Prescription Drugs Are Guaranteed Safe

It sure looks that way on the slick ads that fill the airwaves and magazines. As we noted earlier in this chapter, however, about 10 percent of prescription drugs that hit the market are later discovered to cause serious side effects that didn't turn up in clinical trials. With that in mind, you might think that pharmaceutical companies would want to keep close track of whether people become ill when they take new drugs the companies market. In fact, the FDA requires them to do just that. Yet drug companies fail to perform these follow-up studies 70 percent of the time, says Paul Brown, a consumer health advocate with the US Public Interest Research Group.

That's why Merrill Goozner recommends that you change the channel or turn the page when you see an advertisement for a new drug. Goozner is director of the Integrity in Science project for the Center for Science in the Public Interest (another consumer watchdog group) and author of *The $800 Million Pill: The Truth Behind the Cost of New Drugs*. "There is no place for those ads in the practice of medicine," he says.

That doesn't mean new drugs have no value. If there are currently no medications available to treat your condition, and there's solid evidence that a new medication is effective without causing intolerable side effects, the new drug could offer some hope. However, if a heavily hyped new drug would merely replace a medication that's currently working well for you, then why switch and expose yourself to unknown risk? If your doctor recommends doing so, ask why.

MYTH #4: Hospitals Are Sterile Houses of Healing

It's tempting—and certainly convenient—to believe that hospitals are squeaky clean and sterile. You'd like to think the floors, or at least other surfaces, are so immaculate you could eat off them. But it's simply not the case.

Despite many hospitals' diligent attempts to keep hospital-acquired infections under control, your room and even your doctor probably carry nasty drug-resistant germs that could kill you, or at least make you very sick and keep you in the hospital longer—exposing you to even more germs. Microbes such as bacteria that cause staph infections lurk on bed rails, bedside tables, IV poles, and various pieces of equipment that touch you. According to the Centers for Disease Control and Prevention, 1.7 million people develop infections while staying in, or immediately following discharge from, US hospitals each year. Nearly 100,000 die.

Human error is partly to blame. For instance, doctors all too often neglect to take the simple step of washing their hands between patients, and most don't disinfect the stethoscope that recently touched another patient's chest.

Germs aren't the only deadly dangers. We've already mentioned the disturbing problem of medical errors, which are common enough to be the eighth leading cause of death in the United States. Among the most common blunders that occur in hospitals are mistakes in prescribing and administering medications. For many

DON'T TOUCH THAT REMOTE!

According to one study, the TV remote control in your hospital room probably carries more bacteria than the toilet bowl handle. To help protect yourself from these and other germs, follow a few simple guidelines during your stay.

1. Ask doctors and nurses to clean their hands before treating you. An alcohol-based hand cleaner will do the trick. Ask nicely, but be brave. Failing to ask could put your health in jeopardy. Even if your doctor is wearing gloves, the gloves are probably contaminated if the doctor didn't wash her hands before putting them on.

2. Ask that the stethoscope surface be disinfected. Wiping it with alcohol takes only seconds.

3. Wash your own hands. Do this especially after using the bathroom or handling items that could be contaminated. Wash for at least 15 seconds with warm soapy water.

4. Don't touch your mouth with your hands. Germs that lurk on surfaces you touch can enter your body and cause infection when you touch your mouth.

5. Keep your utensils on your food tray. Putting them on your bedside furniture increases the risk that they'll be contaminated.

in-patients, receiving the wrong drug or an incorrect dose is as much a part of the hospital experience as bad food. According to "Preventing Medication Errors," a recent report by the Institute of Medicine, the typical hospital patient either gets the wrong medicine, receives the incorrect dose, or fails to receive a needed medication at least once per *day*.

MYTH #5: Sleep Isn't That Important

Given the hectic lives we lead today, eight or nine hours of sleep may seem like a delicious indulgence we just can't afford. But research suggests that if you're concerned about your health, you can't afford *not* to get enough shuteye.

Sleep does far more than give you the energy you need to get through the day and help you cope with stress. For one thing, it helps you keep your weight in check. Studies suggest that sleep deprivation leads to increased levels of the hormone grehlin, which triggers hunger, and decreased levels of leptin, which signals fullness. The result: You eat more.

Lack of sleep also affects the immune system. Rats deprived of sleep die, most likely because of an immune system breakdown that allows an influx of deadly bacteria. Sleep deprivation may also increase levels of inflammatory chemicals in the body, and inflammation is now known to contribute to a host of serious diseases, from diabetes to heart disease to cancer.

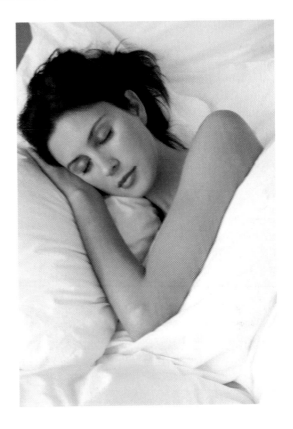

Failing to log enough pillow time can contribute to depression, make high blood pressure worse, and even raise your blood sugar. A Harvard Medical School study found that women who slept five or fewer hours per day were nearly a third more likely to develop diabetes than women who got a more reasonable amount of sleep.

Finally, during sleep, the body appears to repair damaged brain cells and "reorganize" the brain, possibly affecting learning and memory. If you "forgot" to get enough sleep last night, you may be forgetting other things, too.

> If you "forgot" to get enough sleep last night, you may start forgetting other things, too.

MYTH #6: The Placebo Effect Is Negligible

Tell that to your brain, though it probably won't believe you.

The word *placebo*, from the Latin for "I shall please," first turned up in medical texts in the

18th century, defined as a treatment intended to make a patient happy rather than do any actual healing. So why do placebos sometimes *work?*

Placebos are often called sugar pills, and indeed, they're sometimes tablets made of sugar or starch, though a placebo can be any form of faux medical therapy or treatment made to look like the real thing. Scientists include placebo groups in clinical trials thanks to the work of anesthesiologist Henry K. Beecher, MD. In 1955, Dr. Beecher analyzed 15 studies in which patients with various diseases had received placebos and found that about 35 percent of them responded as though they had received real treatments.

This finding had major implications for the study of new drugs and other therapies, since it suggested that about one-third of sick people get better if they *think* they're receiving treatment. As a result, when scientists conduct a clinical trial of a new drug or therapy today, they have to account for the placebo effect. An experimental therapy is usually considered a flop if it fails to treat significantly more than 35 percent of the patients who receive it.

Some recent studies have cast doubt on Dr. Beecher's 35 percent rule and on the concept of the placebo effect in general. However, studies show that placebo treatments are surprisingly effective for a variety of conditions, including Parkinson's disease, depression, and gastrointestinal problems such as irritable bowel syndrome. Conditions with the highest response rates tend to be those with symptoms that are difficult to quantify, such as pain.

Skeptics claim that any response to a placebo is "all in your head." They're right, in a sense. Sophisticated medical imaging shows that people given placebos experience significant changes in brain chemistry. At least 30 studies have shown that when people who are experiencing some form of pain are told they will receive a pain reliever but are given a placebo instead, their bodies nonetheless produce morphine-like compounds called opioids.

More important, placebos seem to diminish pain. In one study, researchers applied heat to the skin of volunteers until it hurt. Then they slathered a phony cream on the sore skin, telling the volunteers that the salve contained soothing medication. More than 70 percent of the volunteers said the placebo cream relieved their pain.

"The brain has the capability to exert control over the rest of the body, but we really don't know how it works," says Columbia University research psychologist Tor D. Wager, PhD, who led the study.

The placebo effect appears to go beyond pain reduction. For instance, in a recent experiment, asthma patients who believed they were receiving the drug salmeterol but were given placebos not only felt better but also had improvement in their lung function, though not as much as people who received the real drug.

Can You Spot the Truth?

How well can you spot a medical myth or outdated belief? Test yourself below. You'll read more about many of these topics later in the book.

BELIEF	THE TRUTH
Eating high-fiber foods prevents colon cancer.	**FALSE.** Doctors once believed that eating a lot of "roughage" kept the colon free of cancer-causing toxins. Several large studies found, however, that neither high-fiber diets nor fiber supplements prevented colon cancer.
Everyone should drink eight glasses of water each day.	**FALSE.** There is no scientific basis for this common recommendation. According to the Institute of Medicine, a man needs about 125 ounces (15 to 16 cups) of water daily, while a woman requires 91 ounces (a little over 11 cups). That amount is easily gotten from a normal diet, since all beverages and many foods contain water. To stay well hydrated, simply drink when you're thirsty.
A "broken heart" is a genuine medical condition.	TRUE. Doctors have shown that people who experience severe emotional trauma, such as losing a loved one, sometimes develop a condition known as stress cardiomyopathy, also called broken-heart syndrome. The condition causes a ventricle, or cavity, in the heart to expand, though it is rarely fatal.
Stress and spicy foods cause ulcers.	**FALSE.** Infections caused by bacteria called *Helicobacter pylori* cause 80%–90% of stomach and intestinal ulcers. Treatment with antibiotics and Pepto-Bismol is usually successful. Most other ulcers are caused by sensitivity to aspirin and other nonsteroidal anti-inflammatory pain relievers, such as ibuprofen.
Washing your hands with antibacterial soaps helps prevent colds.	**FALSE.** Washing your hands frequently is always a great idea, especially during cold season; the rhinovirus, which causes the common cold, can live on your skin for up to three hours. However, since antibacterial soaps don't destroy viruses, they offer no advantage over other soaps.
Foods that are high in cholesterol are the main cause of clogged arteries.	**FALSE.** Cholesterol is a waxy substance found in all animal foods. Studies show, however, that eating modest servings of high-cholesterol foods does not raise blood levels of cholesterol. Saturated fat in meat and dairy foods, as well as the trans fats found in many commercial baked goods, are much greater threats to your arteries.
"Use it or lose it" applies to brain function.	TRUE. Many population studies have suggested that people who regularly engage in activities that require the brain to process information—whether reading, going to museums, or playing checkers—are less likely to develop Alzheimer's and other neurological diseases that lead to loss of mental clarity.

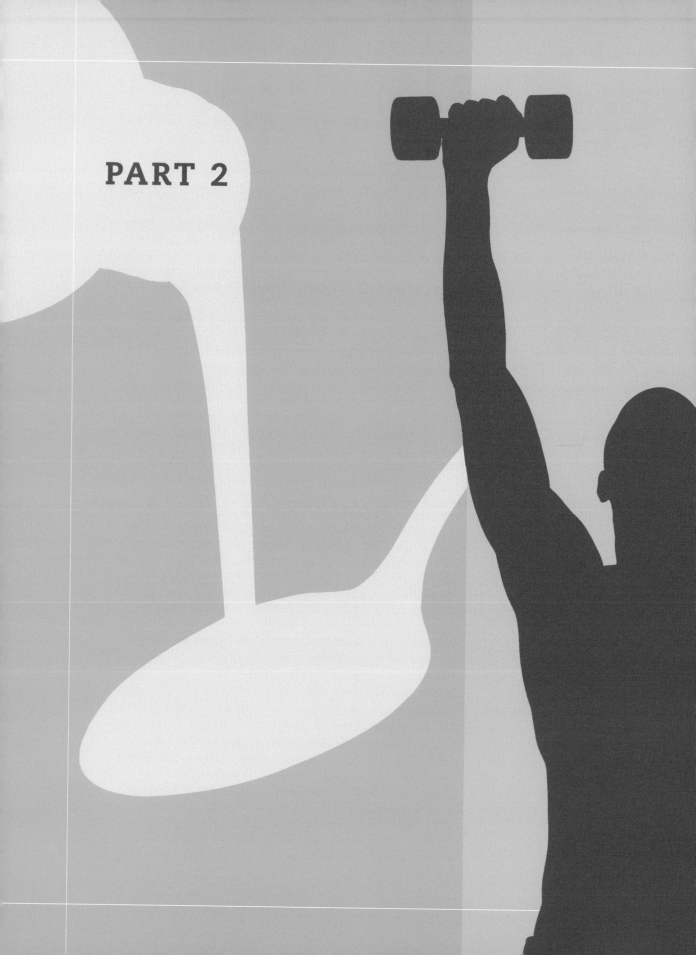

PART 2

your
general
health

looking good

Anti-Wrinkle Creams

Life leaves its mark, sometimes on our faces. And just as surely as we can't turn back time, neither can we erase the creases, lines, and furrows it etches. But it is possible to make them at least slightly less noticeable with the right product (hint: choose wisely, but don't overpay) and plenty of patience.

Do anti-wrinkle creams work?

YES Anti-wrinkle creams reduce the appearance of fine lines and wrinkles, but for noticeable results, you'll need a prescription.

Potions and lotions promising younger-looking skin do one thing well: Generate profits for the companies that sell them. The fact is, almost any moisturizing cream can make your skin look and feel good for a few hours. Some anti-wrinkle creams do more, particularly those that contain retinoids, the vitamin A derivatives in prescription products such as Retin-A and Renova. They won't provide results overnight, but over the course of a few months, you may see an effect.

Used since the 1960s to treat acne, vitamin A derivatives increase skin cell turnover and stimulate the production of collagen, the main protein in skin's connective tissue, which boosts the strength and elasticity of skin. In one study reported in the *New England Journal of Medicine*, sun-damaged skin treated for about a year with tretinoin (the active ingredient in Retin-A) had an 80 percent increase in collagen formation compared to a 14 percent decrease in skin treated with a placebo cream.

Other studies show that tretinoin makes fine lines and wrinkles less noticeable. Australian researchers studied a 0.05 percent concentration of Retin-A in people with sun-damaged skin and found that over 24 weeks, treated skin was less wrinkled, tighter, and smoother. Another study found that the use of a 0.02 percent cream over 24 weeks significantly improved fine wrinkles, coarse wrinkles, and yellowing of the skin compared to a placebo cream.

If you want results like these, though, go to a dermatologist, not a drugstore. Over-the-counter creams—even those containing retinols—may improve the

BOTOX IN A JAR?

We know you've seen them—advertisements for skin creams promising to erase wrinkles (not to mention stretch marks) every bit as well as injections of Botox. StriVectin-SD, for example, is super-expensive, but does it pay off? It contains peptides that supposedly not only firm the skin by boosting collagen production but also penetrate deep into the skin to relax the muscles underneath. But according to Laurie Polis, MD, board-certified dermatologist at Soho Skin and Laser in New York City, while these products are good at hydrating the skin, no over-the-counter cream could penetrate into the muscles and have an effect. Likewise, collagen cannot be delivered topically to any depth where it can have an effect. In one study conducted in Florida, Botox outperformed three of these products hands down, both in the eyes of the researchers who evaluated the wrinkle reductions and in the opinions of the patients.

ANTI-WRINKLE CREAMS

health of your skin, but according to the nonprofit organization Consumers Union and its French counterpart, l'Union Federale des Consommateurs-Que Choisir, the changes are barely visible to the naked eye. In 2006, their study of a variety of creams (including one that cost $335 for one ounce) found that after 12 weeks of use, even the best-performing creams reduced the average depth of wrinkles by less than 10 percent. There was no correlation between the price of a product and its effectiveness.

Do antioxidants in skin creams do any good?

MAYBE The answer depends on the concentration of antioxidants and whether they're "packaged" in a stable form. And that's almost impossible for a consumer to tell.

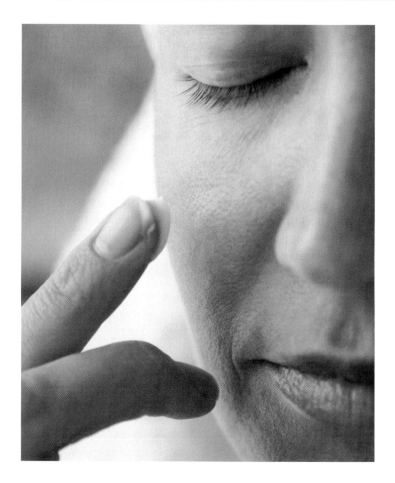

Your skin, especially the outer layer, is naturally endowed with antioxidants that neutralize cell-damaging free radicals caused by the sun's rays and by pollution in the air, among other things. Manufacturers of skin-care products have jumped on nature's bandwagon, adding topical antioxidants like vitamins C and E and green tea extracts to skin creams and sunscreens. It sounds good in theory, and in fact, topical antioxidants can indeed increase skin's immunity to air pollution and sun damage and help it look rejuvenated.

But here's the rub: Not all creams contain antioxidants in high enough concentrations or in forms that are stable enough to be effective once they penetrate the skin, if they can penetrate it at all. (Unlike sunscreens, they're designed to work inside the skin as well as on the surface.) According to dermatologist Laurie Polis, MD, a board-certified dermatologist in New York, the following antioxidants should be among the top few ingredients in skin-care formulations.

Vitamin C: Studies show that applying vitamin C over 12 weeks can make skin look smoother and less wrinkled.

Our BEST ADVICE

Load up on antioxidant-rich foods to help protect your skin from the inside out. Vitamin C plays an important role in collagen production and helps prevent bruising. Vitamin E provides essential oils that moisturize the skin and keep it looking supple and smooth.

The only drawback: expense. "Creams containing vitamin C at a level that would be effective can be expensive," says Dr. Polis. Chances are, if it's a drugstore cream, it doesn't have enough C or doesn't have it in a form that can penetrate the epidermis (ester C is one that does). Other forms labeled "vitamin C" do nothing except make for good marketing. Since it's hard for consumers to know what they're getting, Dr. Polis recommends buying from a dermatologist or choosing a brand-name product from a reputable company.

Vitamin E: Perhaps the most commonly added compound in skin-care products, alpha-tocopherol (the biologically active form of vitamin E) has been shown to effectively maintain skin's defenses against sun damage. Other studies show vitamin E reduced the inflammation that occurs after sun exposure.

Green tea extract: Green tea fights both oxidation and inflammation, at least in test tubes. But in one study in which women were treated with either 10 percent green tea cream plus an oral green tea supplement or a placebo cream and supplement, the skin of those who received the real treatment looked more elastic under the microscope

Our BEST ADVICE

When it comes to skin creams, more is not better (unless it's sunscreen). Creams that contain vitamin A derivatives can temporarily cause redness, dryness, and irritation. To reduce the potential for irritation, wait an hour after washing your face to apply Retin-A, since washing strips your skin of natural oils. You may also need to start with a weak concentration and work up to a stronger one. Be careful in the sun, too. Vitamin A–treated skin is more susceptible to sunburn, so always wear sunscreen.

----

but not noticeably better to the eye after eight weeks.

DMAE: This naturally occurring substance, originally used orally to stave off cognitive decline, has been called a facelift in a jar. It won't give you the face you had 20 years ago, but studies have shown that it does increase skin firmness. In a 16-week study, daily application of 3 percent DMAE (2-dimethylaminoethanol) filled

in lines and wrinkles and improved the appearance of aging skin. And the effects remained after subjects stopped applying the gel for two weeks.

It's not clear how it works, and researchers at the University of Laval in Quebec, who tested it on skin cells, found that it caused swelling in cells that could indicate damage. In fact, that reaction may even be the reason the supplement works.

Coenzyme Q10: Research shows that this naturally occurring antioxidant, ubiquitous in the body, protects against inflammation caused by sun exposure, especially when used with other antioxidants called carotenoids.

Idebenone: Pronounced *eye-deb-eh-known* and related to coenzyme Q10, this is one of the most powerful antioxidants in topical skin products. In one study that assigned oxidation protection scores to a handful of antioxidants, idebenone scored 95 compared to 80 for vitamin E, 68 for kinetin, 52 for vitamin C, and 41 for alpha lipoic acid. ∎

VITAMIN E FOR SCARS?

Plenty of people smear vitamin E oil on cuts and surgical wounds as they heal in the hope that they'll end up with less noticeable scars. So far, though, there's little scientific evidence that it works. In fact, in studies, some wounds treated with vitamin E actually looked worse afterward. And in some people, vitamin E oil can irritate the skin and cause a rash.

Botox

Back in the 1990s, many of the rich and famous seemed to suddenly lose their ability to crack a smile, or even summon a convincing frown. Call it the Botox effect. Injections of botulinum toxin, also called sausage poison because it grows in poorly handled meat products, are now the most popular nonsurgical cosmetic treatment. They block the muscle contractions that cause wrinkles, stopping wrinkles at their source.

Does Botox erase wrinkles?

YES Botox injections diminish facial lines and wrinkles within two weeks.

Two large, well-designed studies involving hundreds of participants concluded that Botox injections improve the look of worry lines, or brow furrows. The peak effect was seen 30 days after injection, when 80 percent of patients showed mild or no furrows while trying to make a sad face, as judged by their doctors. Among the patients themselves, 89 percent reported seeing at least a 50 percent improvement in their brow wrinkles. There have also been studies showing that Botox is effective on crow's-feet, chin wrinkles, and neck lines, though it hasn't been officially approved for these uses in the United States.

Results typically last for less than four months, at which point patients need fresh injections. There is a cumulative effect over time, though; people who get regular injections may see longer-lasting results.

The most common side effects are headache and a temporary look of having pulled an all-nighter (caused by droopy upper eyelids). Both tend to decrease with repeated treatments. A small number of patients also report mild flu-like symptoms lasting a few days. No deaths have been reported among people who used Botox for cosmetic purposes, and the most common complaint in one review study was lack of effect in the treated area. The doctor's skill does come into play; results depend in part on the dosage given and the exact location of the injections.

Can anything make Botox work better?

YES Most dermatologists and plastic surgeons use either Botox or collagen to treat deep lines and wrinkles. According to research, however, they

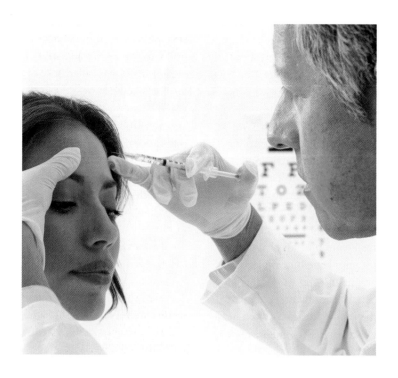

might be better off using both. One study of 65 patients broken into three groups (who received either Botox, collagen, or a combination of the two) found that people who received combination therapy showed significantly greater improvement in worry lines on the forehead than those who received either Botox or collagen alone. What's more, at three months post-injection, the combo patients maintained better improvement than the others. ■

CAN YOU BECOME IMMUNE TO BOTOX?

Yes, but it is very, very rare. Repeated treatments with Botox may cause the body to produce antibodies, proteins that tag foreign objects like cold viruses, and in this case Botox, as bad guys to be neutralized. This reduces the effectiveness of subsequent treatments not only for wrinkles and brow lines but also for other, non-cosmetic uses of Botox, such as treating profusely sweaty armpits. The more frequent the injections and the higher the dose, the more likely it is that your body will develop antibodies.

Cellulite Creams

Cellulite may seem the bane of the overweight, but in fact, 85 to 98 percent of women have dimpled thighs and backsides. It's more visible in some than in others, regardless of weight. Those who are genetically predisposed to dimpling suffer the most.

Can cellulite creams get rid of cottage-cheese thighs?

NO They may temporarily improve an "orange peel" appearance, but there is no evidence that the creams reduce cellulite.

Researchers don't know the exact cause of cellulite, but they do have theories about why women have it and men don't. In women, connective tissue beneath the skin separates fat into channels so it resembles a down quilt. As the fat expands, the connective tissue stays fixed, making the skin appear puckered. But connective tissue in men has more of a crisscross pattern, so when fat expands, the connective tissue expands with it in both directions, and the skin looks smooth. Scientists also think poor circulation plays a role in the development of cellulite.

Cellulite creams promise to reduce the dimples with a variety of ingredients. For instance, emollients hydrate and plump the surface of the skin, and ingredients like caffeine supposedly reduce fluid retention, so the layers beneath look firmer. Retinol, the anti-wrinkle vitamin-A derivative, is often included to, in theory, thicken the outer layer of skin so the fat pockets don't show as much.

While no cream on the market will get rid of cellulite, some may have small temporary effects. Results don't last if you stop using the creams, because the products don't actually treat the layer of fat beneath the skin.

One ingredient purported to actually reduce thigh circumference is a cream version of aminophylline, an oral asthma drug that, when applied topically, is said to stimulate the breakdown of fat. Early studies showed promising results, but more recent studies have shown only modest improvement, if any. ■

COLLAGEN AND WRINKLE FILLERS

Collagen and Wrinkle Fillers

Marketed as quick nonsurgical fixes for sagging, lined faces, wrinkle fillers like collagen, Restylane, and Juvederm allow you to slip into a doctor's chair during your lunch hour and come out looking a few years younger. The catch: For lasting effects, you have to keep going back.

Do collagen injections plump up the skin and reduce wrinkles?

YES But collagen is no longer the gold standard of "facial fillers." Newer fillers last longer.

Collagen injections are mankind's attempt to undo gravity's effects on the face, adding back plumpness and smoothness that nature stole. Derived from connective tissue in cows, collagen has been the primary "line filler" of choice for decades. And it works—but it doesn't last long (three months on average), and some people experience allergic reactions. Newer options may last longer, with less risk of side effects.

Fillers made of hyaluronic acid, a dissolvable complex sugar, last for up to a year. After 4 to 12 months, the filler is broken down and eliminated from the system. Unlike collagen, which comes from cows, hyaluronic acid is not of animal origin, so allergic reactions are highly unlikely.

In a study conducted in six medical centers in the United States, researchers treated 138 patients with Restylane (containing hyaluronic acid) on one side of their faces and collagen on the other. Both were equally effective at first, but after six months, most patients thought Restylane worked better. Another study, at the University of Michigan, suggests that injecting Restylane into the skin stretches fibroblasts, young skin cells that make collagen, so they more closely resemble those of younger skin and are better able to produce collagen. With Restylane, the effects last longer even after the filler dissolves because the stretched fibroblasts continue to produce more collagen.

In 2006, the FDA approved another filler, Juvederm (also containing hyaluronic acid), and the results have been promising. In one study of 439 patients, 90 percent of those who received Juvederm reported significant improvement in the appearance of wrinkles compared to only 36 to 45 percent of those who received collagen. Many other injectables are currently available, and still others are under investigation. Side effects of injections, which include swelling and bruising, are usually the fault of the doctor's technique, not the filler used. ∎

Collagen injections are mankind's attempt to **undo the effects of gravity** on the face.

Hair Regrowth Products

Ask a man if he'd rather lose his hair or his job. The answer may explain the quest for a baldness cure that dates back to the ancient Egyptians. While snake-oil products abound, no holy grail has been discovered, although some products may help you hold on to what you have and maybe even sprout a little more.

Does Rogaine combat male pattern baldness?

YES Rogaine stimulates hair regrowth on the crowns of men's heads. It doesn't work well on a receding hairline.

Rubbing Rogaine into the scalp twice daily has been shown to help regrow hair and prevent further loss. The over-the-counter treatment is available in two strengths: 2 percent and 5 percent (Rogaine Extra Strength). One study that tested both found that after nearly a year, 57 percent of men who used the 5 percent strength had hair regrowth, compared with 41 percent of men who used the 2 percent strength and a surprising 23 percent of men who used a placebo (apparently, belief in the product helps). Hair growth peaked at four months with both products. Other studies have shown less difference in effectiveness between the two concentrations.

Don't expect to regain your old mane, though. New hair may grow in thinner and shorter than the hair you had (think peach fuzz), at least at first. And Rogaine seems to work best on men who treat their hair loss early; it won't regrow hair in areas that are totally bald. According to the package information, it won't repopulate a receding hairline either. Of course, the benefits of Rogaine stop after you stop using it.

Does Propecia work better than Rogaine?

YES A Turkish study involving 65 men pitted the prescription baldness pill Propecia (finasteride), which is taken once a day, against Extra-Strength Rogaine. After one year, the pill came out on top: Eighty percent of the men in the pill group had more hair than they did at the beginning of the study, versus 52 percent of the Rogaine group.

Before it was a treatment for baldness, finasteride was (and still is) a prescription treatment

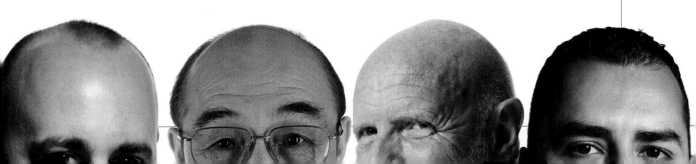

HAIR REGROWTH PRODUCTS

for enlarged prostate, under the brand name Proscar. It prevents the conversion of testosterone into another hormone, dihydrotestosterone (DHT). Having too much of this hormone can shrink hair follicles to the point where no new hair can grow. Like Rogaine, Propecia seems to work best for men with baldness on the crown of the head. It may also work on the middle front of the head, but it's less effective at growing hair on the temples.

Propecia isn't without possible side effects, which may include a decrease in sex drive and breast tenderness. Women can't use the drug or even handle broken tablets because it can cause serious birth defects in male babies.

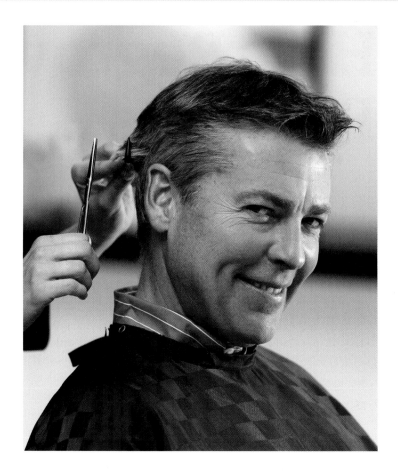

Are there new drugs for baldness in the pipeline?

YES Another treatment approved for prostate enlargement and being reviewed by the FDA for baldness is dutasteride (Avodart). Like Propecia, it affects the hormone DHT, and it may work better than Propecia. One 24-week study of 416 men conducted at Duke University Medical Center tested both drugs and found that men who received Avodart increased target area hair count and had better hair growth than men who took Propecia. Some experts say the drug is likely to work better than any other medication currently available for women with inherited pattern hair loss as well as for men who don't respond to Propecia. According to the FDA, however, women should never take Avodart. Our best advice: Hold off until more rigorous trials are conducted.

Do any folk treatments work?

MAYBE Some natural remedies do seem effective for a patchy hair-loss condition called alopecia areata, also called spot baldness, but there's no telling whether they work for traditional male pattern baldness. For spot baldness, both garlic gel and onion juice have been found to stimulate hair growth. In one placebo-controlled Iranian study in which men used a topical garlic gel twice a day in combination with a steroid cream for three months, the garlic significantly boosted the therapeutic effect of the cream. A similar study conducted in Iraq found that onion juice stimulated hair regrowth after just two weeks, and after six weeks, new hair was seen in almost 90 percent of the men. ■

Laser Eye Surgery

Thanks to laser eye surgery, people too blind to see their alarm clocks in the morning can walk into an ophthalmologist's office and have 20/20 vision 10 minutes later. And with recent advances in technology, the surgical doors have opened to people who were previously turned away due to large pupil size or extremely bad eyesight.

Is LASIK a safe and effective way to correct vision?

YES Studies show that LASIK corrects vision impairments to 20/20 or better for most patients, with few risks.

LASIK is the acronym for laser-assisted in situ keratomileusis, a type of surgery for correcting nearsightedness, farsightedness, and astigmatism. After administering anesthetic eyedrops, the surgeon slices a flap in the outer layer of the cornea, leaving just enough tissue to act as a hinge. He uses a laser to reshape the cornea, then folds the flap back in place. Surveys show that more than 90 percent of patients are satisfied with the results of the procedure.

In a study conducted at the Eye Institute of Utah, postoperative vision correction was 20/20 in 51 percent of eyes and 20/40 or better in 97 percent of eyes. And one year after treatment, 93 percent of patients' vision was within the intended level of vision correction.

The procedure appears to be quite safe: A study of more than 32,000 US Armed Forces members who underwent laser surgery found a vision loss of one line on an eye chart in 1 in 1,250 people. Data from the Oregon Health and Science University Casey Vision Correction Center showed no cases of vision loss greater than two lines after 18,000 surgeries.

Flap complications occur in about 0.2 percent of surgeries. A study conducted in Tokyo found that among 3,751 eyes, 15 required retreatment with a new flap during the six-month study period.

Some people experience side effects such as seeing starbursts or halos at night or not being able to see well in dim light. But the most common complication is dry eyes. In a study of 190 eyes, 20 percent were diagnosed with chronic dry eyes that persisted for six months or more. People who need the most correction are most likely to experience dry eyes.

Does custom LASIK deliver better results?

YES LASIK surgery continues to become more refined—and effective. In wave-front guided LASIK, also called custom LASIK, the ophthalmologist takes several three-dimensional measurements of how your eye processes images, creating a customized map that will guide the laser in reshaping your eye. Each bump, pock, and imperfection in your cornea is reflected on the map, and your cornea is reshaped to correct these irregularities. As a result, the custom surgery poses a lower risk of complications,

Our BEST ADVICE

One review of LASIK procedures found that results were influenced by the humidity in the room and the humidity and temperature outside. Surgeries performed in the summer were more likely to require second surgeries to tweak the outcome. Your surgical room should feel like an icebox. If you have the option, have the procedure on a cold winter day.

LASER EYE SURGERY

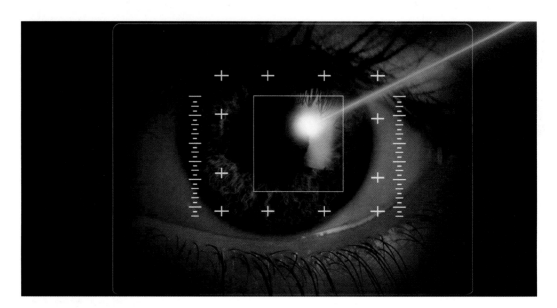

such as halos and difficulty seeing in low light, while achieving better vision correction. A study conducted by the Stanford University department of ophthalmology found that the surgery produced 20/20 or better correction in 74 of 84 eyes treated.

Is bladeless surgery safer and more effective than traditional LASIK?

YES You'll probably get better vision and fewer side effects.

Traditional LASIK requires a surgeon to slice a flap in the outer layer of the cornea, like peeling back the smooth skin of a grape to reveal the softer matter beneath. After the laser reshapes the cornea, the flap is put back in place. Now surgeons have the option of using a second laser instead of a metal blade to create the flap. This "bladeless" procedure (using a brand of laser called IntraLase) can be performed with either "custom" or standard laser surgery.

According to Joseph Dello Russo, MD, an early pioneer of laser vision correction, "In addition to experiencing fewer complications, more patients achieve vision better than 20/20 when the IntraLase is used instead of a blade."

The bladeless procedure creates a smoother, more even surface for the second laser to work on. It also produces a more consistent flap thickness and lets the doctor create a "custom" flap that's just right for your eye. There may be another advantage: Studies suggest that creating the flap with a blade changes the characteristics of the eye, which can compromise the effectiveness of wave-front guided procedures because the measurements that guide the procedure are made before the flap is created. Using the bladeless method doesn't alter the optical characteristics, so results are more precise.

Clinical studies show that more patients get 20/20 vision or better with this procedure than with the traditional one, and fewer complain about their ability to see well in low light. Also, in at least one study, bladeless surgery was found to more accurately correct astigmatism.

Are contact lenses safer than laser surgery?

NO A review of several large studies found a greater risk of vision loss with contact lenses (thanks to infections, corneal scratches, and so on) than with laser correction surgery. ■

Laser Hair Removal

While men struggle to keep every hair on their head, women struggle to get rid of hair elsewhere. Some plunk down serious money for laser treatments to denude their faces, legs, armpits, and bikini lines without waxing, plucking, or razor irritation. Men can even have their back hair zapped. But the treatments aren't for everyone.

Does laser hair removal work?

YES Lasers effectively remove hair, but multiple treatments are required for permanent hair loss, results vary, and darker skin types are more difficult to treat.

Laser hair removal targets melanin, the dark pigment that gives color to hair and skin. The melanin absorbs energy from the laser light, and the heat disables nearby hair follicles, or at least those that are in their active growth phase. (At any given time, between 50 and 85 percent of hair follicles are in this phase.) The darker the hair, the more light is absorbed, and the more hair follicles are disabled. Most physicians repeat treatments every four to eight weeks to allow hairs in the latent phase during the first treatment to become active.

The best results are seen in patients who have fair skin and dark hair. For them, a single treatment can reduce hair by up to 40 percent, three treatments by up to 70 percent, and repeated treatments by up to 90 percent. Results last for up to a year, and longer in some people. More than 70 percent of patients are satisfied with laser treatments, significantly more than those who are satisfied with electrolysis or waxing.

To date, there is no single laser hair removal system that can remove hair for people with all colors (including blonde, gray, and white) and all skin types, though technology is gradually moving in that direction. By using lasers with longer pulse durations and performing multiple treatments, doctors can offer patients with darker skin effective hair removal, but the risk of potential side effects, such as swelling, redness, brown spots, and scarring, is greater.

In one study of 31 patients with darker skin, hair count reduction at six months was 35 percent. One week following treatment, 48 percent of patients experienced hyperpigmentation (brown spots) in areas treated by the laser. The same study found that using a topical corticosteroid cream 10 minutes prior to treatment and five days after treatment may help minimize side effects. ■

The best results are seen in patients who have fair skin and dark hair.

Our BEST ADVICE

Avoid laser hair removal if you have a tan. Tanning alters the skin's pigment and affects how it absorbs laser energy, which can lead to increased side effects.

Liposuction

No matter how much you exercise or cut calories, you can't change a genetic predisposition for accumulating fat in certain areas. Thanks to modern technology, though, you can walk into a doctor's office and leave two hours later with a more pleasingly contoured figure. But don't look to liposuction as a means of losing significant weight.

Does suctioning out fat remove unsightly bulges?

YES Liposuction does remove fat in targeted areas, though you may regain weight elsewhere after the surgery.

With liposuction, in which body fat is literally vacuumed out through a tube inserted through the skin, doctors can remove between 0.5 and 15 pounds of fat from stubborn areas that don't respond to diet and exercise, such as belly pooches, saddlebags, broad backsides, and double chins. The caveat: Weight lost as a result of the procedure can and often does come back, though it's less likely to reappear in the spots that were liposuctioned, since fat cells in those areas are actually removed.

In one study in Dallas, 43 percent of patients gained weight following liposuction, with 56 percent gaining between 5 and 10 pounds six months after the surgery. Yet 80 percent of patients were satisfied with the results, probably because their "trouble spots" still looked smaller.

Is liposuction totally safe?

NO As surgery goes, liposuction is relatively safe, but it's not without risks.

Two surveys peg the mortality rate from liposuction during the late 1990s at about 20 per 100,000, or 1 death for every 5,000 procedures, due to complications such as excessive

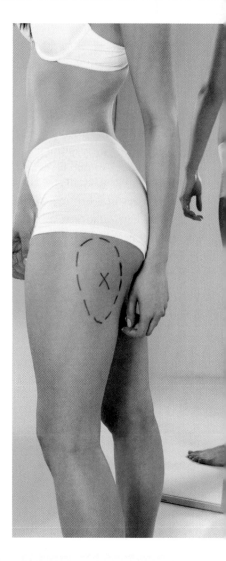

LIPOSUCTION FOR BREAST REDUCTION

Women who want to reduce the weight of their breasts without major surgery or scarring now have the option of liposuction. The procedure can reduce breast size by an average of one cup size, according to one unpublished study. Scars from liposuction are less conspicuous than those from breast reduction, and the surgery takes only a third as long. Women with a lot of fat tissue in their breasts (this often includes those who've gone through menopause) are better candidates than women who have more glandular tissue than fat tissue (this often includes younger women).

blood and fluid loss, infection, and blood or fat clots that traveled to the lungs. People who are obese or have other health problems are at greater risk. Other potential side effects include increased sensitivity or loss of sensation in the treated area and breast enlargement following liposuction of the abdominal wall. One study found that 40 percent of patients who had liposuction of the abdominal wall experienced spontaneous breast enlargement following the procedure.

Is liposuction a miracle cure for fat people?

NO Liposuction won't make an obese person thin. In fact, the more fat removed, the more dangers the surgery poses. And it won't get rid of cellulite or stretch marks. The best candidates for the procedure are people who are at or close to a healthy weight but who have fat deposits that haven't responded to diet or exercise. It helps if they have highly elastic skin to prevent sagging. ■

Lunchtime Facelifts

Think of these as facelifts for the drive-through generation. The procedures typically cost less than traditional facelifts, and you're in and out in no time flat. But do you get what you pay for? Before you drop a lot of lunch money to lift your visage, heed the age-old adage "buyer beware."

Do lunchtime facelifts work as well as traditional ones?

NO Lunchtime lifts just don't "hold up" as well in the long term.

Getting your face lifted, plumped, or otherwise reshaped used to require general anesthesia, sizable incisions, and at least an overnight hospital stay, not to mention a week or two away from the world to recover. Now you can walk into a center on your lunch break and come out an hour later looking years younger.

"Thread lifts" use barbed sutures to lift the sagging areas of the brows, midface, and neck. After making very small incisions, the surgeon inserts a needle threaded with sutures under the skin. The barbs on one end of each thread open up like an umbrella and lift sagging skin, while the teeth on the other end anchor skin to the rest of the facial tissue—and

voilà, you have younger-looking cheeks, jowls, neck, and forehead. The procedure requires only local anesthetic and little recovery time.

Some experts warn against choosing the needle over the knife, however. "Using strings to lift faces and necks works on puppets, not on humans," says Robert Kotler, MD, author of *Secrets of a Beverly Hills Cosmetic Surgeon*. "These procedures have a low incidence of complications—after all, there's no cutting or general anesthesia involved—but they also have a very short life span."

While traditional facelifts last 10 to 15 years, thread lifts are good for somewhere around 2 to 4 years. The results are subtler (read less impressive), and in some cases, "thread migration" may cause an uneven appearance, and threads may even be visible through the skin. Doctors who believe in these facelifts recommend them mainly for younger patients with minimal facial sagging. ■

Sunscreens

Mostly gone are the days when beachgoers and backyard sun worshipers slathered baby oil all over themselves to get a deep, savage burn, er, tan. Today, people are more interested in protecting their skin from the sun's harmful rays than in soaking them up, and there are more sunscreens than ever that promise to do it—as well as a new worry in the form of high-tech "nanoparticles."

Do all "broad-spectrum" sunscreens protect against UVB and UVA rays?

NO If you want optimal sun protection, you have to search the ingredient lists.

Sunscreens these days have gotten pretty sophisticated. Beyond their SPF (sun protection factor) ratings, which suggest how much longer you can stay out in the sun without burning than you could without sunscreen, many claim to be waterproof (though most swimmers know better) and sweatproof. More important, many labels now sport the words "broad spectrum," meaning the sunscreen claims to block both the short-wave UVB rays that cause sunburn and the UVA rays that penetrate the surface of the skin, damaging collagen and elastin fibers and contributing to wrinkles and possibly skin cancer.

But how effective are these products? According to an analysis conducted by the US consumer watchdog organization the Environmental Working Group, 18 percent of sunscreens analyzed that claimed broad-spectrum coverage provided poor UVA protection. According to the analysis, for the best protection against UVA rays, you should look for any of the ollowing four ingredients.

- Avobenzone (also known as Parsol 1789)
- Mexoryl SX (recently approved by the FDA, it's been used for years in Canada and Europe)
- Zinc oxide
- Titanium dioxide

If your sunscreen contains avobenzone, you should know that this ingredient breaks down quickly in the sun, so products that rely on it for UVA protection should also contain a stabilizer like Helioplex, Active Photo Barrier Complex, Dermaplex, Sun-Sure, or AvoTriplex.

Among the products that met the stringent criteria of the Environmental Working Group were UV Natural Sunscreen, Sport (SPF 30+);

SHOULD YOU DOSE UP ON VITAMIN D?

Some people justify soaking up sun with the fact that sunshine prompts the body to make vitamin D. But that logic doesn't pass muster. The truth is that most of us get enough vitamin D during everyday activities like walking to the post office or even driving, assuming we aren't wearing sunscreen. While the health benefits of vitamin D are well established, the downsides of significant sun exposure far outweigh any upside.

Vanicream Sunscreen, Sport (SPF 35); Hawaiian Tropic Baby Faces Sunblock (SPF 60+) ; and Blue Lizard Australian Suncream, Sensitive Skin (SPF 30).

It's also critical to apply sunscreen liberally—much more liberally than you probably do. Experts recommend using a shot glass of sunscreen every time you slather up.

Do I need a sunscreen with more than 30 SPF?

NO Sunscreens with an SPF over 30 provide almost no more protection than you get with an SPF 30 product.

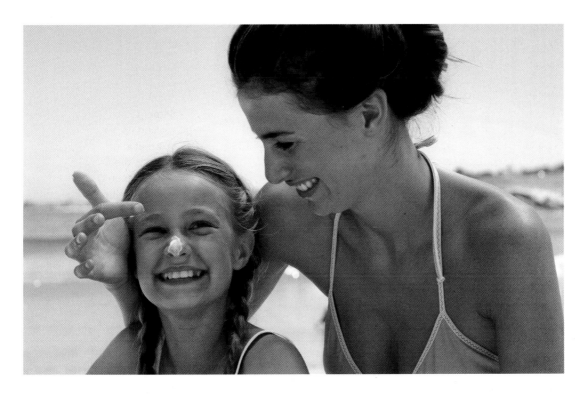

Are nanoparticles in sunscreens safe?

MAYBE According to the available research, there's no telling whether zinc oxide and titanium dioxide nanoparticles can penetrate healthy skin.

Zinc oxide and titanium dioxide are two proven ingredients that block UVA rays. Unfortunately, they also turn your skin white (picture lifeguards' noses). Enter nanotechnology. By shrinking the two chemicals to particles too tiny for the brain to fathom, manufacturers can make the cream clear—and just as effective. Hundreds of sunscreens on the market today contain these particles, called nanoparticles.

Whenever scientists mess with nature, though, questions about safety arise. Reducing chemicals to nano proportions can alter their physical properties, creating a whole new set of rules and reactivity that scientists don't yet understand. Some fear that nanoparticles may pass through the skin and create havoc—for instance, combining with sunlight to produce harmful free radicals, which damage cells. But the weight of the current evidence suggests that zinc oxide and titanium dioxide nanoparticles remain on the surface of the skin, where they can do no harm.

More study is needed, though. No one can be sure how nanoparticles might interact with other ingredients in sunscreens, and little testing has been done. For now, many experts say that any risk is outweighed by the benefits. ■

SUN PROTECTION IN A PILL?

Extracts from a tropical fern called *Polypodium leucotomos* have antioxidant properties that seem to help protect the skin from sun damage when taken orally. Sold in Europe for two decades, the pills recently became available in the United States under the brand name Heliocare. It isn't intended to fight sunburn and shouldn't be used instead of sunscreen.

Supplemental Hormones

It's a fact of life: Our bodies slow down and become frailer as we age. Desperate to retain their strength and vigor, to say nothing of their sex drive, some aging boomers are replacing the hormones that naturally decline with age. But most experts agree these treatments aren't ready for primetime. (To read about testosterone, see the Sex Drive entry on page 98.)

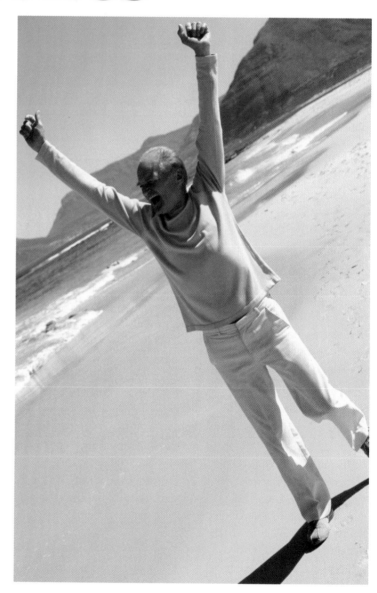

Is there good evidence that taking human growth hormone slows the effects of aging?

NO Hormones have been touted as a remedy for everything from wrinkles to lagging libidos. But experts agree that the market for these products is years ahead of the research.

Sure, the amounts of hormones like human growth hormone (HGH) decline as we age, but replacing them with synthetic versions doesn't necessarily slow the aging process, and it may increase the risk of a variety of health problems and unwanted side effects.

The idea of taking hormones to combat the natural aging process took off in the 1990s after the *New England Journal of Medicine* presented results of a small study finding that men who were injected with synthetic HGH three times a week for six months experienced significant increases in lean body mass, bone mineral density, and skin thickness.

Several studies since then have replicated these findings, but typically in adults who were deficient in growth hormone (injections are currently approved to treat people with growth hormone deficiency but not for anti-aging purposes). For these people, HGH can improve body composition, muscle strength, physical function, and bone density, but the improvements are often accompanied by carpal tunnel syndrome, edema, joint pain, swelling, and possibly an increased risk of cancer.

It isn't at all clear that HGH injections can help the average person look or feel younger, and the long-term risks are unknown. Products that claim to offer HGH in pill form almost certainly have no benefit.

Can DHEA reverse the signs of aging?

NO Taking DHEA is not akin to sipping from the fountain of youth.

Your adrenal glands naturally produce DHEA, which they use to make other hormones, including estrogen and testosterone. As you age, the glands make less and less DHEA, but it's unclear whether that decline

WHAT'S IN THE BOTTLE?

The FDA does not regulate DHEA supplements (or any other supplements), and products may contain wildly varying amounts of the purported main ingredient—some with dangerously high amounts and some with none at all. Repeated blood tests are the only way to determine that you're getting the hormone and at what level. Most DHEA supplements contain extracts of a Mexican wild yam plant that are converted into DHEA in the lab by a series of chemical reactions. But not all of these products contain a usable form of DHEA.

has anything to do with declines in body function. What's more clear is that taking a DHEA supplement (sold over the counter as a "dietary supplement" in the United States and by prescription in many European countries) probably won't make you look or feel younger—and the risks almost certainly outweigh any benefits.

In one study, researchers compared perimenopausal women who took 50 milligrams of DHEA daily for three months with others who got a placebo. The DHEA group didn't experience improvements in mood, libido, memory, or well-being compared to the placebo group. Another study found no beneficial effects on body composition, physical performance, insulin sensitivity, or

quality of life among those treated with either DHEA or testosterone. Side effects can include hair loss or the growth of facial hair.

Since it is a steroid, megadoses of DHEA help develop hard bodies by binding to bone cells that beef up bone density, strengthening muscle fibers, and reducing body fat. But it may also increase the risk of hormone-sensitive cancers such as those of the prostate and breast.

"The idea that DHEA preserves youth and increases libido is a myth," says Geoffrey Redmond, MD, an endocrinologist at the Hormone Center of New York in New York City. What's more, long-term research on the safety of hormone supplementation is lacking. ∎

"The idea that DHEA preserves youth and increases libido is a myth."

Tooth Whiteners

Want to whiten your teeth at home? Good old-fashioned tooth brushing will get teeth clean, of course, by scrubbing away surface stains, but to remove deeper stains, people can turn to a dizzying array of products, from press-on whitening strips to gels that are painted on or used with a mouth guard. Most use some form of peroxide to whiten tooth enamel.

Do at-home whitening strips and gels whiten teeth?

YES These products produce results in yellowish teeth, but not in brownish or grayish teeth.

Researchers from the University of Michigan analyzed 25 clinical studies of at-home bleaching products containing carbamide or hydrogen peroxide and found that after two weeks of use, the whiteners worked better than no whitening treatment, and differences in efficacy were mainly due to differing levels of active ingredients. Many of the studies they examined, however, may have been biased because they were conducted or funded by the manufacturers of the products. Nevertheless, this is the best scientific evidence available.

The quest for a Hollywood smile also comes with a price.

Up to 78 percent of people who use tooth bleaches experience sensitivity in their teeth while using whitening systems, with people who have receding gums faring the worst. Home bleaching gels are more likely to cause irritation than treatments at the dentist's office since the one-size-fits-all trays aren't customized to fit your mouth, potentially allowing peroxide to leak into soft tissue and gums. Overuse of bleaching products can also lead to inflamed gums, rough tooth enamel, splotchy teeth, and a phenomenon known as "skim milk smile" (overbleached teeth that appear translucent blue or gray). Most symptoms disappear once the user stops bleaching. How much is too much? If your teeth become sensitive to cold air or liquids or tingle frequently, you've gone overboard.

For the best whitening results, you may want to see your dentist. Professionally applied whiteners contain amounts of hydrogen peroxide ranging from 15 to 35 percent (home kits have about 10 percent) and are sometimes used with a laser to accelerate the whitening process. And while home-use products are intended for use over a two- to four-week period, professional procedures are completed in about an hour.

Do whitening toothpastes whiten teeth more than regular toothpastes?

NO Some whitening toothpastes contain peroxide; others rely on "polishers" such as baking soda and silica. All toothpastes can make teeth look white by scrubbing off stains, but whitening toothpastes don't seem to provide much extra benefit. Consumer Reports tested 41 brands of toothpaste that claimed to whiten teeth and found none of them performed any better than regular toothpaste. ∎

Our BEST ADVICE

Eat more fruits and vegetables. Raw vegetables and fibrous fruits like strawberries can brighten teeth by removing stains.

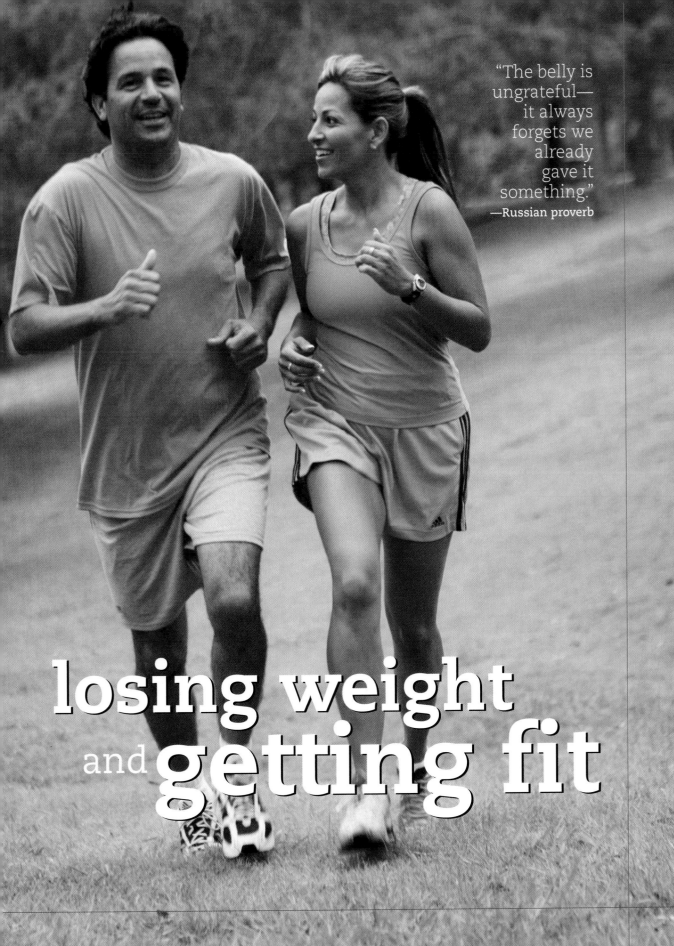

"The belly is ungrateful—it always forgets we already gave it something."
—Russian proverb

losing weight and getting fit

Calorie Cutting

You've heard it before: Calories are the key to weight-loss success (or failure). Consume less than you burn, and the pounds will vanish like last night's cheeseburger. Simple, right? Actually, no. Calorie cutting works—but not as well as you might think. What's more, not all calories are equal. Choose the right ones, and you can potentially eat less without going hungry. Choose the wrong ones, and your food could leave you wanting more.

Will I lose weight if I eat less?

YES Cutting calories leads to short-term weight loss, but the results won't last forever if that's all you do.

Weight loss is a notoriously difficult feat to pull off, and overwhelming research shows that most people who try, fail. According to a review of studies by UCLA scientists, the word on dieting is downright dismal: An average of 41 percent of people gain back more weight than they lost within a year after starting to diet. And the researchers believe this figure is conservative—too low. It doesn't account for people who drop out of studies because they're embarrassed by their expanding waistlines.

   That said, cutting calories does work in the short term, though it's necessary to cut more calories than most people realize (3,500, to be

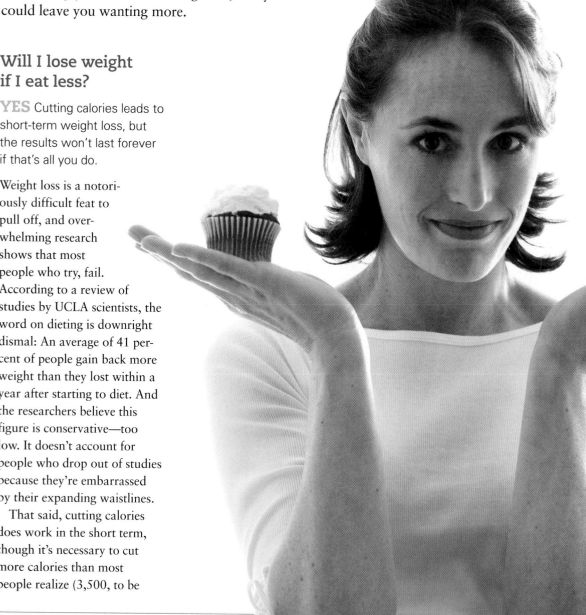

exact) in order to lose 1 pound. According to a review of studies by the National Institutes of Health, going on a low-calorie diet (1,400 to 2,000 calories a day, depending on your current size) can help people lose 8 percent of their body weight over 3 to 12 months.

So why do so many diets fail? There are lots of reasons. First, people are human, and diets are hard to stick with. Second, our bodies work against us: After you've lost some weight, your metabolism slows down so that you have to eat less and less just to maintain that weight loss. It's your body's way of making sure you don't starve.

A third problem: People who are overly anxious to drop pounds sometimes cut too many calories. In the beginning, this can cause intense food cravings, although they eventually wear off. (In fact, in the long run, low-calorie diets have actually been shown to curb hunger.) Finally, if you don't exercise while dieting, you're likely to lose muscle mass, which slows your metabolism even more (see page 64 for details).

Does it matter where your calories come from?

YES Calories are not created equal. Those from fat or refined carbohydrates are more likely to end up on your thighs.

If a cream-filled doughnut and a chicken breast sandwich have the same number of calories, does that mean you can have the doughnut for lunch instead of the sandwich and come out even? Nutritionally, not a chance. But even weight-wise, you're worse off with the doughnut.

Our **BEST** ADVICE

Use the Internet to tally daily calories and track them in a centralized location. You can get calorie counts for thousands of foods at sites like CalorieKing.com and NutritionData.com. Then log them in at tracking sites like FitDay.com.

First, there's the thermic effect of food. You may not remember this from high school biology, but it means that some foods take more energy to chew, digest, metabolize, and store than others. Unfortunately, the body is very efficient at processing fat and expends very few calories doing so—one reason that fatty foods seem to spend "a moment on the lips, a lifetime on the hips." The body is quite good at processing carbohydrates, too. Protein, on the other hand, has to be converted into carbohydrates before it can become fat. That takes a lot of work, burning up as much as 30 percent of the calories in the food you're eating.

Then there's the effect of food on blood sugar. Refined carbohydrates (think white bread, cookies, and fruit drinks) tend to raise blood sugar levels rather dramatically, which encourages fat storage, weight gain, and hunger. On the other hand, fibrous foods

EATING LESS: THE FOUNTAIN OF YOUTH?

Cutting calories will not only help you fit back into your skinny jeans, it may also curb the aging process. Significantly reducing calorie intake has been shown to increase life span, at least in lab animals. As for the human research, studies show that people on calorie-restricted diets have substantially lower levels of inflammatory proteins in the blood. Why is that important? Inflammation plays a key role in virtually every human health condition, from Alzheimer's to heart disease to arthritis. The more inflammatory substances circulating in your bloodstream, the more quickly your body will deteriorate.

like apples, as well as protein foods, not only take more energy to digest but also raise blood sugar less, making them friendlier to your waistline.

Finally, foods that contain a lot of water, such as vegetables and soup, tend to fill the belly on fewer calories, so you'll stop eating them way before you stop eating the Krispy Kremes.

Can keeping a food diary help you lose weight?

YES Jotting down everything you eat keeps you honest and makes you think twice before overindulging.

Most people don't have a clue what they really eat every day. For instance, studies show that dieters tend to underestimate their calorie intake by as much as 50 percent. Keeping a food diary can solve the problem. It doesn't have to be fancy; any notebook will do. Just write down every morsel you put in your mouth while you're trying to lose weight (and whenever the number on the scale begins to climb). Then use a calorie-counter book or Internet site to estimate how many calories

FINDING YOUR CALORIE TARGET

Add a zero to your weight to get your basal metabolic rate, or BMR, the amount of energy you expend at rest. Multiply your BMR by one of the numbers below, based on your physical activity level, to find the total number of calories necessary to maintain your current weight.

Sedentary = 1.2
Low activity = 1.5
Active = 1.75
Very active = 2.2

If you weigh 140 pounds, your BMR is 1,400. If you're sedentary, multiply 1,400 by 1.2, and you find that the number of calories you need each day to maintain your weight is 1,680. Want to lose a pound a week? Slash 500 calories from that number each day for a daily intake of 1,180 calories.

each item contains, total up your daily calories, and tease out your diet saboteurs. Is an afternoon candy bar habit putting you over your calorie max? Are you drinking more calories than you realized with each caramel latte? Are you pouring yourself too much cereal in the morning?

Experts claim food diaries can help dieters slash 500 to 1,000 calories a day by uncovering food traps like high-sugar sodas and juices. In fact, keeping a food diary is one of four key behaviors consistently used by people in the

National Weight Control Registry, an ongoing study of dieters who maintained a weight loss of 30 pounds or more for at least one year.

A good food diary is more than just a list of foods and quantities. Recording where you were, whom you were with, how hungry you were, and how you felt before and after you ate can also help you spot influential patterns. (Does work stress make you gobble up snacks at the office? Do you eat less when your husband is away?)

Don't want to look up calorie counts for every piece of food you pop in your mouth? No problem. Seeing what you've eaten in black and white, even without the numbers, is likely to make you think twice before heading back to the table for a second slice of pecan pie. ■

Keeping a food diary is perhaps the most important strategy for weight-loss success.

Carbohydrates

Even now that the low-carb craze has died down, today's dieters fear potatoes more than last week's mystery meat. But "to carb or not to carb?" is the wrong question. As with most things in life, it's the quality (of your carbs) that counts more than the quantity. Lentil soup, anyone?

Do low-carb diets work?

YES People lose more weight during the first six months of a low-carb diet than they do on other kinds. But after one year, the various diets even out.

There are countless variations of the low-carb diet. Some plans allow all the cheese, bacon, and Béarnaise sauce you can eat, while others limit food loaded with saturated fat in favor of skinless chicken breasts and low-fat cottage cheese. The common denominator: They all restrict carbs and help dieters shed pounds, at least in the short term.

There's little doubt that low-carb diets speed initial weight loss. In one recent study published in the *American Journal of Clinical Nutrition*, after 12 weeks on a low-carb plan, study participants lost an average of 10.8 pounds compared to 5.5 pounds for those on a low-fat diet.

It's little wonder these diets work: A low-carb diet is basically a low-calorie diet with a high protein content. Sure, removing a bun from a burger, eating a salad instead of fries, and opting for diet soda over regular makes for a lower-carb meal, but it's also a lower-calorie meal. What's more, low-carb diets are typically easier to stick with because the protein and fat in these plans help dieters feel full. In one study, during a 12-week phase of unrestricted total calorie intake of a high-protein, low-fat diet, researchers found that people spontaneously ate 450 fewer calories per day and reported feeling more satisfied than those on a high-carbohydrate diet.

But here's the catch: Studies show that at one year, the weight loss on a low-carb diet tends to equal that on a low-cal diet, possibly because people get tired of eating breadless sandwiches and shunning rice.

Are low-carb diets more effective for some people than for others?

YES What it takes to fit back into your skinny jeans is as much about your other genes as about what you put in your mouth.

Why can your best friend hit the bread basket before dinner without gaining an ounce, while the mere thought of crusty rolls causes your thighs to expand? It boils down to the hormone insulin, which escorts blood sugar into cells for energy and storage. Some people are genetically programmed to react to carbohydrates by secreting an oversize dose of insulin—and

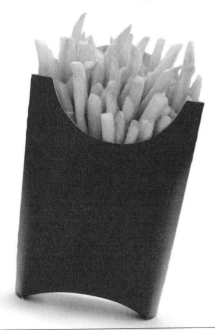

they will probably benefit most from a low-carb diet.

A study published in the *Journal of the American Medical Association* found that after 18 months, high insulin secretors dropped about 13 pounds on a low-carb diet compared to a 2.5-pound drop for high insulin secretors on a higher-carb, lower-fat diet, even though both groups cut out the same number of daily calories (about 400). Lower insulin secretors lost the same amount of weight on either diet.

How do you know if your DNA fits the bill? Look in the mirror. If you store fat in your belly (an "apple" body shape), you're more likely to secrete excess insulin than if you store fat in or around your hips (a "pear" body shape). For a more scientific approach, pull out a tape measure and measure your waist at the belly button. Then measure your hips at their widest part (where your derriere is largest) and divide your waist measurement by your hip measurement. For women, a result of 0.8 or less indicates a normal or low insulin secretor; for men, it's 0.95 or less.

If eating carbs makes you hungrier, or you have frequent cravings for rice, pasta, and the like, that's another sign you're a high insulin secretor. Try cutting back on carbs and replacing white breads, pastas, and grain products with whole grain foods. If your cravings diminish, chances are you've found a winner!

Do low-carb diets stress the kidneys?

NO If you don't already have a kidney problem, you're not likely to develop one from a low-carb diet.

A diet low in carbs is automatically higher in the other two macronutrients: fat and protein. Some experts worry that the extra protein may tax the kidneys; after all, these organs are responsible for breaking down protein. But there's no scientific research to back that theory. In a study of 1,624 women, Boston researchers found no association between high protein intake and declining kidney function in women with healthy kidneys.

That said, people with existing kidney problems should steer clear of low-carb plans. The less work you give the impaired organs to do, the

Processed foods and refined grains may be the primary reason for the obesity epidemic.

better. When the body breaks down protein, it forms substances that change damaged kidneys' structure and function, promoting further damage.

Are diets with a low glycemic index the best approach for most people?

YES More and more experts agree that a low-glycemic diet is an effective way to lose weight.

Not long ago, health experts recommended a low-fat, high-carb diet for optimal health and weight management. But people ballooned, and carbs took the brunt of the blame. Specifically, it was the *types* of carbs people gorged on, like french fries, mashed potatoes, and hamburger buns—in other words, starchy foods and refined grains stripped of their fiber and other nutrients—that were the likely culprits. Because these foods digest quickly and convert easily into glucose, or blood sugar, they cause blood sugar and insulin surges that lead to insulin

resistance and weight gain, or so the theory goes.

Those white buns and white potatoes rank high on the glycemic index (GI), a measure of how quickly a food is broken down into glucose. The reference point is pure glucose, which is arbitrarily scored as 100. The higher the GI, the greater the blood sugar spike a food causes.

Thanks to our penchant for processed foods and refined grains, the GI of our diets has increased dramatically over the past 30 years. In fact, some experts believe this is the primary reason for the obesity epidemic, along with increasing portion sizes.

Australian researchers evaluated several studies comparing low-GI and high-GI diets and found that people who ate a diet with a low GI lost an average of 2.5 pounds more than people who ate a higher-GI diet over periods ranging from five weeks to six months. One likely reason: Low-GI

Our BEST ADVICE

Does eating low-GI mean you have to swear off potatoes, rice, and corn? Certainly not. But you may want to eat less of them and get more of your carbs from non-starchy vegetables, such as steamed spinach and broccoli, and from beans. Instead of rice- or corn-based cereal, choose a bran cereal. And steer clear of most store-bought baked goods (especially those made with white flour), sweetened fruit drinks, and nondiet soda.

---

diets assuage hunger by keeping blood sugar levels relatively steady. In a study of 39 overweight or obese people published in the *Journal of the American Medical Association*, Boston researchers found that participants on a low-GI diet reported less hunger than those on a low-fat diet. Their metabolisms slowed less, too (recall that dieting eventually slows metabolism, so the body burns fewer calories—one reason people have such a hard time losing weight). ■

Exercise

There's no "magic bullet" for weight loss, but one thing is all but certain to work: exercise. Whether you do it in a gym or in your garden, all at once or in short spurts, intensely or moderately, it burns calories, fights insulin resistance, and builds metabolism-boosting muscle. It also builds something else: self-esteem.

Is diet alone enough for sustained weight loss?

NO You'll lose weight in the short term by slashing calories, but exercise is what keeps pounds off for good.

Research shows that while dieting leads to short-term weight loss, the weight, like a boomerang, generally comes back. Adding exercise can change that picture. According to the National Weight Control Registry, an ongoing study of dieters who maintained a weight loss of 30 pounds for at least one year, 90 percent of participants use regular physical activity to keep the pounds off.

Exercise burns calories, of course. It also builds muscle, which takes up less space than fat. The result: Your wardrobe fits better. Muscle tissue also requires more calories to sustain it than fat tissue does. In other words, the more muscle tissue you have, the more calories you'll burn at rest. That's important because while diet alone may be effective at the outset, ultimately you'll reach a plateau when your metabolism slows—and that's when you'll need to get moving.

A study conducted at the Washington University School of Medicine found that people who cut out 230 calories a day for a year and didn't exercise, lost muscle mass, strength, and aerobic capacity. People who exercised *without cutting calories* lost a similar amount of weight without sacrificing muscle mass.

Research from Baylor College of Medicine in Houston confirms that exercise, even without diet, can be more effective for losing weight and keeping it off than diet alone. Researchers assigned 127 people to either a diet-only, exercise-only, or diet-plus-exercise program for one year. All participants lost similar amounts of weight during the first year, but when they were reassessed during year two, the diet-only crew gained 2 pounds over their baseline weight, whereas the groups that included exercise remained 5.5 pounds below their starting point.

Our BEST ADVICE

Instead of hitting the treadmill every day, try mixing things up a bit. You could do yoga on Mondays, walk on Tuesdays, play volleyball on Wednesdays, lift weights on Thursdays, and so on. You can even use cross-training within a single workout. For instance, jog for a few blocks, then stop at a park and do some pushups.

Is there a best time to exercise?

YES If you're simply walking to get healthy or take off some weight, it doesn't matter when you do it as long as you do it. That could mean you're better off exercising in the morning so the task doesn't get bumped from your schedule by a busy day. But if you're an athlete looking for the best-quality workout, choose the late afternoon, when body temperature is highest. Muscles are warm, reaction time is quick, and strength is at its peak. If you push yourself harder as a result, you can burn more calories to boot.

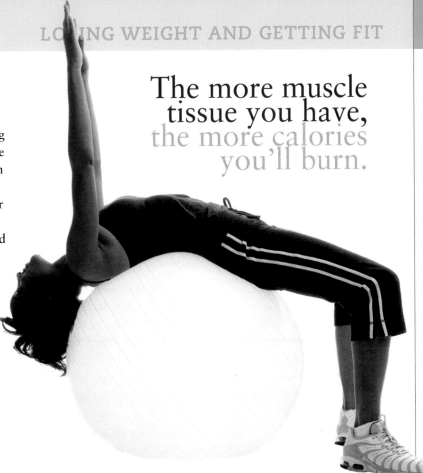

The more muscle tissue you have, the more calories you'll burn.

Does cross-training burn more fat than a steady aerobic routine?

YES Doing several different activities each week burns more calories than doing only one.

If you're someone who does only one form of exercise—say, walking or using an elliptical trainer—you may be missing out on a chance to lose more weight. A study of 72 college students conducted at the University of South Alabama found that women who cross-trained by alternating between activities such as jumping rope, cardio-boxing, lifting weights, and using a medicine ball had less body fat at the end of a 12-week training period than women who only took step aerobics classes. Both groups logged the same amount of workout time. And there was a bonus: The cross-training group felt better about their bodies and reported greater improvements in overall appearance, health, and fitness compared to the people in the aerobics-only group.

Cross-training not only helps you work all your body parts, it also reduces the risk of injury (you're not stressing the same muscles and joints day after day), and it keeps things interesting.

Does interval training burn extra calories?

YES Adding more intense bursts of activity to your regular workout increases its effectiveness.

Here's an idea for beefing up your exercise session without killing yourself: Throw in one block of running for every five blocks of your regular walk. The concept is called interval training—inserting short bursts of intense activity into more leisurely workouts—and it's used by athletes to build

EXERCISE

endurance and improve performance. For regular folks, the biggest bonus may be burning more calories in the same amount of workout time. Using interval training on occasion may even help you burn more body fat on days when you do your regular workout.

A small study conducted at the University of Guelph in Ontario had eight women use interval training on stationary bikes. For an hour every other day, they alternated four-minute bursts of riding at 90 percent effort with two-minute rest intervals. After the two weeks ended, the women burned 36 percent more fat when they cycled normally for

an hour than they did before the interval training.

It's likely that pushing yourself to do short bouts of harder activity recruits new muscle fibers that pitch in even during regular workouts, boosting the calorie and fat burn.

Interval training lets you challenge your muscles in ways that easier workouts don't, without overtaxing muscles and joints and potentially hurting yourself. But if you have heart disease or high blood pressure, check with your doctor before trying any workout that makes you out of breath.

Is hitting the gym better for you than everyday exercise?

NO Most of us hit the gym with a specific goal in mind: To burn calories. But just because you take an aerobics or Spinning class twice a week doesn't mean you'll expend more calories than if you perform basic daily tasks, or "lifestyle activities," like scrubbing the bathtub or tending the garden.

Obesity researchers from Johns Hopkins University studied the question in obese

Our BEST ADVICE

Are you ravenous after exercise? The problem may be what you ate *before* your workout if you loaded up on simple carbohydrates to power you through. The more muscle you have, the more insulin your body absorbs, which means you're in for a bigger postworkout blood sugar crash once the sugar high is gone—and then you're starving! Instead of eating a bagel or a bowl of pasta before your workout, snack on fiber-rich foods like oatmeal or apples for a steadier stream of energy.

women. Some of the women did structured aerobic exercise, while others did moderate lifestyle activities. All followed a low-fat diet with 1,200 calories a day. Both groups lost about the same amount of weight—about 17 pounds—over 16 weeks. What's more, people in the "lifestyle activity" group regained less weight after a year than those in the other group.

Does exercise increase hunger?

NO It's a common misconception: If you burn hundreds of calories during a workout, you'll end up eating more. But research shows that exercise

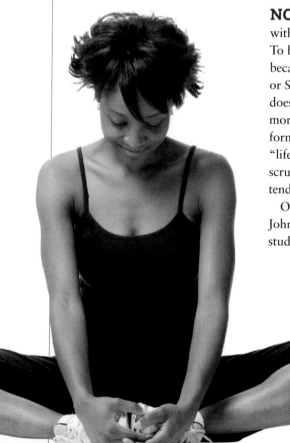

has no effect on food intake. In a study of 23 healthy men, researchers at the Human Appetite Research Unit at Leeds University in the United Kingdom found that hunger was suppressed during and after workout sessions and that exercisers put off eating for longer than people who didn't exercise. But the total amount of food consumed was the same, regardless of whether people worked out at a low intensity, high intensity, or not at all.

These findings don't apply to endurance athletes who exercise for two hours a day or more, who do compensate for the extra calories burned.

Is walking as effective as running?

YES Mile for mile, walking burns almost as many calories as running does, provided you walk briskly.

You'll burn about twice as many calories while running for 30 minutes as you will walking for 30 minutes. But if a runner and a walker cover the same distance, they burn about the same number of calories, so if you're willing to take the "slow route," you'll probably lose just as much weight.

In fact, studies have proved that how *long* you exercise matters more than how *hard* you exercise. This was true in a year-long study at the

Cooper Institute in Dallas, which asked 201 overweight sedentary women to change their diets and follow one of four exercise programs. It found that the duration of the exercise was more important than the intensity of the exercise in terms of weight lost as well as cardiorespiratory fitness. Other studies confirm this result.

Also, of course, you're less likely to hurt yourself when you walk instead of run. Consider this fact: When you run, your foot strikes the pavement with a force equal to 3 to 5 times your body weight. When you walk, the force is only about 1 1/2 times your body weight. The harder your foot strikes the ground, the more likely you are to be injured.

To build more muscle from walking, make sure you pick a route that includes some hills. And to encourage yourself to walk more, use a pedometer, a small gadget that counts the number of steps you take. Studies show that people who wear them walk more—and lose more weight.

One caveat: The more you walk, the more difficult it is to

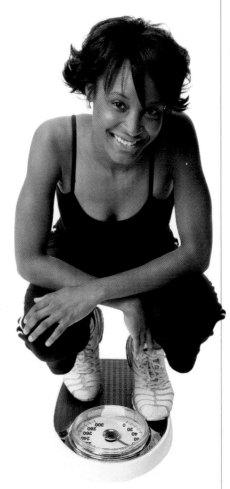

see results. One study at the American College of Sports Medicine found that as 27,596 women increased their weekly walking distance, the amount of weight lost as a result of walking diminished. Thus, when it comes to walking, the most overweight and sedentary people benefit the most.

Duration of exercise is more important than intensity in terms of weight lost.

Exercise
(continued)

Does yoga promote weight loss?

YES There's no doubt that yoga burns far fewer calories than running. Even "power" versions of yoga burn only 238 calories during a 90-minute session compared to 254 calories for a 30-minute run. Nevertheless, researchers from the Fred Hutchinson Cancer Center in Seattle found that among 15,500 overweight baby boomers, those who practiced yoga lost 5 pounds over 10 years, while those who never sprawled out on a yoga mat put on an average of 13.5 pounds during the same period. Researchers postulate that people who practice yoga develop greater body awareness, which may prevent them from overeating—it's much harder to hold the downward dog position after chowing down on pizza. A one-year study of 40 male high school students in India found that yoga helped students reach their ideal body weight while also increasing their strength and endurance. Fat folds and body circumferences were reduced significantly, too. ■

Fasting

One way to jumpstart a diet is simply to stop eating, at least for a few days. Naturopaths view brief fasts as a way to "detoxify" the body. But will it also send those extra pounds packing?

Will fasting help me lose weight faster?

NO Experts agree it's a quick way to drop a few pounds, but they'll probably come right back when you start eating again.

When you fast, your body's metabolism slows in order to conserve energy. That means you burn fewer calories. Any calories you do take in are more likely to be stored as fat. And since you're running without fuel, chances are you won't have any energy to exercise.

Weight loss isn't the only reason people fast. Popular diet books claim that abstaining from food or subsisting only on juice "cleanses" the body of toxins and gives it a break from the hard work of digestion. Yet there's some evidence that fasting actually increases the concentration of toxins in the body. Wildlife researchers at Cornell University's Center for the Environment noted a 293 percent increase in the concentration of PCBs in dogs who fasted for 48 hours.

The likely reason: "Toxins are stored in fat tissue," says weight-loss coach Jonny Bowden, PhD. "When you start releasing those fat cells [by not eating], you're not giving the liver the nutrients it needs to eliminate those toxins. So essentially, your body becomes a toxic waste dump."

There's more. Without carbohydrates, your body turns to stored fat for energy and to muscle tissue for the protein it needs for cell growth and repair. That muscle tissue includes the heart—and blood doesn't flow as efficiently to your other organs as a result. Instead of resting, your organs are actually working overtime. ■

Fiber

What do crunchy carrots, crisp apples, and chewy oatmeal have in common? It's not a nutrient; it doesn't even contain a single calorie because it can't be digested. But it could make the difference between wearing your current pant size and downsizing to a smaller one. "It" is fiber, and most of us consume only half the amount we should.

Can I lose weight by eating more fiber?

YES Fiber is a key player in the battle of the bulge. It slows digestion, adds bulk to the diet, and makes you feel full for longer, so there's less room for "junk."

Cup for cup, fiber-rich foods have fewer calories than their low-fiber counterparts. A cup of apple juice weighs in at 117 calories and 0 grams of fiber, while an apple with skin comes in at just 74 calories and an impressive 3.4 grams of fiber. Since the body can't digest fiber, it runs right through your digestive tract instead of landing on your hips. Chalk up one point in fiber's favor.

Here's a second: Fiber (think bran cereal and whole wheat bread) takes up a lot of room in the stomach, which helps you feel full. It also slows digestion, which keeps a lid on blood sugar spikes that can trigger hunger a few hours later. The soluble fiber found in oats, beans, and apples actually forms a gel in your stomach that acts as a barrier between your meal and the stomach acids that digest it. When a meal is digested slowly, your blood sugar levels increase more gradually—and you stay full longer.

Finally, foods with a lot of fiber take longer to chew, and the slower you eat, the less food you're likely to consume.

The bottom line: You'll lose more weight if your diet contains more fiber. A study published in the *Journal of the American Dietetic Association* found that the main difference between normal-weight adults and their overweight or obese counterparts was the amount of fiber they consumed. Although, according to food questionnaires, the two groups ate about the same amounts of sugar, bread, dairy products, and vegetables, the normal-weight subjects consumed a whopping 33 percent more dietary fiber and 43 percent more complex carbohydrates each day, per 1,000 calories, than those who were overweight or obese. They also ate less fat. Other studies link fiber with lower body weight, body fat, and body mass index.

Experts recommend consuming a minimum of 25 grams of fiber daily. To get your daily dose, gradually bump up your servings of fruits, vegetables, whole grains, and beans—and wash them down with plenty of water to help all that fiber pass through. ■

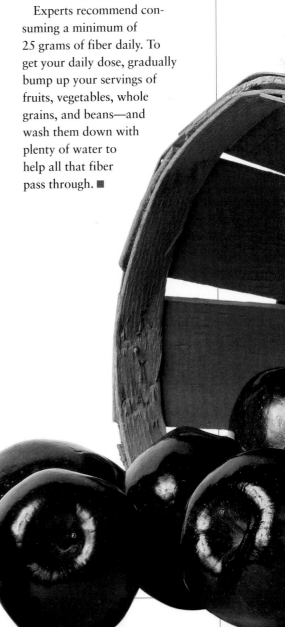

Gastric Bypass

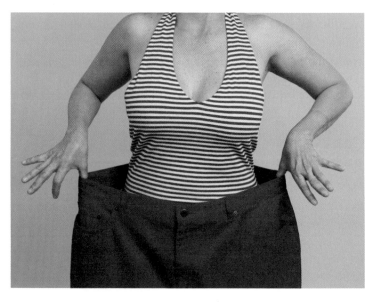

As obesity rates skyrocket, more people are flocking to surgeons to have their stomachs "shrunk." So-called bariatric surgeries staple or otherwise block off a small part of the stomach and connect this new, smaller stomach to the small intestine. The result: People can't eat as much. They also can't absorb as much of the food they do take in because part of the intestine is bypassed. It's a drastic measure, and it produces dramatic results—sometimes.

Does gastric bypass guarantee permanent weight loss?

NO There's no denying that gastric bypass surgeries cause significant weight loss, but the results won't last forever unless patients do their part.

Gastric bypass surgeries, which essentially detour food around most of the stomach, cause significant short-term weight loss for most patients, to say nothing of their ability to ease or even reverse chronic conditions like diabetes, high cholesterol, high blood pressure, and sleep apnea. After surgery, patients can eat only small amounts of food at a time because the new, smaller stomach pouch holds less than 1 ounce of food. Eventually it expands enough to accommodate 4 to 6 ounces of food, still a far cry from the 32 ounces it could hold before. To prevent nutritional deficiencies that could lead to conditions like anemia and bone loss, patients are required to take multivitamin supplements.

Studies show a substantial weight loss in the months after surgery—up to 62 percent of excess body weight—but it's followed by a gradual regain. In one study conducted in Sweden, the average loss 2 years after gastric bypass surgery was 23 percent of the patient's original weight; 10 years after, it was only 16 percent.

Since the stomach is largely muscle, patients can train it to accommodate more food. Unless you change your habits for life, you're likely to regain at least some of the lost weight—and possibly see diseases like diabetes and high blood pressure return.

The procedures don't come without side effects, such as gas, pain, and diarrhea, and can pose significant risks. In the Swedish study, 13 percent of patients had postoperative complications such as bleeding, blood clots, infection, or lung-related problems, and 5 out of 2,010 died shortly after their procedures. Mortality rates from the surgeries range from 0.5 to 2 percent. ■

Low-Fat Diets

Before carbohydrates assumed the role of dietary enemy number one, it was fat that would supposedly consign us all to a lifetime of rolling stomachs and blubbery thighs. But fat's reputation has been rehabilitated. You may even have better luck losing weight if you allow a moderate amount of it into your diet.

Are ultra low fat diets the best way to lose weight?

NO Fat isn't the cause of our obesity problem; overeating is. Diets that reduce fat to less than 15 percent of calories may even backfire.

Many high-profile nutrition experts claim fat has been unfairly implicated in the obesity epidemic. In fact, one likely reason people weigh so much today is that they took the edict to eat less fat a bit *too* seriously, favoring low-fat muffins, crackers, and cakes— and consuming way too many simple carbohydrates in the process.

Good studies today show that diets that are high in protein and either low or modest in carbohydrates result in greater weight loss (at least in the short term) than low-fat diets, which consist mostly of carbohydrates. Unlike carbohydrates, fat has little or no effect on blood sugar, and it's thought that steady blood sugar levels help keep hunger and food cravings in check.

Very low fat diets— those that get less than 15 percent of their calories from fat—are also extremely difficult to maintain, no doubt because humans crave fat by nature. In a study of 120 overweight volunteers conducted at Duke University Medical Center, only 57 percent of low-fat dieters completed the six-month study compared to 76 percent of those on a low-carb plan.

Sure, earlier research showed that extremely low fat diets dramatically reduce the risk of heart attack, stroke, and other chronic diseases, but many nutrition experts believe these benefits may have been due to the high fiber and low sugar content of the diets—not the lack of fat.

That said, cutting a *moderate* amount of fat from your

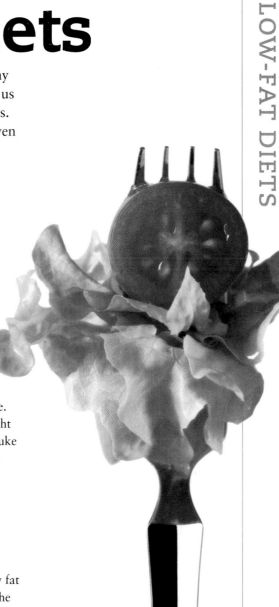

Low-Fat Diets
(continued)

diet is still a good idea, especially if you're getting fat mostly from cheeseburgers and fried chicken instead of from healthier sources such as fish and olive oil.

Do low-fat diets work better than other low-calorie diets?

NO Researchers who examined the results of a handful of well-conducted weight-loss studies found that people on low-fat diets lost about the same amount of weight at 6, 12, and 18 months as people on other low-calorie diets.

A real blow to low-fat diets was dealt by data from a study involving nearly 49,000 women, part of the long-running Women's Health Initiative. It showed that women who tried to reduce their fat intake to 20 percent of their total calories weighed about the same eight years later as women who didn't change their diets at all. One possible reason for the lack of results is that the women didn't quite achieve their fat-cutting goals, getting down only to about 29 percent of total calories. Nevertheless, the moral of the story stands: Losing weight and keeping it off is difficult indeed. ■

Meal Timing

According to some diet gurus, when you eat is almost as important as what you eat. They advocate noshing on mini-meals throughout the day to keep blood sugar steady and metabolism high. Have regular repasts gone out the window? One thing's for sure: Mom was right. Breakfast really is the most important meal of the day.

Can you lose weight by eating three squares a day?

YES While diet experts swear by eating small meals throughout the day, you can still lose weight by eating a regular breakfast, lunch, and dinner.

One of the latest diet trends is noshing on five or six small meals a day instead of three larger ones. Diet gurus claim that spreading calories throughout the day helps keep blood sugar levels (and therefore hunger) in check, metabolism high, and energy up, which means you're more likely to move around. But according to the published weight-loss research, there's no "right" way to approach mealtimes. Whether your body performs better on one meal or six is up for debate, and experts claim it's different for different people (once again, insulin secretion probably plays a role).

A recent Swedish study tested eating plans of three meals per day versus three meals plus three snacks in 140 obese people and found that both groups lost about the same amount of weight after a year (everyone cut calories.) Another study at the University of Missouri involving 100 men and women showed similar results: Both snackers and nonsnackers lost an average of 10 pounds over 24 weeks.

Other studies associate eating more than three times a day with being overweight and obese, but the frequent eaters were noshing on junk foods, not fiber-rich fruits and vegetables. The general consensus: If you need your snacks, make sure they're low in calories and high in nutrients.

Does eating breakfast help you lose weight?

YES Study after study shows that people who lose weight and keep it off eat breakfast every day.

If you think skipping breakfast means taking in fewer calories throughout the day, think again. Studies show that people who skip breakfast usually make up the calories later in the day—and then some. One study published in the *American Journal of Clinical Nutrition* found that when women had breakfast, they ate about 100 fewer calories per day than when they didn't have a morning meal.

Eating breakfast is one habit that people who succeed in losing weight tend to share. Researchers from the University of Colorado Health Sciences Center found that among the nearly 3,000 people who had lost an average of 70 pounds and kept it off for at least one year, almost 80 percent reported eating breakfast every day. In a study of 10,087 Dutch adolescents, those who ate breakfast every day were significantly less likely to be overweight than those who ate breakfast irregularly or never.

Eating breakfast may help even if it doesn't make you consume fewer calories during the day, perhaps because it kicks your metabolism back into high gear after a night of sleep, during which the body conserves energy. In a study of 52 moderately obese women, those who ate three meals a day, including breakfast, lost 17 pounds over 12 weeks. By comparison, women who ate only two meals a day (no breakfast) lost only 13 pounds. Both groups ate the same total number of calories.

Does eating at night make you fat?

NO There's no good evidence that this pervasive belief is true.

A pint of ice cream eaten at 8 p.m. has the same number of calories as a pint of ice cream eaten at 8 a.m. So why do so many people associate evening eating with packing on the pounds? First of all, most of us don't eat ice cream in the morning; we spoon it up at night in front of the TV. If noshing in front of the tube means overeating junk food, you can be sure it will catch up to you (and your waistline). This is probably how the myth

Our BEST ADVICE

To milk the most benefits from eating breakfast, choose your food wisely. Studies show a breakfast that contains more protein and fewer simple carbohydrates will keep you full longer and help banish cravings later in the day. So an egg or two plus a slice of whole wheat toast and a handful of fiber-rich berries is a better choice than, say, a big bowl of cornflakes or a bagel. If you want cereal for breakfast, make it a low-GI choice, such as bran cereal or oatmeal. Stick to the serving size on the box and add fruit to your bowl if you want more food.

about late-night eating got started. But what about healthy meals eaten in late in the evening?

Many people believe that any food eaten at night is more likely to stick to bellies and thighs because there's little opportunity to burn off those calories before sleep, when the body's metabolism slows. But again, it's most likely all about portion sizes. If you haven't eaten since lunch at noon and you sit down for dinner at 10 p.m., chances are you're starving, and you'll end up eating more than you should. Eating late at night may also decrease your desire for breakfast in the morning, and as you just read, skipping breakfast can hamper your weight-loss efforts. ∎

Eating breakfast is one habit that **people who succeed** in losing weight tend to share.

Protein

Protein is the new "it" nutrient. It makes you feel full so you can keep calories under control and helps ensure that when you drop weight, it comes mostly from fat, not muscle. The protein we eat also contains amino acids that are essential to just about every bodily function, such as allowing cells to grow and reproduce.

HOW MUCH PROTEIN DO YOU NEED?

The recommended protein intake is 0.4 gram per pound of body weight if you're moderately active and 1 to 2 grams per pound if you lift like Arnold Schwarzenegger used to. Protein intakes above 2 grams per pound of body weight offer no additional muscle-building benefits.

Does eating enough protein help you lose weight?

YES Eating protein while dieting helps preserve lean muscle mass, which keeps your metabolism from slowing down.

One problem with dieting is that most dieters lose muscle mass in addition to body fat. Since muscle burns more calories than fat does, the result is a slower metabolism. Exercise is key to maintaining muscle mass, but eating enough protein helps, too.

Another perk of protein (think skinless chicken breasts, eggs, fat-free milk, and beans): Among the three macronutrients—carbs, protein, and fat—protein is the most difficult to store as body fat. First, the body has to convert protein into carbs before it can be converted into fat, a process that burns calories. Second, when you eat protein, your body doesn't require much insulin to metabolize it. High insulin levels appear to decrease fat burning, while lower levels mean you're less likely to store excess calories as fat.

A 12-week study of 46 women conducted at Purdue University found that dieters who consumed 18 percent of their calories from protein lost nearly twice as much lean body mass compared to those who got 30 percent of their calories from protein. And even though both groups slashed 750 calories from their usual diets, the higher-protein eaters reported greater enjoyment from their food and felt more satisfied—no surprise, since protein has been shown to curb appetite and help keep hunger at bay between meals.

Don't go overboard, though. "The body can only use about four to eight ounces of protein at a time," says Christine Gerbstadt, RD, MD, national spokesperson for the American Dietetic Association. "The rest is converted into carbohydrate for immediate energy or stored as fat."

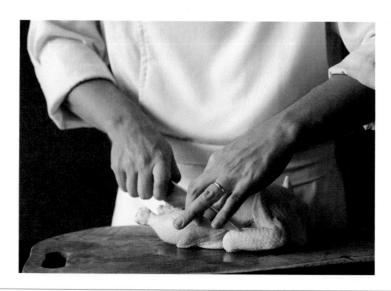

Do protein shakes help add muscle?

YES But mainly after an intense workout. Regular folks probably don't need them.

In order to rebuild muscle tissue that breaks down during exercise, the body needs protein, especially during the first 30 to 90 minutes after a workout. Studies show that eating (or drinking) protein after a workout speeds muscle recovery and supplies the body with the necessary amino acids for muscle growth and repair.

According to a study conducted at Baylor University in Texas, taking whey and casein protein supplements significantly increased muscle mass among 36 men who did heavy weight lifting for 10 weeks. Other studies show that between 20 and 60 grams per day of whey protein improves muscle mass and performance in athletes on a strength-training program.

In elderly patients, protein supplementation has been shown to increase muscle strength, reduce bone loss, and accelerate healing after a bone fracture.

Most people can easily get all the protein they need from a healthy diet. If you do drink protein shakes, remember that they contain calories. Unless you use them to *replace* a meal, you'll probably end up gaining weight from drinking them. ■

Sleep

In today's time-crunched society, only one-quarter of us get the recommended eight hours of sleep a night. No wonder "nap pods" are cropping up in airports and shopping malls—weary folks need mini-siestas to get through the day. Unfortunately, lack of sleep can take a toll, not only on your health but on your waistline, too.

Can getting enough sleep help you lose weight?

YES Skimping on sleep may cause you to develop insulin resistance, which can lead to weight gain.

It doesn't take a PhD to understand why you reach for a doughnut instead of hitting the gym when you're running on four hours of sleep. If you limit the amount of time you spend in deep sleep, the brain thinks you're running low on energy and increases your appetite accordingly.

As part of the Nurses' Health Study, 68,183 women who reported chronic sleep deprivation in 1986 were followed for 16 years using questionnaires every two years. Women who reported sleeping five or fewer hours each night were 32 percent more likely to gain 30-plus pounds than those who slept seven hours a night. By contrast, women who slept seven to eight hours a night had the lowest risk of major weight gain.

A study of 740 adults conducted in Quebec found that people who reported getting 5 to 6 hours of sleep each night were 69 percent more likely to be overweight or obese than those getting 9 to 10 hours each night and 38 percent more likely than those getting 7 to 8 hours. The less the subjects slept, the less leptin they secreted. Leptin is a hormone that signals the brain that you have enough energy and don't need more food. Experts claim that sleep deprivation not only reduces circulating leptin levels but also increases levels of ghrelin, a hormone that stimulates appetite. ■

Our BEST ADVICE

Replace one hour of inactive wakefulness (think watching TV) with sleeping. Research shows that just this one small step is likely to cause a substantial reduction in calorie intake.

Strength Training

Women, take note: Strength training isn't just for men anymore. In fact, it could be your best strategy for losing weight—better even than walking or running. And you'll see the results in the mirror before they show up on the scale. Some bonuses: Lifting weights (or doing resistance exercises) staves off bone loss and improves balance, no bulging biceps or broad shoulders required.

Does strength training burn more fat than aerobics?

YES Strength training boosts metabolism by increasing muscle mass, which leads to weight loss.

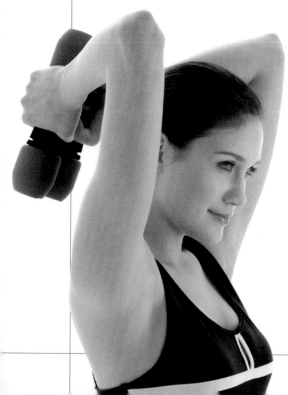

Walking or pedaling a stationary bike will burn calories, for sure, but the body's metabolism quickly returns to preexercise levels, usually within about 40 minutes. Not so with strength training, also called resistance training. According to researchers at Johns Hopkins University, strength training leads to increased calorie burn for up to two hours after the workout ends. It also builds muscles you won't get otherwise, and maintaining muscle mass is key to keeping your metabolism from dipping while you diet.

Working with weights also helps people jiggle less and fit back into clothes that were uncomfortably tight, since muscle takes up less room than fat. In a study comparing strength training with aerobic exercise, researchers at Brigham Young University found that middle-aged women who participated in a home strength-training program three times a week for 12 weeks experienced greater improvements in body image than those who walked at the same frequency and duration. Other studies show that strength training leads to less blood sugar being stored as fat, making people who lift weights, use dumbbells, or do situps and pushups less likely to develop the belly fat that leads to diabetes and heart disease.

Does lifting heavier weights build more muscle?

YES If your goal is building big muscles, you'll want to lift heavier weights.

If you're looking to burn calories during your strength workout, you have a choice:

If you have blubber surrounding rock-hard abs, **all you'll see is flab**, not the six-pack.

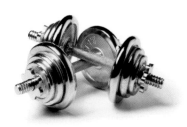

You can lift heavy weights and be done with your workout quickly or lift lighter weights for a longer period of time. Either will burn the same number of calories. If big muscles are your priority, go with the heavier weights if you can safely handle them. You'll challenge your body in new ways and increase the size of your muscle fibers more. Need a visual? Compare the physique of a marathoner with that of a sprinter. The sprinter with huge, powerful legs probably does leg presses with heavy weights. The marathoner, more concerned with endurance and overall toning, probably doesn't—and looks the part.

Do free weights provide a better workout than machines?

YES Unlike weight machines, free weights require you to stabilize your core muscles, such as your abdominals, before you can perform exercises. Not only do you have to work harder (which burns more

calories), you also strengthen muscles beyond those you're specifically targeting. Another bonus: Using free weights more closely matches the way you move in sports and in life. Just shift the way you hold the weight, and you'll work a different muscle.

On the other hand, if you're new to weight training, or if you're trying to strengthen a specific muscle or rehabilitate an injury, machines are a better bet. They require less coordination and allow you to increase weight gradually in small increments. Machine workouts also take less time; you can move from one machine to the next with only the occasional change of weight and adjustment of the seats or pads.

Will spot training shrink problem areas?

NO No matter how many crunches, leg lifts, or torso twists you perform, shrinking trouble zones won't happen with spot training alone.

Got belly flab? Get cracking on those situps. Saddlebags? Do lots of leg lifts. Or so many people think. Alas, they're wrong.

The problem they're ignoring is simple: fat. Though situps, leg lifts, and the like will certainly tone the muscles under your problem spots, it won't get rid of the fat that

hides those muscles. If you have a layer of blubber surrounding rock-hard abs, all you'll see is flab, not the six-pack. To lose fat, you need to cut calories and gain muscle mass all over your body to increase your metabolism. There's no way around it.

According to the American Council on Exercise, the best way to reshape a problem area is to incorporate strength and toning exercises with aerobic exercise to burn calories. Doing ab work will give you a stronger girdle to hold things in. Quadriceps and butt exercises will give you a higher, rounder derriere—and your thighs won't jiggle as much. Work your biceps and triceps, and you can effectively rid yourself of chicken wings. ■

Our BEST ADVICE

Use both aerobic exercise and strength training to get the most benefits from exercise. According to guidelines set forth by major health organizations, people should do strength exercises at least twice a week. Short on time? Work the big muscles first— your thighs, calves, butt, and biceps—to get the greatest metabolic boost, since larger muscles consume more oxygen and burn more calories.

Stress

Stress can seem relatively benign—after all, everyone's under stress, and no one dies from it. Or do they? When you consider that chronic stress raises blood pressure and suppresses the immune system, it no longer seems so harmless. The effects of chronic stress on weight aren't harmless either.

Does stress promote weight gain?

YES Chronic stress encourages an ever-expanding waistline. Acute stress, on the other hand, promotes weight loss, at least in some people.

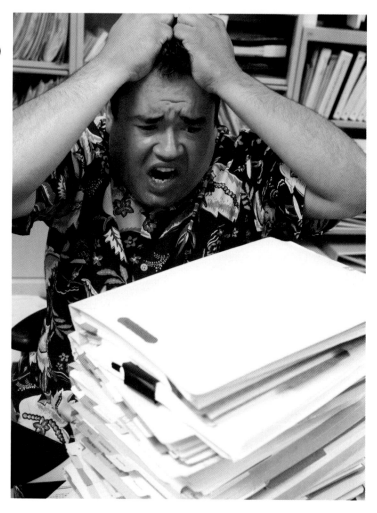

When you're under stress, your body releases so-called stress hormones, including adrenaline, which makes you feel keyed up, and cortisol, which makes you … fat. Cortisol is a powerful appetite stimulant. Blame it, in part, for the fact that people under stress make frequent trips to the fridge and the candy jar.

Some people handle stress better than others, and they tend to secrete less cortisol during tense times. A study conducted at the University of Leeds in the United Kingdom found that people who release a lot of cortisol when they're stressed eat more food—hence the reason some people gain weight when they're under pressure and others don't.

Chronically elevated cortisol levels appear to stimulate the growth of fat cells in the abdomen, triggering the worst kind of weight gain (abdominal fat is strongly linked to heart disease and insulin resistance). In one study, Australian scientists fed stressed and unstressed mice a diet high in fat and sugar and watched the stressed mice balloon twice as much as the unstressed mice,

developing portly bellies and a host of health problems, like high blood pressure, prediabetes, and high cholesterol. In the animals' fat tissue, researchers discovered sharply elevated concentrations of a molecule called neuropeptide Y (NPY), which is released by the body when it's under pressure. NPY unlocks receptors in the fat cells, prompting them to grow in both size and number. The effects of stress appear to be similar in humans. ■

Stretching

Stretching *sounds* so very good for you, and for decades we've been told it *is* good for you. Yet almost everything you believe about stretching is probably wrong. Is stretching an essential part of any fitness activity, a way to reduce the risk of injury and prevent soreness? Or could stretching actually do more harm than good?

Does stretching prevent injuries?

NO There's some evidence that stretching, especially when it involves bouncing, may even contribute to injury by causing tears in the muscle.

People have the idea that they should stretch before working out, mostly because they've heard it thousands of times. When it comes to activities like jogging, cycling, and strength training, though, there's no scientific data showing benefits from stretching. An Australian study of 1,538 men in the army who participated in 40 sessions of physical training over 12 weeks found that those who performed five minutes of stretching had the same number of leg injuries as those who went without stretching.

Stretching not only fails to prevent injuries, it can also reduce performance by pushing the body beyond its comfort zone. The result: Your muscles tighten up. It's called the stretch reflex. After about two seconds of holding a stretch, the muscle contracts, creating a tug of war.

In a study of 22 college students, stretching before weight training reduced performance by almost 25 percent. Students who stretched before workouts tired more quickly and performed fewer repetitions.

Is stretching worthwhile?

YES Both static stretching (holding a stretch) and ballistic stretching (stretching with a bounce) increase range of motion. While ballistic stretching can cause muscle tearing if done inappropriately or before muscles are warm, it can increase range of motion when done correctly. And maintaining full range of motion is critical, especially as we age. Researchers at Johnson State College in Vermont assigned 29 men to either a static stretching, ballistic stretching, or no-stretching group. After four weeks, the men in both stretching groups had greater range of motion and a higher stretch tolerance than those who went without stretching.

Stretches should be held for 15 to 30 seconds and repeated two or three times—and they shouldn't hurt. Ease your body into a comfortable stretch, and your muscles will relax into the position rather than tear. And be sure to stretch after, not before, exercising, when your muscles are already warm.

Does stretching prevent soreness?

NO Soreness is an indication that your muscles are getting bigger and stronger. It usually occurs 24 to 48 hours after exercise, so feeling some tenderness in your body after exercise is a good thing—one that stretching won't counteract. Researchers at the University of Sydney in Australia reviewed five scientific studies related to stretching and muscle soreness and found that stretching before or after exercise didn't prevent muscle soreness. Other studies have yielded similar results. ■

Our BEST ADVICE

Warm up before you exercise instead of stretching. The trick, experts claim, is to use the same muscles you'll use during your workout. Save stretching for after your workout when your muscles are already warm. Ease into the stretch—it shouldn't hurt.

VEGETARIAN DIETS

Vegetarian Diets

You'd be awfully hard-pressed to find a doctor or nutritionist who would argue against eating more fruits and vegetables. There are several major health benefits to vegetarian eating if you do it right, as you'll read on page 101. Controlling weight is definitely one of them.

Does going vegetarian help with weight loss?

YES Studies show that the less meat you eat, the less weight you gain over time.

Vegetarians tend to be slimmer than meat eaters, and they have a much easier time shedding pounds. Their body mass indexes are, on average, 3 to 20 percent lower, and obesity occurs in only 0 to 6 percent of vegetarians compared to 5 to 45 percent of nonvegetarians. So it's not surprising that data from 87 studies found that following a vegetarian diet is highly effective for weight loss—and not because vegetarians are exercising or counting calories. For one thing, vegetarian foods tend to be more filling.

In a study conducted at George Washington University School of Medicine, 64 overweight postmenopausal women consumed either a vegan diet (meaning no animal products, including eggs and dairy) or a control diet low in saturated fat and cholesterol, both without portion control or calorie limits. The results: Women on the vegan diet lost significantly more weight than those in the control group.

Other studies link vegetarian diets with reduced body weight. Researchers at the University of Oxford in the United Kingdom looked at nearly 22,000 people in four different groups—meat eaters, fish eaters, vegetarians, and vegans—over five years. The meat eaters gained the most weight. More surprising, people who switched to a diet containing less animal food gained the least weight of all. Another study of more than 55,000 Swedish women found that meat eaters were more likely to be overweight or obese than vegetarians or vegans. ■

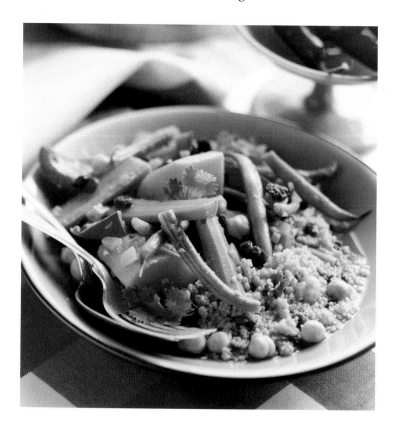

Water

Who hasn't been drowned by the admonition to drink 8 to 10 glasses of water a day? Turns out, that advice doesn't hold water (see page 107). But that hardly makes water worthless. After all, our bodies consist mostly of water, which makes up as much as 70 percent of our body weight. Water makes up 80 percent of our muscles and 75 percent of our brains. We need it to lubricate our joints and organs, regulate body temperature, and transport nutrients. But can it help you lose weight?

Does drinking water suppress the appetite?

YES Studies show that drinking water, either with a meal or incorporated into the food (think soup), helps dieters feel full.

Some people swear by drinking lots of cold water because they say the body burns calories trying to warm the water. Studies have confirmed that drinking cold water does temporarily increase the body's calorie burn, but not by enough to make any difference.

The real reason water may facilitate weight loss is that it helps people feel full, although no one knows how long the effects last or how much water is needed to keep you away from the fridge.

A very small study conducted at the University of Kuopio in Finland found that when eight healthy women drank two glasses of water while they were eating breakfast, they felt less hungry than when they dined without water. A larger study conducted by Barbara Rolls, PhD, author of *Volumetrics*, and her colleagues found that consuming water as part of a food, as in chicken soup, appears to be more effective for curtailing appetite for the next meal than drinking water with the food.

Do I need more water if I do heavy exercise?

MAYBE Most people will replace the water they lose during a workout over the following 24 hours. But if you're intent on making sure the amounts match up, weigh yourself before and after you exercise. For each pound you've lost, drink 16 ounces of fluid. And unless you've worked out for more than an hour in hot weather, skip the sports drinks. Heat and exhaustion are the two factors that make you lose large amounts of electrolytes through sweat. If you haven't experienced those two things, the food you eat afterward will restore any lost electrolytes.

Can you drink too much water?

YES The average person's kidneys can rid the body of nearly a quart of water per hour. But if you consume extremely large quantities of fluids, exceeding the kidneys' ability to excrete them, you can drink to excess.

Water overload, or hyponatremia, is a rare condition seen almost exclusively in marathon runners and ultra-endurance athletes when they drink too much fluid and lose excessive sodium through sweat. This combination dilutes the sodium concentration in the blood, causing a potentially lethal condition that starts with symptoms like headache, confusion, vomiting, and fatigue. If severe enough, hyponatremia can lead to seizures, coma, and even death, but it usually requires three to four hours of fairly continuous exercise and continuous consumption of fluids. ∎

Weight-Loss Groups

Big-gulp drinks, double bacon cheeseburgers, super-size fries—it's no secret that portion sizes have ballooned in recent years and that options for quick food fixes are seemingly limitless. How can anyone navigate all of that alone? The solution: Team up. Studies show that having support enhances self-control and self-esteem and provides motivation to keep going strong.

Do weight-loss groups help people lose more weight?

YES The studies are unequivocal: People who attend support groups as part of a comprehensive weight-loss program lose more weight than those who go it alone.

Some things are hard to do alone. Riding a seesaw is one of them, and so is losing weight. That's not surprising, considering how difficult it can be to cut calories and stay motivated enough to keep doing it, day in and day out.

Having some help works. In one study of nearly 50,000 postmenopausal women, one group was given educational materials with specific advice about how to cut calories by eating less fat and more fruits, vegetables, and whole grains. The other group participated in 18 individual or group sessions during which they received the same advice—plus support and encouragement. Guess which group lost more weight? That's right. The women who attended the meetings lost an average of five pounds during the first year, about four pounds more than the other group.

The more meetings you attend, the better your results. Researchers at New York Obesity Research Center found that among 423 men and women, those who participated in a commercial weight-loss program with group support lost more weight during the first year (10 pounds compared to 3 pounds) and dropped more inches than those who lost weight without participating in a program. Another study found an association between attendance at group meetings during the year following weight-loss surgery and the amount of weight lost.

Want help from the comfort of your living room? Internet-based support is effective, too.

Does having a weight-loss buddy help?

YES Get a group of friends together who also want to slim down, and not only are you more likely to lose weight, but you also have a better chance of keeping it off.

Researchers at the University of Pennsylvania recruited 166 people to participate in a weight-loss program either alone or with three friends or family members. Among those who embarked on the program with friends, 95 percent completed the program compared to only 76 percent of those who dieted solo. After 10 months, 66 percent of the group dieters had maintained their weight loss compared to only 24 percent of those who were on their own. ∎

The more meetings you attend, **the better your weight-loss results.**

Weight-Loss Pills

How often do we say, "If only there were a pill for that!"? Well, there are pills for people who weigh too much—quite a few, actually. But they won't make the pounds magically disappear. Today's diet drugs are safer and more effective than older drugs, but side effects and safety concerns remain. Plus, experts agree that drugs should be used as a last resort, together with changes in diet and exercise habits.

Do weight-loss pills work?

YES Over-the-counter and prescription weight-loss pills help you lose weight, but they won't work without diet and exercise, and data on long-term effects is lacking.

Most weight-loss pills work in one of two ways: Either they curb your appetite by releasing chemicals such as epinephrine that speed up your metabolism—often causing jitters—or they inhibit the breakdown and absorption of the fat in the food you eat—often causing loose, oily stools and other, even more unappealing side effects such as "anal leakage." The drugs are meant to be used along with, not

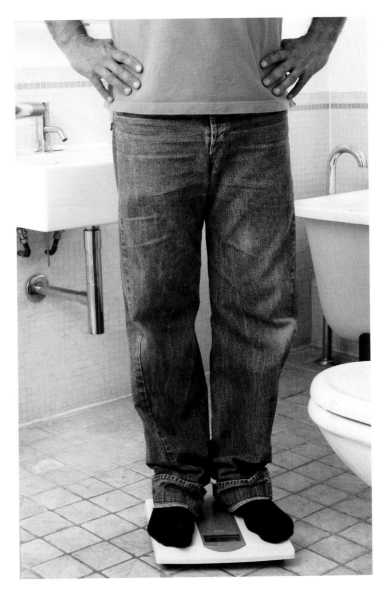

instead of, dietary changes and exercise. Hardly the "magic bullet" many people hope for.

The drugs work, at least in the short term, but researchers say they don't meet the unrealistic expectations of patients or healthcare professionals. A

meta-analysis of a variety of different prescription weight-loss drugs showed an average weight loss of about 11 pounds after one year.

Most of these drugs are meant for short-term use only. Once you build up a tolerance

WEIGHT-LOSS PILLS

Who's Who of Weight-Loss Drugs

DRUG	ABOUT THE DRUG	BUYER BEWARE
Rimonabant (Acomplia)	Acomplia blocks cannabinoid receptors in the brain, which helps control calorie intake by making overeating less pleasurable. Available in some countries, this drug has not been approved by the FDA due to safety concerns and is not sold in the United States.	Increases the risk of suicidal thoughts and behavior.
Sibutramine (Meridia)	One of two prescription medications approved by the FDA for long-term weight loss, Meridia helps trigger a sense of fullness by altering levels of feel-good brain chemicals, including serotonin and norepinephrine.	Can cause blood pressure to spike, so if you have hypertension or are at high risk for heart disease, steer clear.
Orlistat (Xenical)	The second FDA-approved diet drug, it works in the gut, inhibiting the breakdown and absorption of dietary fat. The drug blocks 30% of the fat you take in.	Can cause embarrassing side effects such as gas, diarrhea, and sudden loss of bowel control, especially if you eat too much fat. May prevent the absorption of important fat-soluble vitamins A, D, and E.
Orlistat (Alli)	This is the only FDA-approved over-the-counter weight-loss pill. It's the same drug as Xenical, but the dosage is lower. It comes with an online plan to help you change your diet.	See Orlistat (Xenical).

to the drug and stop feeling an effect, you're not supposed to increase the dose. In fact, many experts argue that the role of these drugs is to give patients an opportunity to learn to eat better and make time for exercise. The appetite suppressants modify patients' brain chemistry so it's easier for them to stick to a diet, resist compulsions to eat, and build confidence that they can lose weight.

Do these drugs have downsides?

YES Drugs that speed the metabolism also raise the risk of high blood pressure and may cause a rapid heartbeat, dizziness, and restlessness. Drugs that block the absorption of fat also block the absorption of fat-soluble vitamins such as beta-carotene and vitamins D and E, so people who take those drugs should

also take a multivitamin several hours before or after. And with either type of drug, unless you've made lasting lifestyle changes, your weight will go right back up once you go off the medication.

Do any available weight-loss supplements work?

MAYBE There's a variety of ingredients in some of these

pills that may curb appetite and burn a few extra calories, but there's no telling what's actually in your pill bottle.

More "fat-burning" supplements line the shelves than you can shake a carrot stick at. About 20 percent of American women have tried one at some point, and some of the pills may even help—a little.

One ingredient that does work is the stimulant ephedra, or ephedrine, the stuff in some cold medicines and decongestants. Researchers found that people who took weight-loss formulas containing it lost about two more pounds per month than those who were taking a placebo. Supplements that contained ephedra plus caffeine were slightly more effective, but users also had two to three times the risk of problems like anxiety, nausea, vomiting, and heart palpitations. Because of the potential for abuse of ephedra, the FDA has banned sales of dietary supplements that contain it.

Since then, manufacturers have turned to ingredients such as bitter orange (a natural source of a mild stimulant chemically similar to ephedrine), green tea, and guarana (a source of caffeine), purported to boost metabolism and suppress the appetite. All of these have some effect in the body, but clinical studies have been scant, results have been mixed, and no studies have assessed their long-term effects. And remember: Since there's no regulatory body that governs supplements, there's no telling for sure what's really in the bottle you buy. Formulas vary widely in terms of the quantity and quality of their effective ingredients.

Does hoodia work?

YES Not all weight-loss pills are stimulants. Hoodia originates from a cactus-like plant in South Africa and Namibia and has been long praised for its ability to help tribes make long treks through the desert with little food. Experts agree there's something in it that suppresses appetite; it's thought to trick the brain into thinking you're full. A British pharmaceutical company had licensed the effective ingredient, a molecule known as P57, and is investigating it in an anti-obesity drug. But you won't find P57 at your local store. There's a very limited supply of hoodia, so what claims to be the real thing may be nothing more than a water pill. There are no peer-reviewed human studies on hoodia, so side effects and long-term effects are unknown. ■

There's no telling for sure **what's really in the bottle** you buy.

"We are most alive when we are in love."
—John Updike, author

family matters

Breastfeeding

Breast milk is nature's perfect baby food. It's easy to digest, enhances newborns' ability to fight off infections, and contains exactly the right balance of nutrients during the most critical developmental phase of their lives. It's no wonder then that experts encourage new moms to breastfeed—and the moms are following doctors' orders. The latest data shows that 74 percent of women breastfeed during the early postpartum period compared to 68 percent in 1999.

Does breastfeeding give kids long-term benefits?

YES But some benefits may have been overblown. According to sibling studies in which one child was breastfed and the other was not, the only long-term benefit of breastfeeding is a slight edge in brainpower.

Researchers looking at data on 2,734 sibling pairs found that kids who were breastfed at any point had higher IQs (by 3 points) than formula-fed infants, and the effects persisted into adolescence. But the authors suggest that other long-term benefits of breastfeeding, such as reduced risk of becoming obese or developing heart disease, have been overstated. Any perceived benefits, they claim, are likely to be products of the breastfeeding mothers' lifestyles, behavior, and childrearing practices, not mom's milk.

As for short-term effects, hundreds of studies show that nursing helps prevent diarrhea, respiratory tract infections, ear infections, urinary tract infections, and other conditions, but only while the child is being breastfed.

Does it improve mom's health?

YES Breastfeeding not only helps you bond with your baby and prevent postpartum depression but also protects you from several chronic diseases.

Breastfeeding releases hormones such as oxytocin and prolactin that promote relaxation and help moms feel more nurturing. Breastfeeding exclusively also puts your menstrual cycle on hold (so you're much less likely to get pregnant), helps you shed pounds after pregnancy, and causes estrogen levels to drop, which protects against osteoporosis,

hormone-related cancers, and diabetes.

Research shows that women who breastfeed are less likely to develop breast cancer than their nonnursing counterparts. The practice also has a similar effect on ovarian cancer. In a study of 149,693 women, Harvard researchers found women who nursed for 18 months or longer had an almost 40 percent reduction in risk of ovarian cancer compared to women who never breastfed. Other studies show that women who breastfeed for more than 6 months are less likely to develop type 2 diabetes. The longer women nurse, the lower their risk.

Of course, it doesn't hurt that breastfeeding burns about 500 calories a day. That too has long-lasting effects on health and well-being. But perhaps the greatest benefit to breastfeeding moms is extra sleep. Research shows that parents of infants who nurse at night get about 45 more minutes of precious shuteye than parents who give their little ones formula. ■

Childbirth

Making health decisions for yourself is complicated enough, but add an arriving baby to the mix, and the list of dos and don'ts becomes daunting. While some of the most important issues may be beyond your control (for instance, despite your ardent desire to give birth the old-fashioned way, you may need a C-section if nature doesn't cooperate), others are personal decisions that can affect your long-term health and your baby's.

Do episiotomies prevent tears?

NO Episiotomies do not prevent tears, and they may cause problems that could have been avoided without the procedure.

During childbirth, doctors sometimes perform an incision called an episiotomy to enlarge the vagina and make delivery easier for mom and baby. Worldwide, it is one of the most common procedures performed on women, used in about one-third of vaginal births. But are doctors making the right move? Maybe not. As it turns out, there's an extensive body of research showing that episiotomies may cause the same problems physicians are trying to avoid.

A review of more than 40 scientific studies shows that routine use of episiotomies doesn't prevent tearing of tissue between the vagina and the anus and that natural tears as a result of childbirth are typically smaller than episiotomy incisions. In April 2006, the American College of Obstetricians and Gynecologists posted recommendations that called for restricted, not routine, use of episiotomies, claiming the procedure does not benefit moms or newborns and may actually increase the risk of further tears and painful sex.

There are instances when an episiotomy is required, such as when the baby's head is too large for the opening, its shoulders are stuck, or a delivery happens too quickly for the vagina to stretch naturally. Doctors may also resort to episiotomy for vacuum and forceps deliveries. But new research is calling even that practice into question. One study found an increased risk of tears with the use of episiotomies during "special deliveries."

Does having an episiotomy affect your sex life?

YES Pain during sex is more common among mothers who've had episiotomies. Some women even find that intercourse is less pleasurable because sexually charged nerve endings may be replaced with scar tissue after the procedure.

Is banking cord blood good insurance against future disease?

NO The idea that banking baby's cord blood provides a safety net for the future is not worth banking on.

Many people view stem cells as potentially lifesaving miracle cures, and companies that offer new parents the chance to bank their babies' umbilical cord blood, which is rich in stem cells, prey on that belief—and their fear of the unknown. But people who spend the money for this "insurance for the future" are very likely wasting their cash, and a lot of it, say experts.

Stem cells have the unique ability to transform into heart, skin, lung, and other tissue, and doctors today sometimes use stem cells extracted from bone marrow or cord blood to treat various forms of cancer as well as sickle cell disease and certain other genetic conditions. Stem cells from cord blood have the advantage of youth: Because they're younger than mature stem cells and are "immunologically naive," they can be transplanted into unrelated people with less risk of rejection than stem cells derived from bone marrow.

Still, there's precious little chance—verging on none—that if your baby did go on to develop a serious disease, the cord blood stem cells would come to the rescue. Experts say few life-threatening conditions would benefit from the patient's cord blood stem cells as opposed to bone marrow stem cells. What's more, most conditions the child might develop cannot be treated with the patient's *own* stem cells at all, since the genetic mutation that caused the disease is in the stem cells, too. ■

Our BEST ADVICE

If your child has an older sibling with a condition (cancerous or genetic) that can be treated with cord blood, banking your newborn's blood could save your other child's life. Want to be altruistic? Donate your newborn's cord blood to a public cord blood bank and potentially save a stranger's life. A bonus: Scientists test cord blood for genetic and infectious diseases. If abnormalities are found in your baby's cord blood, you'll be notified.

Circumcision

To circumcise or not to circumcise? That's the decision parents of newborn boys must make. During circumcision, surgeons remove the foreskin of the penis, usually shortly after birth. Some religions call for the procedure, and up to 85 percent of men in the United States have had it. But the reasons for circumcision extend beyond religion or aesthetics. Studies show it protects against penile cancer and sexually transmitted diseases.

Does circumcision lower the risk of infection?

YES Boys who are circumcised are less likely to contract sexually transmitted diseases when they grow up.

During the first year of life, uncircumcised boys have 10 to 20 times as many urinary tract infections as circumcised boys do. And the health-related perks of this procedure extend well into adulthood. Studies show that uncircumcised men are nearly three times more likely to get human papillomavirus (HPV), the primary cause of cervical cancer in women, and more than twice as prone to acquiring HIV, the virus that causes AIDS, compared to circumcised men.

Foreskin contains a higher density of Langerhans cells, which HIV cells latch onto, than the surface of the penis. Researchers think the smaller number of infection-prone cells in circumcised men also lowers the risk of sexually transmitted diseases. New Zealand researchers followed 510 men for 25 years and found that circumcision reduced the risk of STDs like syphilis, canchroid, and herpes by up to one-half.

Another reason to consider the procedure: It also protects women. An international study from five different countries found that chlamydia is three times more common in women whose partners are uncircumcised than in the partners of circumcised men. Other studies suggest male circumcision could markedly reduce the number of women who contract cervical cancer. ■

CONTRACEPTIVES

Contraceptives

Thousands of years before the advent of "the Pill," men and women were improvising ways—some ineffective, some downright risky—to thwart Mother Nature's intended outcome of sex. Today there are a handful of effective options to choose from. When they don't work, it's often because they weren't used properly, though no method (besides plain old abstinence) is foolproof.

Are birth control pills the most effective method?

NO IUDs are more effective than oral contraceptives (99 percent compared to 97 percent).

More than 80 percent of women use oral contraceptives during their lifetimes, and many never even consider other options. But studies show that due to human blunders (like forgetting to take one of your pills), oral contraceptives are only up to 97 percent effective compared to a 99 percent effectiveness rate for intrauterine devices, or IUDs. Another method, the vaginal ring, which is inserted into the vagina and releases estrogen and progestin to protect against pregnancy, is just as effective as oral contraceptives but provides lower exposure to hormones, more consistent estrogen levels, and better control over menstruation, according to Swedish research.

On the other hand, the pill is more effective than the patch, condoms, diaphragms, and other forms of contraception, and many women prefer it to other methods. In one study of 1,230 women, researchers reported that more women discontinued using the patch than the pill, and some patch users reported skin irritation and site reactions. The patch also delivers more estrogen—and accompanying side effects like bloating, breast tenderness, and increased risk of blood clots—than low-dose birth control pills.

Does long-term use of the pill cause infertility?

NO More than 25,000 studies show that using the pill, for any period of time, has no permanent effects on a woman's menstrual cycle or her ability to have children. Only high-dose pills (which are rarely prescribed today) delay fertility after women stop taking them.

Do pills increase the risk of blood clots?

YES Birth control pills are safe for most women, but they do increase the risk of blood clots among smokers, women over 35, and those who are predisposed to clotting.

After the pill was introduced in the early 1960s, doctors began noticing an increased risk of cardiovascular disease, stroke, and blood clotting among women taking it. To lower these risks, drug companies dropped the amount of estrogen in the pill. Today's formulations contain less than 35 micrograms of estrogen—a dose that's two to three times lower than in pills from previous generations—yet they're safe and effective for most women. But those who are over 35, overweight, or smoke, or who are predisposed to clotting, may want to steer clear, since the pill does increase the risk of clotting for these groups.

One study of 324 women conducted in Italy found that taking oral contraceptives further increased the risk of stroke in women predisposed to the condition. And the impact is even greater in patch users. A study published in *Obstetrics and Gynecology* found a twofold increase in the risk of blood clots among patch users compared to oral contraception.

Is the morning-after pill a guarantee against pregnancy?

NO These pills won't prevent all pregnancies.

A night of unexpected passion, a failed attempt at contraception—sometimes it happens. Enter emergency contraception, a pill (or pills) containing the same hormones found in birth control pills but in a higher dose.

Researchers aren't sure exactly how it works. Studies suggest the pills interrupt ovulation, but it's not clear whether they have any effect on the fertilization or implantation of the egg. According to Planned Parenthood, progestin-only pills are 89 percent effective if started within 72 hours of unprotected intercourse; combination pills that include estrogen are 75 percent effective.

How effective emergency contraception is for you may depend on where you are in your menstrual cycle when you take it. The results of an Australian study indicate that emergency contraception is highly effective when taken before ovulation but that it does nothing to avert fertilization or implantation after ovulation.

For best results, emergency contraception should be taken within 24 hours of unprotected intercourse (as the hours pass, the pill becomes less effective). Main side effects include nausea and vomiting. In the case of the latter, you may need another dose. Nausea and vomiting are less common with progestin-only pills.

Our **BEST** ADVICE

Want to skip your period during a vacation or special occasion like a wedding? If you're taking regular birth control pills, talk to your doctor about skipping the last seven inactive pills and moving right on to the next pack of pills instead.

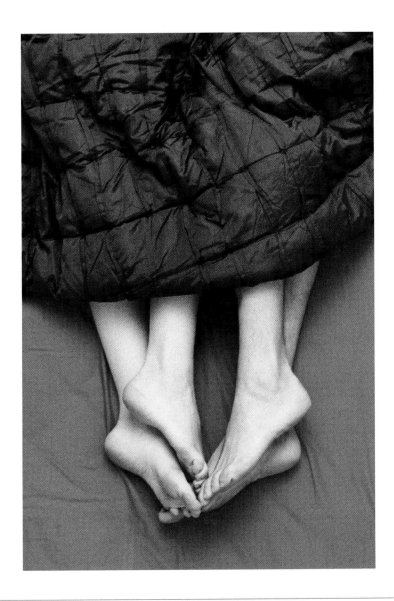

CONTRACEPTIVES

CONTRACEPTIVES

Is it safe to go without periods?

YES Several studies show that extended-cycle pills safely and effectively eliminate menstruation.

Extended-cycle pills like Seasonale reduce menstrual periods to only four a year. They work just like regular birth control pills and contain the same hormones, but the inactive pills that allow women on the regular pill to menstruate every month are taken only after 84 days of active pills.

Infrequent periods (when not on the pill) may be a warning sign of an underlying hormone disorder, but intentionally going without a period by taking a pill appears to be harmless. Researchers from the clinical trials that led to the approval of Seasonale concluded that it was similar in safety and efficacy to traditional oral contraceptives. Using continuous hormone pills to suppress menstruation isn't even new. On the advice of their doctors, some women using regular oral contraceptives have skipped the inactive pills to stem periods in order to ease conditions such as endometriosis or even to avoid their periods during special occasions such as a wedding or honeymoon.

When the pill is used on an extended cycle, the endometrium, or lining of the

How effective emergency contraception is may depend on **where you are in your cycle.**

uterus, becomes very thin. It's not that menstrual blood doesn't exit the body but rather that it doesn't form in the first place. Once the pill is discontinued, the endometrium returns to normal.

Women often experience some spotting and bleeding in their first few months on extended-use formulas, but those problems diminish over time.

A study of 111 women conducted at Texas A & M University found that women who were on extended-cycle pills experienced improved mood, fewer headaches, and less pelvic pain than those on traditional pills.

Are IUDs safe?

YES Although not especially popular, modern IUDs are a safe and effective form of reversible contraception.

An intrauterine device (IUD) is a small T-shaped piece of flexible plastic that's implanted

by a doctor into a woman's uterus. Some IUDs are hormone-free. The ParaGard IUD is a piece of plastic wrapped with copper. It can be left in place for up to 10 years. It's unclear how it works, but it does—in fact, it's more effective than the pill.

A second type of IUD continuously releases a small amount of the hormone progestin, which thickens the

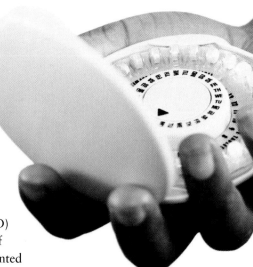

cervical mucus so sperm can't get through. It also reduces the frequency of ovulation and thins the endometrium. This type can be left in place for up to five years.

Recent studies debunk many women's fears that IUDs cause pelvic infections or sterility. But the devices do come with an unpleasant side effect: More bleeding. One German study of 1,466 women found that up to 65 percent of IUD users experienced heavier, prolonged, and more painful periods after an IUD was inserted. ■

Birth Control: Compare the Methods

METHOD	PROS	CONS
IUD 97%–99% effective	Intrauterine devices are highly effective at preventing pregnancy for up to 10 years, depending on the type.	Some women notice increases in menstrual flow and cramping.
Oral contraceptives 97% effective	When used correctly, the pill is highly effective for preventing pregnancy.	Pills don't protect against STDs, and they're not recommended for women who are smokers or are over 35 years of of age, or who have high blood pressure, an increased risk for blood clots, liver disease, heart disease, or diabetes, or who've had a stroke.
The patch 97% effective	You don't have to remember to pop a daily pill. Instead, you put on a patch and change it once a week. After three weeks, you go patchless, and your period comes during that week.	The patch delivers more estrogen than low-dose pills, which may increase the risk of blood clots. Then there's the heat factor. Direct sunlight or sweat can increase and then lower the amount of estrogen released from the patch.
The ring 97% effective	The ring has the same advantages as the patch, but it stays in place for three weeks.	Some women are uncomfortable with the idea of pushing a ring all the way up their cervix.
Depo-Provera 97% effective	Depo-Provera, injected every three months, provides long-term contraceptive protection during that period.	Many women who use Depo-Provera experience severe mood changes. The injections also lower estrogen levels, which can cause vaginal dryness and bone loss. Also, if you use it for two or more years, you may not be able to get pregnant for up to a year after you stop the injections.
Condoms 80%–89% effective	Condoms and other barrier methods are the only forms of contraception that protect against sexually transmitted diseases.	They can—and do—break.

Erectile Dysfunction

Nearly 40 percent of 40-year-old men and almost 70 percent of 70-year-old men experience some difficulty getting and/or maintaining erections. But today, pills provide better sex through chemistry. Even men who aren't experiencing erectile dysfunction are turning to the "thrill pills" to spice up their sex lives, although experts discourage it.

Do impotence drugs work?

YES Drugs can help restore erections for men who have trouble getting and maintaining them.

Impotence drugs like sildenafil (Viagra) inhibit an enzyme called PDE-5, letting muscles in the arteries of the penis relax and widen. As a result, blood flows south to create an erection.

Given that millions of men experience erectile dysfunction, it's no wonder that competitors of the original impotence drug, Viagra, have cropped up in recent years. Vardenafil (Levitra) takes effect more quickly and reportedly has fewer side effects, while tadalafil (Cialis) lasts longer, allowing couples more spontaneity in their lovemaking. All three drugs have been proven effective. A study of 7,560 men conducted in nine European countries found that Viagra, Cialis, and Levitra all improved erectile function and sexual satisfaction after six months of treatment.

The caveat: None of these drugs will give you an erection if you don't have the sexual stimulus or desire. If you're having relationship issues, or you're not turned on by your partner, don't look to a pill to solve your problem.

Are there vitamins or supplements that improve erectile function?

MAYBE Despite the growing number of products

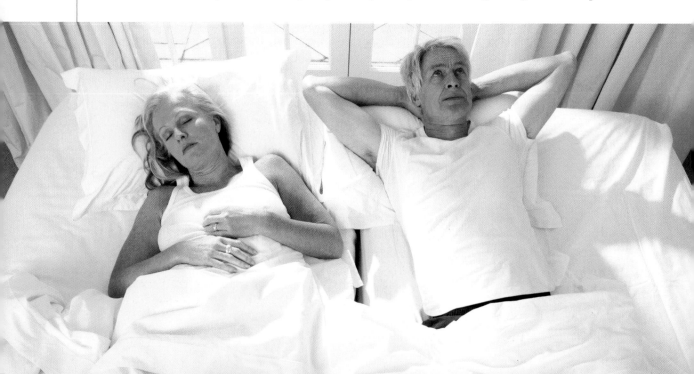

promising to help men get (and maintain) erections, most supplements haven't been studied thoroughly enough to confirm or deny their claims. For example, some studies show good results with L-arginine, an amino acid that converts to nitric oxide, a molecule that helps men get an erection. But a German study found no improvement in erectile function among 30 impotent men who were given 500 milligrams of L-arginine three times a day.

Certain nutrients and spices, such as omega-3 fatty acids and chile peppers, improve circulation, which could help increase blood flow where it's needed. Others, like zinc, reportedly boost testosterone production. Some plants and herbs, namely yohimbe, panax ginseng, maca, and ginkgo biloba, even have some scientific evidence showing they work, though no one knows whether the positive results are caused by the supplements or the placebo effect. Then again, if previously impotent men are getting erections, does it really matter why? ■

Fertility

About 10 percent of couples struggle with infertility—no big surprise considering all the biological stars that have to align to conceive a child. For a woman in her early forties, the chances of getting pregnant without help plummet to 10 percent. It's no wonder that more and more people are flocking to treatments, both ancient and high tech, to boost their odds.

Does acupuncture boost fertility?

YES Based on the available research, acupuncture seems to promote fertility without any negative side effects.

An increasing number of infertile women are using alternative therapies in conjunction with conventional treatment such as in vitro fertilization (IVF). One of them is acupuncture, which involves placing needles in the major pressure points of the body to create, as Eastern thinking goes, an appropriate energy balance for conception and improved blood flow down south. And it seems to work.

In 2002, a German study found that women undergoing IVF who received acupuncture treatments for 25 minutes before and after embryo transfer were more likely to get pregnant than those who did IVF without acupuncture (43 percent compared to only 26 percent). A second study

conducted in China found that among 240 infertile women, 65 percent of those who received acupuncture treatment became pregnant compared to only 45 percent of those who received the fertility drug clomiphene (Clomid). And when Swedish researchers reviewed studies exploring the effectiveness of acupuncture used in conjunction with IVF or fertility drugs, they found that three out of four studies showed significantly higher pregnancy rates in the acupuncture groups than in the control groups.

Acupuncture also seems to mobilize inactive sperm. At least three studies have found that acupuncture improved sperm quality and swimming speed among men struggling with infertility.

Does stress contribute to infertility?

YES Chronic stress dramatically affects a woman's ability

FERTILITY

to get pregnant and a man's ability to produce sperm.

If you're trying to get pregnant, relax—literally. When you're chronically stressed, your body churns out excess stress hormones like adrenaline and cortisol. In large amounts, both of these hormones can prevent ovulation. Add to that the fact that people under pressure tend to gorge on comfort food, smoke more, exercise less, and have less sex, and you have a recipe for infertility.

Research shows that women who perceive their jobs as stressful and demanding are less likely to get pregnant than those who are comfortable with their workload. Other studies show that sperm count and semen quality drop significantly when men are under stress. Researchers in Turkey assessed semen samples from 27 healthy male medical students and found that when the men were under stress from final examinations, their semen contained fewer sperm, and those that were present didn't swim very far.

There's even evidence implicating stress in failed attempts at in vitro fertilization. In a study of 168 women conducted in the Netherlands, researchers found that those who had lower concentrations of adrenaline in their urine during both egg retrieval and embryo transfer were more likely to get pregnant. Another study in Denmark's fertility clinics found that women who reported more personal and marital stress required more treatment cycles to conceive than women reporting less stress.

Does freezing eggs increase the chances of a successful pregnancy?

NO Women who freeze their eggs at age 33 hoping to put the biological clock on hold for nine years are no better off than if they underwent a fresh IVF cycle (if necessary) at 42.

Women who want to freeze their eggs for future use first take fertility drugs to boost their egg supply, then a doctor

Our BEST ADVICE

Visit a shrink. Research from Emory University in Atlanta shows that psychological counseling helps women cope better with stress, which in turn helps restore ovulation. In a study of 16 women who stopped ovulating due to stress, almost 90 percent of those who received cognitive behavioral therapy (which strives to change detrimental behaviors and attitudes) started ovulating again, compared with just 25 percent of those who didn't seek professional help.

retrieves as many eggs as possible—which is also how the process of in vitro fertilization begins. But instead of being fertilized and implanted, the eggs are frozen until the day the woman is ready for that procedure. Many women prefer this approach to freezing embryos.

Freezing eggs appeals to some single women and those scheduled to undergo chemotherapy, among others.

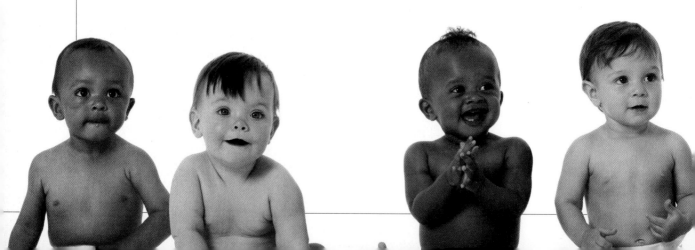

But will it work? Probably not. Even the most optimistic estimates offer patients only a slim chance of pregnancy.

Cornell University researchers reviewed 30 scientific studies and found that freezing eggs for later implantation is four to five times less successful than standard IVF, which creates a viable pregnancy in fewer than 30 percent of treatment cycles. Since eggs are mostly water, they're much more fragile than embryos. The water tends to crystallize on freezing, which can damage key structures within the cell, and eggs often fail to survive the freezing-thawing process. Another caveat: According to the American Society for Reproductive Medicine, the number of babies born from frozen eggs is too low (a few hundred) to be sure the procedure doesn't increase the risk of birth defects.

Scientists believe the procedure will become a more viable option in coming years. For now though, you'll pay a hefty price for the process ($10,000 to freeze your eggs, plus the cost of medication and a $300 to $400 annual storage fee), and it isn't all that likely to put a baby in your belly.

Do vaginal lubricants interfere with fertility?

YES The research is conclusive: Even in small amounts, most lubricants impair sperm's ability to reach and fertilize an egg.

Lubricants may improve your sex life and make intercourse more comfortable, but they also act like spermicide, so if you're looking to get pregnant, try extra foreplay instead. Researchers at the University of Texas Southwestern Medical Center mixed four popular lubricants (K-Y Jelly, Astroglide, Replens, and Touch) with donor sperm and then measured the effects on the swimmers after 60 minutes. The results: All four lubricants inhibited sperm's swimming speed by 60 to 100 percent, which in turn affects their ability to fertilize an egg. Other studies found similar results.

Our BEST ADVICE

Avoid activities that overheat your nether regions. If you want to get your partner pregnant, stay away from the sauna and hot tub and keep the laptop off your lap. It's also a good idea to avoid wearing Spandex during a workout (yes, we're talking to the cyclists out there). Spandex traps heat.

Does wearing briefs lower sperm count?

NO For years researchers have speculated that wearing briefs overheats the scrotum, causing a dramatic drop in sperm count. And while several studies show that excessive heat from, say, hot tubs can affect semen quality and fertility, there's no evidence to suggest that wearing briefs will render you sterile. ■

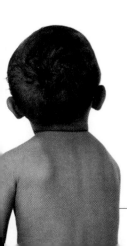
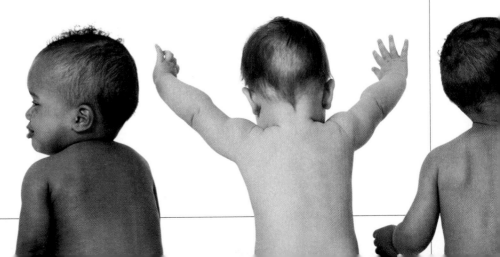

Sex Drive

Sex lets partners feel closer together, releases powerful feel-good chemicals, and may even reduce the risk of chronic diseases like high blood pressure, heart disease, and various cancers. And it burns up to 360 calories per hour. But when our hormones flag, so do our libidos. According to studies in the United States, the United Kingdom, and Sweden, 40 percent of women have significant complaints about their sex lives, mostly about low sexual desire.

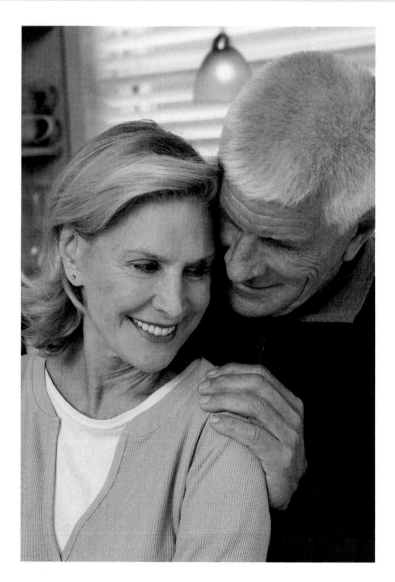

Can testosterone revitalize a woman's desire?

YES Testosterone can boost sexual desire in women, but it doesn't enhance libido for women who were never interested in sex, and the therapy is not without risks.

Testosterone is primarily a male hormone, but women produce smaller amounts in their ovaries. And it's a major sex driver for both genders. When women's testosterone levels start to decline, usually in conjunction with menopause, they often struggle with waning desire, lack of sensation, and decreased ability to climax. Enter testosterone therapy.

Intrinsa, the testosterone patch, has been used in Europe for decades to boost sex drive after menopause. Studies have consistently shown that using the patch along with estrogen therapy increases desire, responsiveness, and sexual activity among post-menopausal women. In a study of 318 women in Los Angeles, testosterone therapy increased sexual desire and the frequency of satisfying sexual activity. A study in Texas found the testosterone patch significantly improved sexual desire and activity among 533 women who underwent surgical hysterectomy.

Nevertheless, the FDA denied approval of Intrinsa due to concerns about long-term safety (most studies have been conducted for less than a year), and experts agree that testosterone is potentially dangerous when given inappropriately. No one knows whether it increases the risk of breast cancer, heart disease, or blood clots or how it will affect women who are not simultaneously taking estrogen. Scientists do know the bad things testosterone can do to women's bodies: It can cause acne, increased growth of facial and body hair, and thinning scalp hair.

Despite the drawbacks, women are clamoring for the hormone, and they're getting it. Since doctors use testosterone for other medical reasons, they can and do legally prescribe it to boost sex drive. But it's usually given as a last resort, in the lowest dose, for the shortest time necessary to achieve desire, and only in combination with estrogen.

Do certain foods boost sex drive?

NO In 1989, the FDA declared there is no scientific proof that any over-the-counter aphrodisiacs work to treat sexual dysfunction. But don't let that stop you from eating oysters, scallops, strawberries, licorice, chocolate, and other foods purported to ignite passion in the bedroom.

If you expect them to work, they just might. After all, the mind is the body's largest sexual organ.

Some foods earned reputations as aphrodisiacs because of their suggestive shape (think asparagus), sweet fragrance (vanilla, cinnamon) or opiate-like effects (chocolate). Others, like oysters and nuts, are praised for their zinc. While zinc won't affect your libido, it does contribute to overall health and may have appeared to work during times when people's diets were deficient in the mineral. Chocolate, once perceived as exotic, largely lost its libido-enhancing status when it became widely available. In an Italian study of 163 women, researchers found no differences in sexual arousal, satisfaction, or depression between chocolate eaters and abstainers.

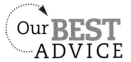

Our BEST ADVICE

If you and your doctor decide testosterone therapy is right for you, make sure you use a patch or gel formulation. Oral forms of the hormone may harm the liver and negatively affect cholesterol levels.

Do arousal gels work?

YES At least one of them does, or appears to. According to one very small study of 20 women, those who used Zestra (a mixture of botanical oils that dilate blood vessels) reported increased arousal, genital sensation, and ability to have orgasms compared to those who used a placebo oil. Apparently the mixture of

SMART MOVES FOR BETTER SEX

You may have heard that exercise is good for your sex drive, but we have something more specific in mind. They're called Kegel exercises, and studies show that regularly performing them enhances arousal, delays ejaculation, and intensifies orgasms for both partners. Kegels target the pubococcygeus (PC) muscle, which stretches from the pubic bone to the tailbone in both sexes. It's this muscle that allows a man to move his penis up and down while it's erect and allows a woman to grip her partner's penis during intercourse. The muscle weakens with age and with pregnancy and childbirth.

To learn to perform Kegels, first stop your urine flow in midstream; you've just used your PC muscle. To exercise the muscle, practice clenching and unclenching it, gradually increasing the length of time you hold the contraction.

SEX DRIVE

plant oils and extracts boosts circulation and enhances sensation in the nether regions. The study was financed by the manufacturers of Zestra, and the company is currently conducting a second clinical study to determine Zestra's effectiveness among 200 women who are experiencing problems in the bedroom.

Does Viagra increase sexual desire in women?

NO Sure, Viagra can make blood flow to your clitoris, but it doesn't work on arousal or desire, at least for the vast majority of women. Pfizer, the drug company that makes Viagra, conducted its own studies on 3,000 women and found the drug was no more effective than a water pill for improving symptoms of sexual dysfunction. The reason, claim the drug makers, is women's complex biology. For most women, sex is inextricably linked with emotion, and desire stems from their brains, not their genitals. ■

MEDICATIONS THAT REDUCE SEX DRIVE

You may be sabotaging your sex drive by taking your meds. Research shows that a variety of commonly used drugs can interfere with sexual function in both men and women, causing low sex drive, inability to get or maintain an erection, and decreased lubrication in women.

If you're taking one of these medications, and your sex drive is low, ask your doctor what your options are.

Selective serotonin-reuptake inhibitors (SSRIs)

Antipsychotic drugs

Appetite suppressants

Blood pressure medications

Cholesterol-lowering medications (statins)

Oral contraceptives

Diazepam (Valium)

Antacids

food, drinks, and
your diet

ALCOHOL

Alcohol

Once scorned as the devil's drink and a crutch for the weak of will, alcohol has undergone a major reputation rehabilitation. Today doctors say that an occasional drink or two protects the heart and may provide other health benefits, though the upside of sipping the sauce must be weighed against the risks.

Does alcohol prevent heart attacks?

YES Years of research confirm that moderate drinking reduces the risk of heart disease and certain other conditions.

The science is overwhelming: More than 100 studies have shown that moderate alcohol consumption—usually defined as two drinks per day for men, one for women—lowers the risk of heart disease as well as for diabetes and strokes. Much remains mysterious about how alcohol safeguards the heart, but this much is not in doubt.

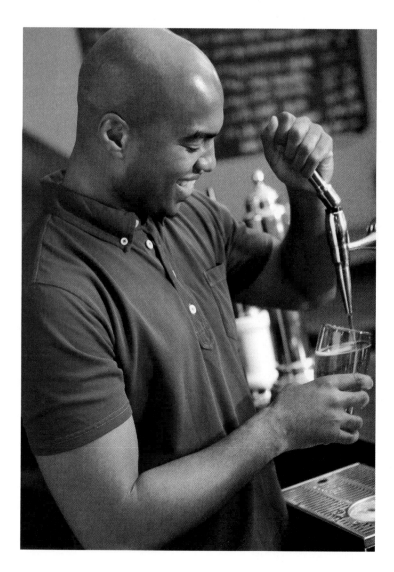

Alcohol raises "good" cholesterol. Scientists have been trying for years to develop safe medications that raise blood levels of HDL cholesterol, the kind that lowers the risk of heart disease by removing excess LDL, or "bad" cholesterol, from the blood. Yet you can find a reasonably effective HDL booster on your wine rack or in your liquor cabinet. Studies show that having one or two alcoholic beverages per day increases the blood concentration of HDL by about 12 percent. Each 1 mg/dl increase in HDL lowers the risk of heart disease by 2 percent in men and 3 percent in women.

Alcohol prevents blood clots. When disk-shaped cells called platelets clump together in the blood, they form clots that can block arteries and cause heart attacks and strokes. Alcohol makes these platelets less "sticky" and therefore less likely to form clots.

Alcohol may help the heart in other ways. For example, animal studies show that small doses of alcohol relax the blood vessels, which improves circulation. (Drinking too much, however, seems to have the opposite effect.) And some alcoholic beverages, such as red wine and dark beer, are rich sources of antioxidants that some scientists believe have important benefits for the heart.

Moderate drinking may help prevent other conditions, too, such as cognitive problems that arise later in life. For instance, one study found that people who sip one to six drinks per week are half as likely to develop Alzheimer's disease or other types of dementia as nondrinkers.

Small doses of alcohol relax the blood vessels, which improves circulation.

PUTTING MORE RESVERATROL IN YOUR GLASS

Disease-fighting resveratrol keeps grapes healthy by fighting fungus. Because fungus grows more aggressively in humid weather, a grape's resveratrol level is influenced by where it's grown and even what day it's picked. Also, some grapes are more vulnerable to fungus than others, so they naturally produce more resveratrol. All that makes selecting resveratrol-rich bottles a bit tricky, but following these rules will help you get a healthy dose, according to Leroy Creasy, professor emeritus of horticulture at Cornell University.

Drink red wine. It contains much more resveratrol than white.

Try some pinot noir. On average, it has two times more resveratrol than other reds. In one analysis of California wines, pinot noir came out on top, followed by merlot and cabernet sauvignon. Keep in mind, however, that the resveratrol content varies from one bottle of pinot noir, or any red wine, to the next.

Drink a variety of reds. Since resveratrol content fluctuates so much, the best way to get a steady diet of this antioxidant is to sip many varieties of red wine from different vintages and producers.

Avoid the cheap stuff. Many large wineries modify levels of bitter-tasting compounds called tannins in their products to ensure that each vintage tastes the same. In the process, wines lose much of their resveratrol. Ask your wine merchant for the names of smaller producers who make wines that fit into your budget.

If you don't drink wine, you can get the benefits of resveratrol straight off the vine: Grapes (as well as grape juice) have about as much of this antioxidant by weight as wine does. Since resveratrol resides in grape skins, any grape variety will do.

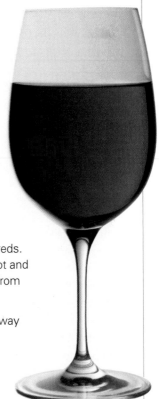

ALCOHOL

The key word, of course, is *moderate*. While studies consistently show that people who have a drink or two per day tend to be healthier than abstainers, those who routinely exceed the two-drink limit have an increased risk of liver damage, high blood pressure, and other diseases as well as car accidents, not to mention social and personal problems.

Is red wine better for you than white?

YES All wine benefits the heart, but red wine has the highest levels of antioxidants, including one that extends longevity, at least in lab animals.

It's known as the French paradox—Parisians and their compatriots adore cigarettes, creamy sauces, and other pleasures that make cardiologists cringe, yet they have surprisingly low rates of heart disease. Many scientists point to the French passion for wine as one explanation.

Ever since evidence for alcohol's heart benefits began to pile up in the 1990s, wine has come out ahead of other forms of alcohol. One review of 26 studies, for instance, found that beer drinkers cut their risk of heart disease by 22 percent, while wine sippers slashed theirs by 32 percent. Some research suggests that drinking either red or white is good for the heart. For

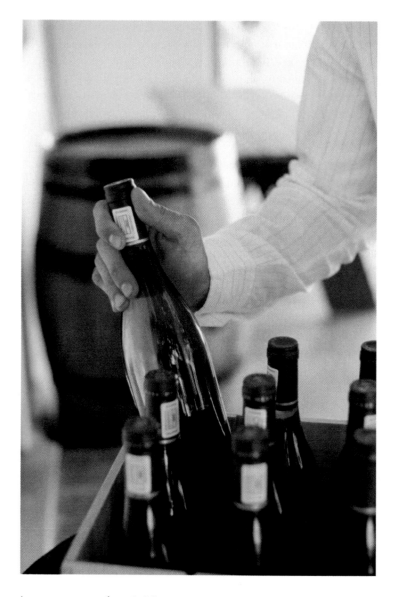

instance, researchers in New Zealand showed that drinking white or red wine improves the function of blood vessels with equal effectiveness.

Nevertheless, it's cabernet sauvignon and its crimson counterparts that have garnered the most attention from the scientific community. The reason? Red wine has higher levels of antioxidants. That's because it's made by crushing

grapes and allowing the resulting juice to ferment with the grape skins, rich in an antioxidant known as resveratrol, in place. To make white wine, the grape skins are removed from the juice, which is light in color. Scientists have extended the life spans of yeasts, flies, worms, fish, and mice with high doses of resveratrol. A recent study published in the journal *Nature* found

ALCOHOL

that mice fed junk food became fat, yet they remained nimble and healthy looking if they received resveratrol, too, and they lived 15 percent longer than other mice.

Granted, you would need to drink 300 glasses of red wine a day to get the same dose of resveratrol. Supplements containing resveratrol are available, but their benefits and safety in humans are unknown. For now, most experts agree that the more modest dose in a glass of red wine may help, and certainly won't harm, your health.

Does alcohol cause cancer?

YES The health benefits of moderate drinking must be balanced against known threats, which include an increased risk of certain cancers.

The studies have piled up over the years, and there's no longer much doubt that regular drinking makes you more vulnerable to cancers of the mouth, throat, liver, colon, rectum, and, in women, breast. No one is sure why drinking alcohol increases cancer risk, but there are some clues. The body breaks down alcohol into a chemical called acetaldehyde

SHOULD YOU DRINK ALCOHOL?

Should you sip a glass of wine or beer now and then to protect your heart? Or is it better to swear off the sauce because it raises the risk of certain cancers? Only you and your physician can decide, though it's important to keep a few things in mind. Despite how terrifying cancer can be, heart disease is a far greater threat. More people die of heart attacks than of all forms of cancer combined. Ask your doctor to evaluate your personal disease risk. You might also consider using one of the various risk-assessment calculators available on the Internet. For example, the Harvard Center for Cancer Prevention's "Your Disease Risk" Web page (www.yourdiseaserisk.harvard.edu) features a questionnaire that calculates the likelihood that you will develop the major forms of cancer, as well as heart disease, stroke, diabetes, and osteoporosis.

Knowing your risk can help you make an informed decision about alcohol. If you currently do not drink, though, the verdict is easy: Don't start drinking for your heart's sake. There are other, less risky ways to get the same heart benefits. Exercising more will increase HDL cholesterol, for instance, and taking a low-dose aspirin every day (with your doctor's okay) can help prevent blood clots.

(pronounced *as-sih-TEL-dih-hide*), which may damage DNA. Drinking booze produces cell-damaging free radicals, too. Alcohol raises estrogen levels, which may increase the risk of breast cancer. It could also make cancer-causing compounds in tobacco more destructive, which may explain why smokers who drink have an extra-high cancer risk.

While heavy drinkers have the greatest likelihood of developing cancer, research

suggests that temperate tippling increases the threat, too. For example, according to the American Cancer Society, the average woman has a one in eight chance of developing breast cancer in her lifetime. Having one alcoholic beverage per day increases the risk to one in seven. Drinking seems to increase the threat of cancer whether or not you have a family history of the disease or were born with cancer-causing genes. ■

Beans

Beans have been part of the human diet for more than 7,000 years, providing an inexpensive source of nourishment for populations all over the world. They contain more protein than any other plant food, and with more than 100 varieties to choose from, beans are as versatile as they are good for you. These humble seeds are packed with nutrients that safeguard overall health.

Are beans good for the heart?

YES Beans may lack glamour, but studies show they protect against both heart attacks and strokes.

Kids joke about their aftereffects. Some food snobs scorn them. But medical researchers have heaped a hill of praise on beans. Along with peas and lentils, beans belong to the family of foods known as legumes. Densely packed with an impressive lineup of vitamins, minerals, and other critical compounds, legumes defend against heart disease and reduce the risk of other health hazards, according to recent studies.

The soybean has received the most scientific interest of late for its power, albeit modest, to lower cholesterol. But if you're not a fan, fear not: People who frequently eat legumes of *all* kinds have low rates of heart disease and other conditions caused by blocked arteries, such as strokes. A major study by the National Institutes of Health involving more than

Our BEST ADVICE

If you replace meat with beans in a meal, have a side dish of leafy greens, sliced red bell peppers or tomatoes, or some other source of vitamin C. The body doesn't absorb the iron in plant foods very well, but vitamin C makes the absorption process more efficient. (Low levels of iron in the blood can cause anemia.) If you're adding beans to your diet, start slowly and increase your intake over time; the bacteria in your digestive system need time to adjust to larger amounts of fiber.

....

9,600 men and women found that people who eat beans and other legumes four or more times a week cut their risk of heart disease by 22 percent.

Filling up on beans may simply crowd out fatty meats and other foods that are less heart healthy. But beans do pack a wallop of nutrients known to fight cardiovascular disease, including the following.

Fiber: Diets high in fiber guard against heart disease. A half cup of cooked beans contains, on average, six grams of fiber. One-third of it is soluble fiber, the kind that lowers cholesterol. Soluble fiber also helps prevent type 2 diabetes, a major risk factor for heart disease.

Folate: This B vitamin helps maintain healthy levels of homocysteine, an amino acid in the blood that has been linked to heart disease. One study found that women who consume a lot of folate (about 700 micrograms a day, on average) and vitamin B_6 (4.6 milligrams daily) cut their risk of heart disease by nearly 50 percent. Other research suggests that folate from dietary and supplemental sources may help prevent high blood pressure, which can cause heart attacks and strokes. One cup of cooked black beans provides 256 micrograms of folate.

Minerals: Legumes are rich in minerals, particularly potassium. Men who get 4.3 grams of potassium per day may lower their risk of strokes by as much as 38 percent. The benefit is even more pronounced among people with high blood pressure.

Antioxidants: You don't know beans if you aren't aware that legumes are a top source of antioxidants. When the USDA identified the 20 common foods with the highest levels of antioxidants, small red beans ranked number 1, closely followed by red kidney beans and pinto beans (numbers 3 and 4, respectively). Black beans (number 18) are an excellent choice, too. ■

Bottled Water

With their images of snow-capped mountains and crystalline streams, the labels of the bottled water you buy in stores or from vending machines promote the idea that the H_2O inside is all-natural, pure, and unspoiled. This clever marketing appears to work: Surveys indicate that many consumers believe bottled water is safer and healthier than their water at home.

Is bottled water better for you than tap water?

NO Bottled water is no cleaner or safer than the H_2O from your faucet. The main difference: It costs much more.

Surprise: In many cases, bottled water *is* tap water. A study by the US-based nonprofit organization Natural Resources Defense Council estimated that about one-quarter of the bottled water sold in the United States comes not from lakes or springs but from public reservoirs. Some bottlers put the water through additional processes to purify it, but your city or town does the same thing to the water that pours from the spigots in your kitchen and bathroom. Chemists have compared samples of bottled water and the variety that comes from a tap in blind tests and have been unable to tell one from the other.

Bottled water *is* unhealthy for your bank account and the environment. Gallon for gallon, bottled water can cost more than gasoline. If you care about the well-being of the planet, it's hard to justify buying water in bottles. According to the Earth Policy Institute, it takes about 1.5 million barrels of oil to produce the plastic used to make all of the bottles of water sold each year in the United States alone.

If you don't like the taste of your tap water, filters can help (see page 178 for detailed information).

Do I really have to drink eight glasses of water a day?

NO Keeping your whistle wet with water is smart, but don't bother counting cups; most people consume all the H_2O they need.

BOTTLED WATER

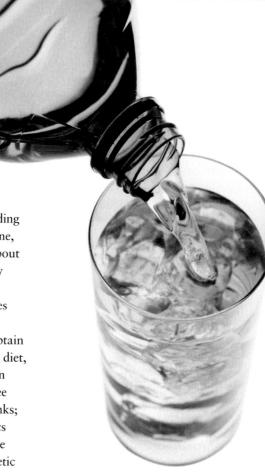

Doctors and dietitians alike once spouted this advice: Drink eight glasses of water a day to avoid dehydration. Many still recommend the "8 x 8" rule, shorthand for "eight 8-ounce glasses of water per day." Yet this dietary directive is all wet.

First, the facts. Water makes up one-half to two-thirds of your body weight. A 150-pound man has about 10 gallons of water in his body. Yet you lose water every day—up to several gallons in urine and another pint or so through perspiration and your breath. Obviously, you must replace that water to keep

Our BEST ADVICE

How much water should you drink? Some authorities have suggested that pale urine is an indication that you're imbibing enough water. However, some foods and vitamins turn the urine a light color, and dark urine isn't necessarily a sign of dehydration. A better rule of thumb: Drink enough water and other fluids to ensure that you have a full bladder at least every four hours or so.

your cells healthy. According to the Institute of Medicine, the average man needs about 125 ounces of water daily (15 to 16 cups), while a woman requires 91 ounces (a little over 11 cups).

However, it's easy to obtain that much from a normal diet, since all beverages contain water. That includes coffee and other caffeinated drinks; although they are diuretics (meaning they increase the need to urinate), the diuretic effect is brief, so these beverages still battle dehydration. Even alcoholic beverages count. And don't forget, solid foods contain a great deal of water; some vegetables are up to 90 percent water.

So where did the 8 x 8 rule come from? No one is sure, but it may be a misinterpretation of standard recommendations for the amount of water hospital patients require relative to

their calorie intake. In fact, people who are ill may require extra water to stay hydrated. The same holds true for people who exercise vigorously, especially in hot climates. But a scientific review found no evidence to indicate that a healthy person with a typical activity level needs to drink eight glasses of water every day. ■

Bread

It's been called the staff of life. To be sure, bread symbolizes sustenance, among other things. It also tastes great slathered with peanut butter or dipped in good olive oil. Yet many diet gurus would have you believe that bread is no better than cake or candy. Are they right, or does their advice fall flat?

Can bread make you fat?

YES White bread raises blood sugar and does a poor job of satisfying appetite. But bread can still fit into your diet if you choose well.

Many popular weight-loss diets use a system called the glycemic index (GI) to help you decide what to eat (see page 139 for more details). Foods that rank low on the GI fight hunger because they take a long time to digest, leaving your appetite satisfied between meals. High-GI foods, on the other hand, are rapidly absorbed during digestion, causing a blood sugar spike that's followed by a crash, which causes hunger pangs to return soon after you eat.

If you have ever gone on a low-carbohydrate diet, you know that bread is one of the first foods to be crossed off your daily menu, at least in the early stages. The reason: White bread and most other popular varieties are high-GI foods. To produce most types of white bread, bakers use flour made from grains that have been stripped of much of their fiber and pulverized into powder. The resulting bread is easy to digest—too easy, since it causes blood sugar to soar, then drop again, making your stomach roar.

A few types of bread have low or moderate GI values. In general, look for bread that has a coarse texture and intact seeds and includes the word *whole* in the first ingredient on the label. That means it was baked with flour made from entire cereal grains, which take longer for the body to digest. Sourdough bread is another alternative. Although it's a white bread, sourdough is highly acidic, which helps to prevent blood sugar spikes. Look to a bakery for real sourdough bread; some manufacturers use sour flavoring agents instead of bacteria to ferment the dough. It's the bacteria that produce the acids that make sourdough better for your blood sugar.

Are all wheat breads better for you than white?

NO If the package says "wheat bread," it's probably just white bread with a dye job. Look for the word *whole* on the ingredient label.

They often sit side by side in your grocery store: One loaf marked "white," the other "wheat." The latter looks healthier—but it may not be.

The fact is that many "wheat" breads *are* white breads. After all, even white bread comes from wheat. Some so-called wheat breads may have been baked with caramel coloring or some other additive to give them a dark, earthy-looking hue—but that doesn't make them any better for you.

Look for bread that has a coarse texture and the word *whole* in the first ingredient.

BREAD

What makes a bread good for your health is the presence of whole, unrefined grains, including the grain's tough outer shell, or bran, and its germ, or seed, both of which are removed to make white bread. The milling process also removes most of the grain's fiber and lots of vitamins and minerals, though manufacturers add back some of the nutrients.

How can you tell whether you're getting true whole wheat bread or white bread that has been dyed brown? Read the package labels—both sides. The words *100 percent whole wheat* or *100 percent whole grain* splashed on the package are a good sign. But always check the ingredient list, too. The first item should include "whole," as in "whole wheat flour." And choose coarse-looking bread with lots of texture; that's an indication that the wheat has been less finely ground, which means the bread should have less impact on your blood sugar. ■

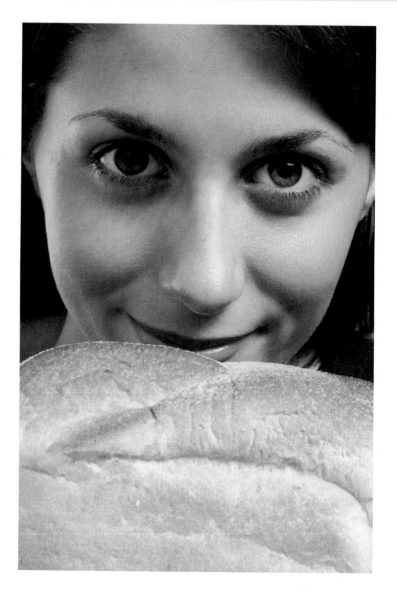

If the package says "wheat bread," it's probably just **white bread with a dye job.**

Chocolate

Yesterday it was a sinful indulgence that rotted teeth, padded hips, and caused acne. Today chocolate is practically a health food, said to boost moods, protect hearts, and even help fight cancer. As if we needed more reasons to like it! But is chocolate too good to be true?

Is dark chocolate good for you?

YES Unlike milk chocolate, dark chocolate is rich in chemicals that fight heart disease. Just make it an occasional treat.

If you've always preferred milk chocolate over dark chocolate, it may be time to give the dark stuff another try.

The cacao beans used to make the chocolate liquor, cocoa butter, and cocoa powder found in chocolate products are chock-full of flavonoids. These powerful antioxidants neutralize free radicals, which damage cells and cause disease. Other good sources of flavonoids include tea, grapes, and grapefruit. Dark chocolate contains far more flavonoid-rich cocoa particles than milk chocolate.

The flavonoids in dark chocolate increase the body's levels of nitric oxide, a gas that causes blood vessels to relax and expand, which in turn promotes healthy circulation and low blood pressure. In fact, some research suggests that frequent servings of dark chocolate may reduce high blood pressure as effectively as commonly used medications. In one study, researchers asked 10 men and women with high blood pressure to eat 3.5 ounces of dark chocolate every day. (A typical chocolate bar is 1.5 ounces.) A similar group of volunteers ate a daily serving of white chocolate, which has no flavonoids. After 15 days, the groups switched to the other variety of chocolate. The researchers discovered that eating dark chocolate—but not white—produced a 12-point drop in systolic pressure (the first number in a blood pressure reading) and a 9-point dip in diastolic pressure (the second number).

Other studies show that eating dark chocolate reduces inflammation, another risk factor for heart disease, and makes the body more sensitive to the hormone insulin, which could help prevent type 2 diabetes.

You may wonder: How can candy be good for me? Dark chocolate has slightly less sugar than milk chocolate, but it has more fat and plenty of calories, so overindulging will make you gain weight. But the fat in chocolate doesn't raise cholesterol levels; about a third of it is in the form of oleic acid, the healthful monounsaturated fat found in olive oil. ■

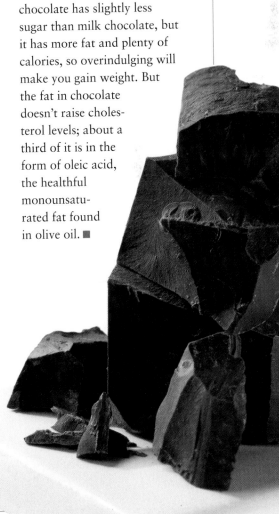

Coffee

It's a great time to be a coffee lover. Espresso cafes are springing up in big cities and small towns faster than you can say "double tall caramel macchiato." Supermarkets that once sold a few varieties of bland brew now offer an array of high-quality beans from exotic locales. And best of all, you can quit worrying that drinking a cup or two of coffee every day is slowly nudging you toward an early grave.

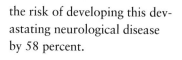

Is coffee good for you?

YES Population studies suggest that coffee confers various health benefits to people who drink it regularly.

Research suggests that a cup of Joe may do more for you than keep you awake during that mind-numbing meeting or endless car trip. Coffee contains potentially valuable compounds, including disease-fighting antioxidants that mop up dangerous free radicals in the body. Scientists who study health trends in broad populations say that people who indulge a coffee habit appear to gain protection against several diseases, including the following.

Type 2 diabetes: Caffeine raises blood sugar levels, which ratchets up the risk of type 2 diabetes. Yet, oddly enough, several large studies have found that consuming coffee appears to protect against this all-too-common disease. One analysis of studies involving more than 193,000 people and published in the *Journal of the American Medical Association* found that heavy coffee drinkers—people who drink up to seven cups per day—seemed to cut their risk of type 2 diabetes by up to 35 percent. In a few studies, people who drank decaffeinated coffee seemed to lower their risk even more.

Gallstones: A 1999 study found that men who drink two or three cups of java per day reduce their risk of developing gallstones by 40 percent. Some scientists believe caffeine blocks development of these painful masses, which form in the gallbladder and bile ducts.

Parkinson's disease: One study of more than 47,000 men found that downing several cups of coffee a day may cut the risk of developing this devastating neurological disease by 58 percent.

Alzheimer's disease: Here's another potential bonus for your brain: Some preliminary research suggests that coffee may protect against Alzheimer's, too. A 2007 analysis of four studies found that coffee drinkers had a 30 percent reduced risk for the most common form of dementia.

Memory loss and other cognitive problems: Cognitive problems are a symptom of dementia, but let's face it: Many otherwise healthy people lose mental sharpness and become more forgetful after middle age. Coffee may help. In one French study, women over 80 who drank three cups or more per day were 70 percent less likely to have memory decline than those who drank one cup or less.

Does coffee cause cancer?

NO Time and good science have turned this old concern on its head. Coffee may even *fight* cancer.

Preliminary research back in the 1970s and 1980s linked coffee drinking and caffeine consumption to breast and pancreatic cancers. Could one of the world's most popular beverages be silently fueling countless cases of cancer?

Fear not, fans of French roast: After the early scares, larger and more sensitive studies failed to find an association between the brew and any form of cancer. Quite the opposite: More recent research suggests that coffee may actually *protect* against certain cancers.

A review of studies determined that people who drink coffee (regular or decaf) or tea regularly reduce their risk of colon cancer by 24 percent. What's more, studies involving more than 241,000 subjects show that people who sip just two cups a day slash their risk of liver cancer by 43 percent. Most scientists who study coffee today have dismissed

How Jolting Is Your Diet?

Consuming moderate amounts of caffeine appears to be safe for most people. Some experts, however, recommend limiting your daily caffeine intake to 300 to 400 milligrams. Tally up your intake using the chart below.

BEVERAGE	CAFFEINE CONTENT
Brewed coffee, 8 oz	72–130 mg
Espresso, 1 shot	58–76 mg
Caffe latte, 12 oz	75 mg
Brewed tea, 8 oz	20–90 mg
Iced tea, 8 oz	9–50 mg
Cola, 12 oz	30 mg
Milk chocolate, 1 oz	1–15 mg
Dark chocolate, 1 oz	5–35 mg
Energy drink, 8 oz	30–77 mg on average; some contain much more

Sources: *Journal of Analytical Toxicology*, American Beverage Association, Starbucks.com

concerns about cancer and begun to focus on how this popular drink might promote health.

Does coffee cause high blood pressure?

NO Drinking coffee or other caffeinated beverages produces a rise in blood pressure, but the effect is mild and fades quickly.

Drinking too much coffee can set your nerves on edge or leave you staring at the ceiling in bed at night, but several major studies have failed to find any link between a coffee habit and chronically elevated blood pressure.

Caffeine increases levels of stress hormones, which are known to raise blood pressure. Not surprisingly, studies show that drinking caffeinated beverages causes blood pressure to rise, but the effect is modest and tends to wear off quickly. And after a few days of regular

COFFEE

coffee drinking, caffeine has no effect on blood pressure. One large study of more than 155,000 women found no connection between coffee drinking and the risk of developing high blood pressure.

Population research suggests that a hot cup of Joe is no tale of woe for your ticker as long as you don't go crazy. Although there is some evidence that drinking five or more cups a day increases the risk of heart attacks, large studies in the United States, Scotland, and Finland have failed to find any link between coffee drinking and cardiovascular disease.

Does coffee really keep you up?

MAYBE That depends on whether or not your body is used to the caffeine.

Drinking too much coffee can cause almost anyone to have trouble falling asleep at night. But why are some people who drink coffee all day, and may even top off their dinner with a cup of espresso, able to nod off as soon as their heads hit the pillow?

Caffeine gives its jolt by blocking a chemical called adenosine. When adenosine attaches itself to receptors in the brain, it triggers changes that make you sleepy. Caffeine is similar in structure and shape to adenosine, and when it "parks" in the adenosine

receptors, voilà—you stay awake. Unless, that is, you're a frequent coffee drinker. Research has shown that consuming caffeine on a regular basis increases the number of adenosine receptors, which partially offsets the effects of caffeine.

The amount of caffeine needed to have an effect varies from one person to another, depending on sensitivity to the chemical, body size, and other factors. Experts say that regular caffeine fiends may still experience sleep disturbances, such as struggling to fall asleep and having poor quality of rest.

Should you switch to decaf?

MAYBE Ask your doctor if it's safe to drink caffeinated coffee if you fall into any of these categories.

You are pregnant. Research shows that drinking moderate amounts of coffee (up to three cups a day) doesn't seem to cause miscarriages, though a few studies suggest that greater amounts could increase the risk.

You have high blood pressure or any other heart condition. Drinking coffee doesn't appear to cause chronically elevated blood pressure, but all the same, doctors often advise patients who already have the condition to cut back on caffeinated drinks.

Our BEST ADVICE

If you use a French press to make coffee, consider switching to a drip-style coffeemaker. Boiled coffee, which includes brew made with a French press as well as Scandinavian and Turkish coffee, contains compounds called diterpenes that can raise total cholesterol by up to 23 mg/dl and LDL ("bad") cholesterol by as much as 14 mg/dl. Filters used in drip coffeemakers remove diterpenes.

You have fibrocystic breasts. Some research suggests caffeine may promote the formation of cysts in the breast, which may cause discomfort. This theory remains controversial, though some women say that cutting back on caffeine helped relieve the problem.

You take certain medications. Caffeine can alter the way your body metabolizes certain drugs. If you take prescription medication, ask your doctor whether it can interact with caffeine.

You have chronic insomnia, headaches, or nervousness. Some people are highly sensitive to caffeine. Eliminating it may help with these problems, though if you're a regular coffee drinker, quit gradually to avoid unpleasant withdrawal symptoms. ■

Dairy Foods

The words *wholesome* and *milk* are practically joined at the hip—a bone you may think you're less likely to break if you drink milk regularly. But as scientists have learned more about milk and other dairy foods, the picture of their nutritional value has become more complex.

Are milk and calcium pills the best things for your bones?

NO Your bones need calcium, but drinking several glasses of milk and popping calcium pills every day may not be necessary.

For years, it was nutritional gospel: For stronger bones, drink lots of milk. If you dislike dairy, take calcium pills every day. But the science supporting this advice is surprisingly shaky.

First, what's not in dispute: Your bones need calcium, which, along with a few other minerals, makes up about 65 percent of your skeleton; the rest is mostly collagen. Most of the calcium in your diet goes toward rebuilding bones, but your body needs this mineral to build healthy nerves, regulate heart rhythm, and perform other important functions, too. If your diet doesn't provide enough calcium, your body borrows some from your bones. Osteoporosis, the "fragile bone disease," occurs when bones lose calcium faster than they can replace it.

Current dietary guidelines advise all adults to consume at least 1,000 milligrams of calcium per day until age 50, when the recommendation jumps to 1,200 milligrams. Dairy foods are among the richest sources of calcium, so you might assume that milk drinkers have the strongest bones, right?

Not exactly. Studies have failed to show consistently that dairy devotees have healthier bones. In fact, several large studies have found that milk drinkers have just as many bone breaks as people who disdain dairy. For example, when Harvard researchers examined the diets of more than 72,000 postmenopausal women over an 18-year period, they found barely any difference in the risk of hip fractures among women who drank at least a glass or two of milk every day and others who sipped one glass or less per week. In another study of nearly 61,000 subjects, Swedish scientists found that women who consumed 1,200 milligrams of calcium per day were just as likely to sustain broken hips as women who got less than 400 milligrams.

The bottom line: A little dairy is probably a good thing, but more may not be better.

Can dairy help you lose weight?

MAYBE Intriguing evidence suggests that dairy foods speed up weight loss, but more research is needed.

Several studies conducted by a team at the University of Tennessee suggest that dairy

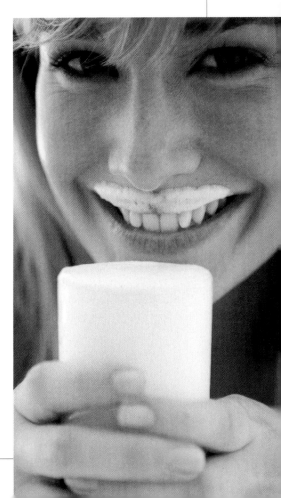

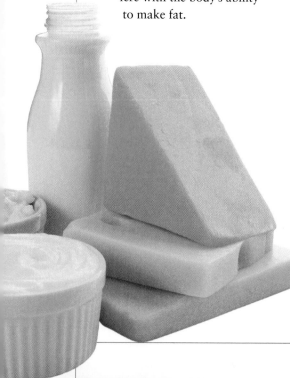

DAIRY FOODS

can give dieters an edge. In one trial, nutritionist Michael B. Zemel, PhD, and his colleagues put obese volunteers on one of three low-calorie diets: One was low in dairy and calcium, one was low in dairy but included calcium supplements, and the third was high in dairy from three servings of low-fat milk or other foods per day. After six months, people in each group lost a significant amount of weight (remember, all three diets were low in calories), but the dairy group slimmed down the most.

In another study by the same team, people who adopted low-calorie diets and consumed several servings of dairy each day lost twice as much weight as volunteers in a similar group whose diets included little dairy. Dr. Zemel and others believe dairy foods contain compounds that interfere with the body's ability to make fat.

These studies included just a few dozen subjects, however, which raises the question of whether their findings would apply to most people. Furthermore, other studies have failed to show that adding dairy or calcium to a daily menu speeds weight loss.

Do low-fat dairy foods lower blood pressure?

YES A major study showed that consuming low-fat dairy products can help lower blood pressure.

People who consume dairy foods regularly tend to have healthy blood pressure. Why? Researchers once thought that calcium might be the key, which made sense. After all, the mineral plays a role in regulating blood pressure. But in studies, taking calcium supplements often failed to lower blood pressure in people with hypertension. Today some researchers suspect that vitamin D is a factor; most milk products are enriched with this vitamin, which appears to create metabolic changes that lower blood pressure. What seems clear is that adding low-fat dairy to a healthy diet does help keep pressure in check.

In the DASH (Dietary Approaches to Stop Hypertension) Trial, which involved 459 men and women, researchers compared a group of people

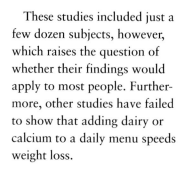

Our BEST ADVICE

Take other steps to protect your bones. Weight-bearing exercise, such as walking or jogging, strengthens bones and can cut the risk of fractures by more than 40 percent among older women. It's also critical to get adequate vitamin D, which helps the body absorb and retain calcium. Supplements may help, although spending a few minutes in the sun each day stimulates production of D. Finally, don't smoke or abuse alcohol; both habits seem to weaken bones.

who were told to eat more fruits and vegetables with a group instructed to do the same and to eat three daily servings of low-fat milk, yogurt, or other dairy foods while cutting back on saturated fat. A control group ate a typical Western diet—high in fat and low in dairy foods, fruit, and vegetables.

After two months, people in the fruits-and-vegetables group who had hypertension lowered their pressure by an average of 7.2/2.8 points more than the control group. Not surprising, since produce is rich in potassium and magnesium, both important for regulating blood pressure. But people who also ate low-fat dairy foods improved more, lowering their blood pressure by 11.4/5.5 points on average. ■

Eggs

Eggs are delicate; drop one, and you'll need a sponge, not a spatula. Yet their reputation as heart wreckers is amazingly strong. Despite being excellent inexpensive sources of protein, not to mention B vitamins and minerals, they are best known for their cholesterol content. But it seems that experts who warned that omelets cause heart attacks now have egg on their faces.

Do eggs raise cholesterol levels?

NO Not enough to worry about, anyway. Studies show that eggs don't deserve their reputation as artery cloggers.

Eggs are loaded with cholesterol. A single large egg contains more than 200 milligrams of the waxy stuff, which is two-thirds of the maximum daily total recommended by the American Heart Association. So it's hardly surprising that doctors started telling patients to go easy on eggs in the early 1970s, as studies showed that people with high blood levels of cholesterol have an increased risk of heart disease.

Good intentions, but questionable science. Researchers now know that cholesterol in food has only a slight effect on the levels of cholesterol in your blood. Saturated fat and trans fat are the real offenders. When you gobble up bacon, doughnuts, or other foods laden with these fats, your liver churns out cholesterol, which can gum up blood flow and cause heart attacks.

Of course, many foods that are high in cholesterol are also bursting with saturated fat, so this distinction doesn't matter much in some cases. Consider, for example, that a fast-food double cheeseburger may have up to 24 grams of saturated fat. But one egg contains only a modest amount of saturated fat: just 1.6 grams.

Several major studies have helped to rehabilitate eggs' reputation in the minds of most physicians and nutritionists. For instance, the long-running Framingham Heart Study found no association between eating eggs and heart attacks. Likewise, Harvard researchers failed to find any connection between eggs and heart disease when they analyzed the diets of nearly 118,000 healthy men and women.

The American Heart Association still recommends eating no more than one egg per day and cutting back on other foods that are high in cholesterol on days that you choose to eat an egg. But the research shows a two-egg omelet isn't likely to kill you.

Are eggs enriched with omega-3 fatty acids worth the price?

NO Most omega-3 eggs on the market won't provide the same heart protection you get from eating fish.

For people who can't bring themselves to eat seafood twice a week, as most health guidelines recommend, eggs and other foods enriched with omega-3 fatty acids—which protect the heart and have other important health benefits—seem like a gift from the grocery gods. However, there are less expensive ways to get

Harvard **researchers failed** to find any connection between eggs and heart disease.

EGGS

the benefits of fish oil, and these "designer" eggs may promise more health benefits than they deliver.

First, fish-oil capsules are much cheaper alternatives to the pricey eggs. You'll pay about two cents per standard capsule, which usually contains 300 milligrams of the omega-3 fatty acids DHA and EPA. That's up to 20 times more of these valuable fatty acids than you get from an omega-3 egg, says University of South Dakota nutritionist William S. Harris, PhD, an authority on omega-3 fatty acids. Some brands of omega-3 eggs can cost more than $3 per dozen.

Second, most omega-3 eggs do not contain DHA or EPA,

the omega-3's in fish, but rather ALA, which comes from flax and other plant foods fed to hens. Some research suggests that ALA has health benefits, too, though they are less well understood. Your body converts ALA to DHA and EPA, but very inefficiently, so eggs from flax-fed chickens won't give you anywhere near the same benefit as eating fish.

If you can find eggs that contain DHA and EPA, your budget can handle the expense, and you don't want to eat fish or take fish-oil capsules, "it's probably worth paying a premium for these products," says Dr. Harris. Otherwise, it's hard to rationalize shelling out extra cash for omega-3 eggs. ∎

Our BEST ADVICE

Before buying eggs enriched with omega-3 fatty acids, find out what the hens that laid them were fed. Only chickens that eat some form of fish oil will produce eggs that contain DHA and EPA, the omega-3's linked to the most health benefits. Unfortunately, carton labels usually don't include this information, so you may need to contact the farm. If the label says the chickens received a vegetarian diet, their feed probably contained flax, not fish oil.

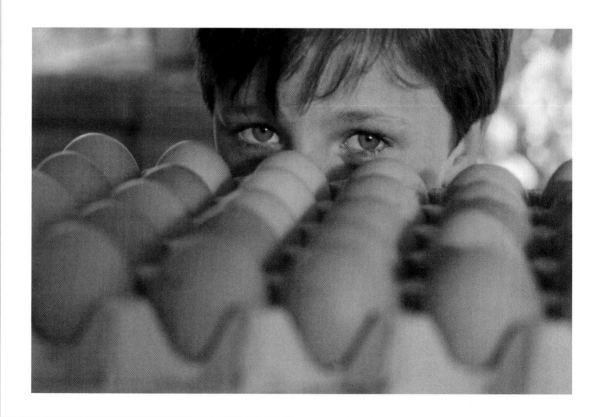

Energy Bars and Drinks

In the middle of a long day, when your fuel reserves dip, the idea of a magic bar or elixir to restore your spirits and provide pep can seem pretty appealing, which helps explains the explosion of energy bars and drinks on the market. But do these products deliver? Don't buy the hype.

Are energy bars healthy snacks?

NO For a quick snack, you're much better off with a piece of fruit or a handful of trail mix—and so is your wallet.

What'll it be for your afternoon snack—a juicy red apple or a candy bar? The makers of energy bars want you to believe you can have the best of both worlds: a healthy treat that tastes like candy or cookies. How well they please the palate is a matter of opinion (though comparisons to flavored cardboard are not uncommon). In terms of nutrition, however, most dietitians agree: While energy bars are better belly fillers than bonbons, they're no replacement for fruit, nuts, and other healthy snacks.

Like candy, energy bars are a conveniently wrapped source of quick calories. However, many energy bars are packed with much more protein than the typical candy bar, so they do a better job of quieting a growling stomach. Chalk one up for energy bars. And unlike candy bars, most energy bars are fortified with vitamins and minerals. That's a plus, too, though if you eat a balanced diet, you may not need these added nutrients (and taking a multivitamin is far cheaper). If you're trying to add soy to your diet, you can find energy bars that contain soy protein and probably taste better than tofu.

On the other hand, some energy bars contain stuff your diet doesn't need, such as saturated and trans fat, high-fructose corn syrup, and other ingredients that have been linked to health problems, including palm kernel oil, maldodextrin (a type of starch that often contains MSG), and acesulfame potassium (an artificial sweetener that some experts say has not been adequately studied).

Keep in mind, too, that *energy* is another word for "calories." If you're looking for a light snack, bars that contain 200 or 300 calories may bust your calorie budget for the day. On the other hand, if you're looking for a meal replacement, energy bars may fall short on calories—not to mention the vegetables and other foods a meal should contain. Counting carbs? Beware: Some bars top 40 grams

Are energy drinks a good source of energy?

NO Despite their exotic-sounding ingredients, what you're really getting is sugar and often a hefty dose of caffeine.

These days, it's not just New York City that never sleeps. If the popularity of so-called

Keep in mind that *energy* is another word for "calories."

ENERGY BARS AND DRINKS

Buying a Better Energy Bar

If you like the convenience of energy bars, shop carefully to find one that gets the job done right. Look for a bar with ingredients that fall within the ranges below.

CHECK THE LABEL FOR:	LOOK FOR THIS MANY GRAMS:	NOTES
Protein	5–15	A bar without enough protein won't keep you full for long.
Carbohydrates	20–50	Choose a bar with a lower carb content if you want a snack to satisfy your appetite; go for more carbs if you want a preworkout energy boost.
Fiber	2–5 or more	Along with protein, a good dose of fiber helps keep hunger at bay.
Calories	No more than 250	If you're using an energy bar for a light snack, keep calories below 200.
Fat	5 or fewer	Fat should preferably be mono- or poly-unsaturated. Avoid bars with saturated fat and trans fat/hydrogenated oil.

energy drinks is any indication, lots of people have scaled back their shuteye. With names like Juiced, Xenergy, and Enviga, the various concoctions contain a wide array of ingredients, including herbs, amino acids, and other natural compounds with purported health benefits. But many of these products have two ingredients in common: sugar and caffeine.

Sugar is a source of calories, so technically it provides energy. Ounce for ounce, the popular energy drink Red Bull has more sugar than Coke. Caffeine provides temporary energy since it increases alertness and seems to rev up energy systems in the body. Some energy drinks have as much caffeine as a shot of espresso. The beverages may contain sources of caffeine even if caffeine's not listed on the label—guarana, yerba mate, green tea extract, and other herbs are natural sources of the chemical. Many drinks also contain the amino acid taurine, which may enhance the effects of caffeine, though this has not been proven.

A big dose of sugar and caffeine may snap you out of midday doldrums, but nutritionists agree there are better ways to stay well supplied with energy: eat a balanced diet, exercise regularly, and yes, get plenty of sleep. ■

Fiber

It has no calories and isn't even considered a nutrient because it isn't digested. Yet the sturdy stuff that gives plants their structure is a dietary star. Fiber helps keep you "regular," of course, and it helps people lose weight. Eating a diet rich in high-fiber foods can have other important benefits, too. But at least one old idea about "roughage" has gone soft in recent years.

Does fiber fight colon cancer?

NO A high-fiber diet can keep your digestive system running smoothly, but it won't keep colon cancer at bay.

It seemed like a logical idea: Eat roughage, stay regular, and keep your colon clear of nasty toxins that cause cancer. The theory that a high-fiber diet prevents colon cancer dates back at least to the early 1970s, when doctors reported that cancers of the gastrointestinal tract were rare among Africans who ate plenty of whole grains, fruit, and vegetables. Scientists began to study fiber's potential by comparing the diets of healthy people with the diets of people who had developed colon cancer. A survey of 13 such studies found that people who ate the most fiber seemed to slash their risk of colon cancer by nearly 50 percent.

This type of study has a few built-in catches, however. For instance, many people change their diets over the years, and when a researcher asks about your diet, it can be awfully hard to remember what you ate a decade ago. When scientists put fiber to some tougher tests, they chewed up its reputation as a colon protector. In one study sponsored by the National Cancer Institute, researchers randomly assigned 2,079 male and female colon cancer survivors to eat either a high-fiber meal plan or to stick with their usual diets. Four years later, almost exactly the same percentage of people in both groups had had

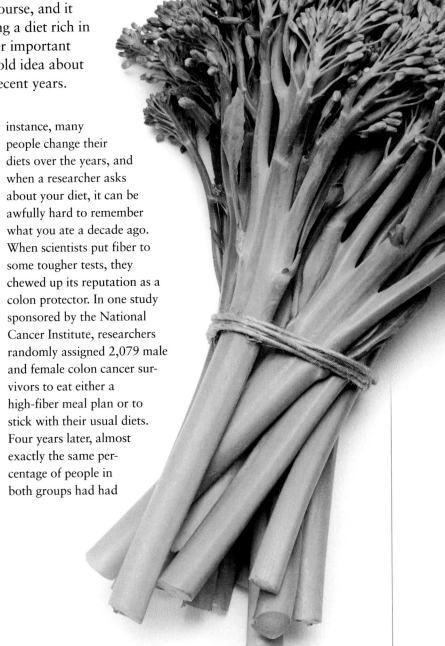

FIBER

Easy Ways to Add Fiber to Your Diet

Most people eat too little fiber. The Institute of Medicine recommends consuming 14 grams of fiber for every 1,000 calories in your diet. For the average person, that means 25 to 30 grams of fiber daily. Here's how much fiber you'll get from a typical serving by making some simple changes.

EAT THIS	NOT THIS	AND GET...
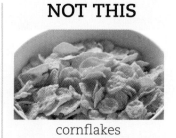 bran cereal	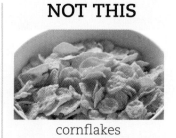 cornflakes	**5.0** grams more fiber.
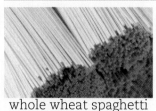 whole wheat spaghetti	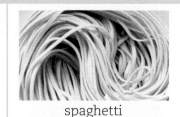 spaghetti	**3.9** grams more fiber.
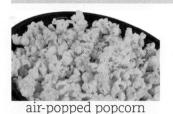 air-popped popcorn	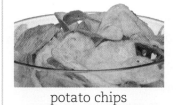 potato chips	**2.9** grams more fiber.
brown rice	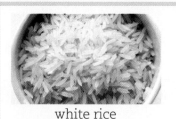 white rice	**2.9** grams more fiber.
baked potato with skin	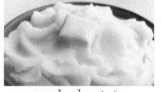 mashed potato	**2.7** grams more fiber.

Source: *Bowes and Church's Food Values of Portions Commonly Used* (Lippincott, 1998).

recurrences of colon cancer. Another large study using fiber supplements yielded similar results.

In the final blow, scientists reviewed 13 studies in which participants were asked about their current diets, then were followed for up to 20 years. The investigators determined that fiber had no benefit.

That doesn't mean there's no reason to eat more fiber; there are plenty of them, as you'll read shortly.

Does fiber guard against heart disease?

YES Eating the recommended 25 to 35 grams of fiber daily can reduce several risk factors for heart attacks.

A number of studies have found that people who eat plenty of fiber tend to have a low risk of heart attacks. For instance, one survey of nearly 44,000 men found that those who ate 29 grams of fiber a day were 41 percent less likely to develop heart disease. Another large study found that women who ate 23 grams of fiber daily had half the risk of heart attacks when compared with others who ate little fiber. Experts recommend that adults eat between 25 and 35 grams of fiber a day, but most people don't come close.

There are two types of fiber, soluble and insoluble. Oat bran and oatmeal are perhaps the best known sources of soluble fiber, but it's also found in beans, peas, rice bran, barley, citrus fruits, strawberries, and apples. When you eat these foods, their soluble fiber passes slowly through the digestive tract, gradually turning thick and gummy. This gel binds with cholesterol particles, trapping them so they can't pass through the intestinal wall and into the bloodstream. Instead, they're whisked out of the body as waste.

Even so, soluble fiber's effect on cholesterol is small. Eating three bowls of oatmeal a day will lower total cholesterol by only about 5 points, which would reduce the risk of heart disease by about 4 percent. That means that a high-fiber diet must provide some other heart benefit. One possibility: People who eat lots of fiber—both soluble and insoluble, the kind in fruit skins and most vegetables—eat less food, period, probably because fiber is filling. Fiber helps keep your weight down, too, which in turn helps to control several risk factors for heart disease that have been linked to obesity, including high blood pressure, low levels of HDL ("good") cholesterol, and elevated levels of blood fats called triglycerides.

Does fiber help prevent diabetes?

YES Many high-fiber foods can help prevent surges in blood sugar that can raise the risk of type 2 diabetes.

When you eat an apple or a carrot, it takes a while for your body to digest it. The story's completely different when you eat a slice of white bread: Almost magically, it's dissolved. In general, foods that are digested slowly cause a smaller rise in blood sugar than foods that are digested quickly. The less a meal raises blood sugar, the less insulin the body must churn out to get that blood sugar into cells.

Insulin resistance, a problem at the core of type 2 diabetes, happens when the body must repeatedly produce a lot of insulin to handle meals full of fast-digesting carbohydrates—usually carbohydrates low in fiber.

While several studies have shown that people who eat high-fiber diets are less likely to develop insulin resistance, soluble fiber—found in oatmeal, beans, and barley, among other foods—may offer the most protection. The gel formed by soluble fiber creates a barrier between the digestive enzymes in your stomach and the starch molecules in food; as a result, it takes longer for your body to digest the meal and convert it to blood sugar. ■

Fish

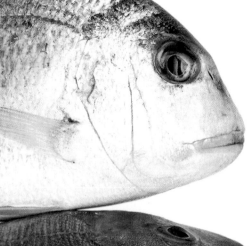

There are more than 20,000 species of fish in the world's waters, although we eat only a small number of varieties. And we don't eat them often enough, doctors say: Solid research shows that people who eat seafood regularly have healthy hearts—and minds. But does fish come with side effects that stink?

Is eating fish worth the risk?

YES High levels of toxins in some seafood represent a genuine concern. But fish's benefits outweigh the threat.

Just a few years ago, this would have been a no-brainer: *Of course* you should eat fish. People who eat at least a few servings of fish per week have far fewer heart attacks, fewer strokes, and fewer fatal arrhythmias, or irregular heartbeats, than people who don't eat fish. What's more, developing brains require the fatty acids found in fish. One recent study found that children born to women who ate at least 12 ounces of fish a week during pregnancy had higher IQs, were better behaved, and were less likely to have other developmental problems.

Unfortunately, the sea of good news about fish has turned murky in recent years. Several high-profile reports revealed that some varieties of fish contain high levels of contaminants, including mercury

and the industrial toxins dioxins and polychlorinated biphenyls (PCBs). Studies have linked exposure to these toxins to cardiovascular problems, damage to the nervous system, and other health threats. Suddenly, many consumers found themselves pausing at the fish counter or hesitating before opening a can of tuna, wondering: "Is this stuff safe?"

To find the answer, a pair of Harvard researchers combed through stacks of studies, government reports, and other scientific literature on fish and human health, then published their findings in the *Journal of the American Medical Association (JAMA)*. The bottom line: Eating fish far outweighs any accompanying risks. The *JAMA* study determined that people who have just one or two servings of fish each week lower their risk of a fatal heart attack by 36 percent and have a 17 percent reduced risk of dying from any cause, compared to people who don't eat seafood.

Should certain people limit their fish consumption?

YES The FDA and EPA advise women who are pregnant or may become pregnant, as well as young children, to limit themselves to two servings of fish (for a total of 12 ounces) per week. They should also avoid fish that tend to contain high levels of mercury, which include king mackerel, shark, swordfish, and tilefish. Likewise, people in these groups should eat no more than six ounces per week of canned albacore tuna, which is moderately high in mercury. (Canned light tuna is low in mercury.)

Does eating fish fight depression?

YES Scientists have observed that rates of serious depression are lowest in countries where fish plays a prominent role in the cuisine.

Major depression causes more disability than any other condition, according to the World Health Organization, but it's possible that the right diet can offer help.

Neurologists point out that the brain is about 60 percent fat, much of it in the form of the omega-3 fatty acids found in fish, known as DHA and EPA. Research suggests that omega-3's make brain cells more fluid, allowing them to deliver signals more efficiently. People who become depressed tend to have low blood levels of DHA and EPA.

Doctors have attempted to treat various psychiatric disorders with fish oil in recent years. While fish oil's benefits for certain conditions are still not clear, a panel of experts assembled by the American Psychiatric Association (APA) recently determined that DHA and EPA significantly improve major depression and bipolar

Safe Omega-3 Sources

Eat a variety of fish, but choose fatty varieties most often to get the most omega-3 fatty acids in your diet. Here are 10 top sources of omega-3's that are also low in mercury.

FISH OR SHELLFISH	OMEGA-3'S*
Salmon	0.68–1.83 grams
Herring	1.71–1.81 grams
Oysters	0.37–1.17 grams
Halibut	0.40–1.00 grams
Tuna (canned, light)	0.26–0.73 grams
Pollock	0.46 grams
Flounder or sole	0.43 grams
Lobster	0.07–0.41 grams
Crab	0.34–0.40 grams
Shrimp	0.27 grams

*Per 3-oz. serving

Source: The American Heart Association.

depression (sometimes called manic depression). For some people, fish oil could literally be a lifesaver: Several studies have found that suicidal patients given DHA and EPA supplements are less likely to harm themselves.

While these types of studies typically use large doses of DHA and EPA, the APA's expert panel nonetheless suggests that all adults can bolster their emotional and mental health by eating fatty fish at least twice a week.

Does eating fish fight inflammation?

YES Seafood rich in omega-3 fatty acids cools chronic inflammation, a risk factor for a long list of conditions.

Inflammation is one of the, well, hottest topics in medicine these days. Your immune system produces inflammation to heal injuries and battle germs. Scientists have long known that out-of-control inflammation causes autoimmune disorders such as

FLAXSEED

Fish
(continued)

rheumatoid arthritis and lupus. In recent years, however, researchers have linked chronic, low-grade inflammation with a host of chronic health conditions.

Fortunately, turning down the heat may be as simple as having a few servings of seafood each week. Studies consistently show that people who consume diets rich in omega-3 fatty acids—especially the kind in fish oil—tend to have low blood levels of inflammatory chemicals such as C-reactive protein (CRP), which many cardiologists now consider a major risk factor for heart attacks. In a recent study of nearly 1,000 men and women, Japanese scientists reported that people who ate the most seafood had the lowest levels of CRP compared to others who rarely dined on fish and shellfish.

Other studies show that people who eat plenty of seafood are less likely to develop diabetes, cancer, asthma, and allergies. Interesting, though preliminary, research suggests that eating fish may prevent and provide relief from other diseases caused by inflammation, including rheumatoid arthritis and inflammatory bowel disease (though in most of these studies, patients took fish oil in the form of supplements). ■

Flaxseed

Not long ago, the only flax you were likely to find in most homes had been spun into linen tablecloths or napkins or processed into linseed oil and used as a wood finish. Today, flaxseed can be found in the kitchen cabinets and refrigerators of health-conscious people looking to lower their risk of heart disease and cancer. Do the seeds live up to their promise?

Is eating flaxseed a good substitute for eating fish?

NO Flaxseed contains a type of omega-3 fatty acid, but the fatty acids in fish pack more punch.

If you don't like fish but want the health benefits of omega-3's, flaxseed may seem like the solution. After all, it's a rich source of omega-3's, too—but alas, not the same ones found in fish.

The omega-3's in flaxseed and other plant foods, like walnuts and tofu, come in the form of ALA (alpha-linolenic acid). Human cells need ALA to function properly, and your body can't manufacture the stuff, which means you have to get it from food. If you've never tasted flaxseed or let tofu pass your lips, you may wonder how you've survived this long. The fact is, ALA is also present in smaller amounts in many common foods, including bread, pasta, beef, pork, and chicken.

The omega-3's in fish oil, docosahexaenoic acid (DHA) and eicosapentaenoic acid (EPA), are the ones that are good for the cardiovascular system and have other well-established health benefits. Your body can turn ALA into DHA and EPA, but very inefficiently. Some estimates suggest that less than 1 percent of the ALA you consume becomes EPA, while an even tinier

Our BEST ADVICE

To add flaxseed to your diet, buy it in bulk at a natural foods store—and pick up a coffee grinder while you're at it. A study in the *Journal of Nutrition* found that eating crushed or ground flaxseed raises blood levels of lignans two to four times higher than eating whole seeds. Sprinkle ground flaxseed on breakfast cereal or salads or add it to baked goods.

portion—less than 0.1 percent—converts to DHA.

Nevertheless, organizations such as the American Heart Association want you to keep eating flaxseed, tofu, walnuts, and other ALA-rich foods. They have few downsides, and some evidence suggests they may have benefits of their own. For instance, several studies have found that people who have high levels of ALA in their blood tend to have lower levels of inflammatory chemicals.

Does flaxseed prevent cancer?

MAYBE The research is promising, but scientists still can't say whether flaxseed lowers the risk of breast cancer or any other form of cancer.

Like humans, plants have hormones. Flaxseed is nature's richest source of plant hormones called lignans, which the body converts to compounds that mimic estrogen. In fact, flaxseed contains 75 to 800 times more lignans than any other plant food. Researchers are studying whether lignans and other phytoestrogens ("phyto-" is Latin for "plant") have a role in preventing cancer. In theory, lignans block the effects of estrogen, which can fuel the growth of malignant tumors, notably some common forms of breast cancer.

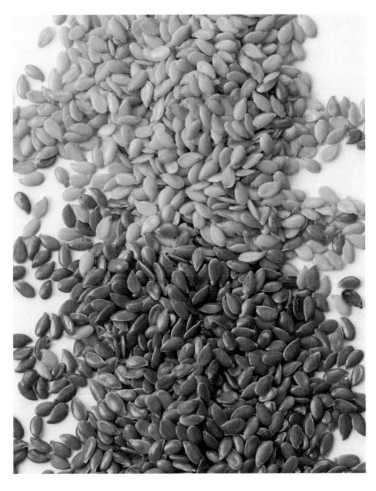

Intriguing evidence suggests that flaxseed and other foods rich in lignans (which include barley, oatmeal, and wheat bran) are potent cancer fighters. For example, studies show that feeding flaxseed to lab mice prevents breast cancer and slows the growth and spread of malignant tumors. Animal research shows that flaxseed also appears to increase the effectiveness of tamoxifen, a drug that reduces the risk of breast cancer by interfering with estrogen. Some studies suggest that flaxseed may also prevent other forms of cancer that are fed by hormones, including prostate cancer.

While the research is exciting, most of it has involved animals. A few studies have found that women who consume the most lignans have a lower-than-expected risk of breast cancer, though the benefit may be limited to women who have not reached menopause. Until more studies are completed, it's not possible to say with certainty that flaxseed fights any form of cancer. ∎

FRUIT JUICE

Fruit Juice

To some people, drinking a glass of chilled juice with breakfast can seem like a way to balance the scales, serving as a nutritious counterweight to the bacon or doughnut they eat with it. But while fruit juice is sweet, delicious, and, yes, nutritious, you're pouring a lot of calories into that glass.

Is drinking juice as good for you as eating fruit?

NO Juice has some but not all of the nutritional benefits of whole fruit, and some drawbacks, too.

There's no easier way to get one of your five daily servings of fruits and vegetables than gulping down a cool, refreshing glass of juice.

No washing, no peeling, and no tossing out rotten bananas that turned brown before you could eat them. No guilt, either, since the USDA says you can count a glass of 100 percent fruit or vegetable juice as one serving.

Don't be fooled, however: Biting into a crisp apple or a tart wedge of grapefruit provides more nourishment than sipping their liquefied counter-parts. That holds true even if you purchase juice labeled "all natural" or "100 percent fruit juice." One reason is simple: Produce is peeled and pulverized when it's processed into a beverage, which strips away important ingredients.

For example, eating a large apple provides a heart-healthy 5 grams of dietary fiber for a mere 72 calories. Drinking a cup of apple juice, on the other hand, provides just a trace of fiber but will set you back 117 calories. If you drink orange juice for your daily dose of vitamin C, you'd be better off eating an orange, which, calorie for calorie, provides about 60 percent more of this vital nutrient.

Beware of sugar, too. A medium white grapefruit only has about 8.6 grams of sugar, but a cup of unsweetened

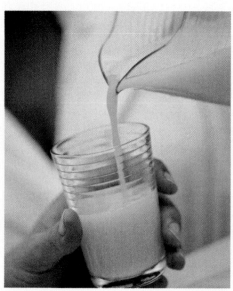

Where Juice Falls Short

Calorie for calorie, fruit is more nutritious than fruit juice. Consider the difference between an orange and a five-ounce glass of orange juice with the equivalent number of calories (69).

NUTRIENT	ORANGE	JUICE
Vitamin C	83 mg	51 mg
Fiber	3.1 g	0.3 g
Calcium	60 mg	16 mg
Folate	48 mcg	28 mcg

Source: USDA Nutrient Data Laboratory.

grapefruit juice has 22.5 grams. Not surprisingly, drinking juice tends to raise blood sugar more than eating raw fruit.

You don't need to swear off fruit juice, but choose wisely (look for 100 percent fruit juice with no sugar added) and watch portion size. Nutritionists consider 4 to 6 ounces an appropriate serving.

Do I have to give up grapefruit juice if I take medication?

NO The juice does contain compounds that boost blood levels of certain drugs, but that doesn't mean you have to stop drinking it.

The news came as a shock: Sipping a tart, bracing glass of grapefruit juice with your breakfast can make your meds go haywire. That was the accidental finding of a 1989 study, in which blood levels of a hypertension drug rose two to three times higher than expected in volunteers who drank grapefruit juice.

Scientists eventually discovered that grapefruit interferes with an enzyme in the intestines that helps break down certain drugs. If the enzyme is inhibited, too much of a drug may enter the bloodstream. Studies have shown that consuming grapefruit or grapefruit juice can decrease levels of the enzyme by nearly 50 percent and that the effect of a single glass can last up to three days. Some of the major categories

Grapefruit and Your Meds: What's the Risk?

The medications below may interact with grapefruit or grapefruit juice. If you're a fan of the fruit, talk to your doctor or pharmacist about your options.

Calcium channel blockers (for high blood pressure)

Drug	Serious	Moderate	Minimal
Amlodipine (Caduet, Exforge)			✓
Diltiazem (many brands)			✓
Felodipine (Plendil)		✓	
Isradipine (DynaCirc)		✓	
Nicardipine (Cardene)		✓	
Nifedipine (many brands)		✓	
Nimodipine (Nimotop)		✓	
Nisoldipine (Sular)		✓	
Verapamil (many brands)			✓

STATINS (for high cholesterol)

Drug	Serious	Moderate	Minimal
Atorvastatin (Lipitor)		✓	
Cerivastatin (Baycol and others)		✓	
Fluvastatin (Lescol)			✓
Lovastatin (Mevacor and others)	✓		
Pravastatin (Pravachol)			✓
Simvastatin (Vytorin, Zocor)	✓		

IMMUNE SYSTEM SUPPRESSANTS

Drug	Serious	Moderate	Minimal
Cyclosporine (many brands)		✓	
Tacrolimus (Prograf)		✓	
Sirolimus (Rapamune)		✓	

SEDATIVES AND ANTI-ANXIETY DRUGS

Drug	Serious	Moderate	Minimal
Alprazolam (Xanax)			✓
Buspirone (Buspar)	✓		
Clonazepam (Klonopin)			✓
Diazepam (Valium)		✓	
Lorazepam (Ativan)			✓
Midazolam (Versed)		✓	
Temazepam (Restoril)			✓
Triazolam (Halcion)		✓	
Zaleplon (Sonata)		✓	
Zolpidem (Ambien)			✓

(continued on page 130)

FRUIT JUICE

(continued from page 129)

OTHER DRUGS FOR PSYCHIATRIC CONDITIONS

Drug	Serious	Moderate	Minimal
Carbamazepine (many brands)		✔	
Trazodone (many brands)		✔	
Nefazodone (Serzone)		✔	
Quetiapine (Seroquel)		✔	
SSRI antidepressants (such as Prozac)			✔
Clozapine (Clozaril)			✔
Haloperidol (Haldol)			✔

ANTIHISTAMINES

Drug	Serious	Moderate	Minimal
Terfenadine (Seldane)	✔		
Astemizole (Hismanal)	✔		
Loratadine (Claritin)		✔	
Fexofenadine (Allegra)			✔
Ceterizine (Zyrtec)			✔
Diphenhydramine (Benadryl)			✔

PROTEASE INHIBITORS (FOR HIV/AIDS)

Drug	Serious	Moderate	Minimal
Saquinavir (Invirase, Fortovase)		✔	
Ritonavir (Norvir)		✔	
Nelfinavir (Viracept)		✔	
Amprenavir (Agenerase)		✔	
Indinavir (Crixivan)			✔

HORMONE TREATMENTS

Drug	Serious	Moderate	Minimal
Ethinyl estradiol		✔	
Methylprednisolone		✔	
Prednisone			✔
Prednisolone			✔

OTHER DRUGS

Drug	Serious	Moderate	Minimal
Amiodarone (Cordarone)	✔		
Sildenafil (Viagra)		✔	
Cisapride (Propulsid)		✔	
Clarithromycin (many brands)			✔
Erythromycin (many brands)			✔
Quinidine (many brands)			✔
Omeprazole (Prilosec)			✔

Source: *Pharmacy Times.*

of drugs that may be affected include medications used to treat heart rhythm disorders, high blood pressure, high cholesterol, psoriasis, depression, erectile dysfunction, allergies, anxiety, arthritis, and HIV/AIDS.

There's probably little reason, however, for most people to stop eating grapefruit or drinking the juice. To begin with, the majority of prescription medications in use today are *not* affected by this citrus fruit. Also, even if a drug you take has the potential to interact with grapefruit, that doesn't mean it will. Grapefruit doesn't inhibit the enzyme needed to metabolize these drugs equally in everyone; in some people, it may have no effect at all. Finally, if a drug you take interacts with grapefruit, and you're reluctant to stop eating it, in most cases there are alternative medications that don't pose a problem.

If you love grapefruit and must take a prescription drug, ask your doctor or pharmacist about a potential interaction or check the literature you receive when you pick up the medication. If there is a potential interaction, talk with your doctor about what to do, whether it's taking another drug or being vigilant for problems that might arise. ■

Garlic

If you love garlic, you probably don't care about its health benefits—you'll eat it no matter what. Still, the "stinking rose" has been used as a medicine by traditional healers for more than 5,000 years. Papyrus documents from 1550 BC show that Egyptian doctors prescribed it for many different conditions. It's been used to treat bubonic plague, cure snakebites, and ward off evil spirits. Today scientists are most interested in garlic's influence on the heart and immune system.

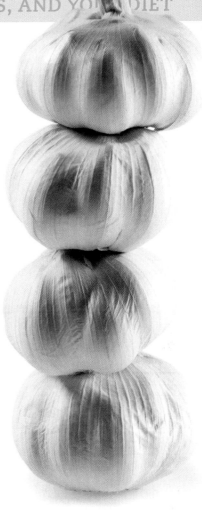

Is garlic good for the heart?

YES While you can't expect miracles, including garlic in your daily diet or taking garlic pills offers modest heart protection.

Some nutritionists believe that the liberal use of garlic in the traditional Mediterranean diet helps to explain why this cuisine appears to protect against heart disease. A recent review of 10 studies found evidence that garlic pills may reduce LDL ("bad") cholesterol by about 11 percent, on average. That's a modest drop; statin drugs, such as atorvastatin (Lipitor) and simvastatin (Zocor), can lower LDL cholesterol by up to 60 percent. Furthermore, some studies found that garlic had no effect on cholesterol.

However, research shows that garlic may do more for the heart than lower cholesterol. The herb makes cell fragments in the blood called platelets less

Our BEST ADVICE

Always chop or crush a peeled garlic clove and let stand for 10 or 15 minutes before adding it to a recipe to let its healing compounds form. Otherwise, the heat will render the garlic impotent. Another option is to eat your garlic raw.

....

likely to clump together and form artery-blocking clots. Again, garlic's impact on blood platelets is modest. Taken together, though, its heart-healthy actions add up to a good reason for including a clove or two—or four—in your daily diet.

Does garlic boost the immune system?

MAYBE There's no question that garlic contains potent chemicals, but whether they can fight colds or cancer is still unclear.

Rates of certain cancers are low in countries where the cuisine features generous amounts of garlic.

NUTS

Garlic
(continued)

Garlic contains potent compounds that make life miserable for bacteria, viruses, fungi, and cancer cells. The presence of these compounds, especially the sulfur compounds that give garlic its characteristic odor, seems to cause cancer cells to self-destruct. In theory, this should mean that eating garlic slows or prevents the formation of malignant tumors.

To be sure, rates of certain cancers are unusually low in countries where the cuisine features generous amounts of garlic. In particular, a few studies show that people who consume plenty of garlic and its plant cousin, the onion, have low rates of oral, throat, and gastrointestinal cancers. A review in the *American Journal of Clinical Nutrition* found that people who eat about five cloves of garlic per week cut their risk of colon and stomach cancer by 30 and 47 percent, respectively. Garlic may protect against stomach cancer by destroying *Helicobacter pylori*, the bacterium known to cause ulcers and damage the stomach lining.

Most of the studies on garlic for colds were done with garlic supplements, not fresh garlic. See page 202 for details on whether the supplements can indeed fight colds and other viral illnesses. ∎

Nuts

Salty peanuts. Crunchy almonds. Buttery walnuts. Nuts seem like the guiltiest of gustatory pleasures, the savory equivalent of jellybeans or gumdrops. Yet the scientific evidence clearly shows that nuts are anything but junk food. Packed with fiber, protein, and healthful fats, not to mention vitamins and minerals, nuts can help satisfy your appetite while they protect your heart.

Are nuts fattening?

NO Your grocer may stock them next to the candy, but don't be fooled. Nuts may even help you control your weight.

Study after study paints the same picture: Nibbling on nuts won't make you fat. In fact, it may even have the opposite effect. If you know anything about the composition of nuts, that may sound, well, nuts.

After all, by weight, one-half to three-quarters of a nut is fat. And doesn't eating fat make you fat?

Not in this case. Several major population studies involving thousands of people have looked for evidence that nuts lead to weight gain, and they found none. To the contrary, studies have shown that people who eat nuts (including peanuts, which are technically legumes) as part of their

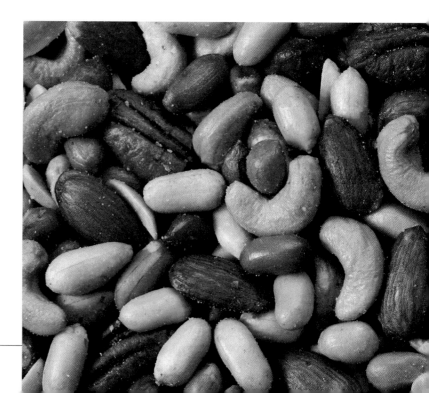

regular diet weigh less than people who don't eat them. One US government diet survey of more than 12,000 people found that the typical nut eater had a body mass index (BMI, a measurement of weight relative to height) that was 5 percent lower than that of the average non–nut eater.

It's possible that the results are skewed by other factors: Perhaps nut lovers simply live healthier lives than people who don't eat nuts, and perhaps some of the obese people surveyed began to avoid nuts after they already had a weight problem. What's clear is that nuts contain an ideal mix of fiber, protein, and fat that helps fill you up and keep you full. Snacks that don't contain protein—and many don't—tend to satisfy hunger for shorter periods.

Furthermore, some of that fat in nuts will never find its way to your thighs or hips. Your body doesn't absorb chewed nuts efficiently during digestion, so a portion of their fat is excreted. Finally, peanuts contain resveratrol, the antioxidant that's also found in red wine and that animal studies suggest may help prevent obesity.

Moderation is essential, of course. Nuts are quite high in calories, but most dietitians say that one ounce of nuts per day—as a snack or as a replacement for meat in an entrée—can fit into most meal plans.

How to Choose a Nut-ritious Snack

Nuts are a top source of healthful fats and fiber, but they can break your calorie budget if you're not careful. An asterisk indicates nuts that are relatively low in saturated fat and high in healthy monounsaturated fat or omega-3 fatty acids.

NUT	CALORIES**	NUTS**	FIBER
Almonds*	169	22	3.3 g
Brazil nuts	186	6	2.1 g
Cashews	163	18	0.9 g
Hazelnuts*	178	21	2.7 g
Macadamia nuts	204	10–12	2.3 g
Peanuts	166	35	2.3 g
Pecans*	201	15 halves	2.7 g
Pine nuts	191	167	1.0 g
Pistachios	169	49	2.4 g
Walnuts*	185	14 halves	1.9 g

**per 1-oz. serving

Sources: *American Journal of Clinical Nutrition*; USDA Nutrient Database; *Nutrition Reviews*.

Do nuts fight heart disease?

YES The research is clear: Nut lovers have healthy hearts, thanks to the bounty of "good" fat and other nutrients in these satisfying snacks.

Can a hankering for hazelnuts help your heart? No fewer than five large population studies have found that cardiovascular disease is far less common among people who consume nuts on a regular basis. For example, one survey showed that older men and women who eat nuts at least five times a week cut their risk of a fatal heart attack by 39 percent.

OLIVE OIL

Nuts
(continued)

Any kind of nut seems to boost cardiovascular health, though the hazelnut happens to be one of the best sources of heart-friendly monounsaturated fat. Studies show that adopting a diet that's high in monounsaturated fat can lower total cholesterol by 10 percent and cut LDL cholesterol, the "bad" kind, by 14 percent. Walnuts are relatively low in "monos," but they're rich in the omega-3 fatty acid ALA, which some research suggests may have cardiovascular benefits.

Nourishing fats are just one reason to eat nuts for heart health. For example, an ounce of dry-roasted peanuts provides a generous dose of nutrients known to protect the cardiovascular system, including folate, niacin, vitamin E, and others. Peanuts are also rich in plant sterols, which help prevent cholesterol from entering the bloodstream.

While doctors have long recommended low-fat diets to prevent heart disease, adding nuts to your diet makes sense. According to Harvard researchers, eating nuts instead of fatty meats and other sources of saturated fat could reduce your odds of having a heart attack by up to 45 percent. ■

Olive Oil

The cuisine of the Mediterranean region is as diverse as its people. The cooking of southern Italy features herbs, garlic, and tomatoes, for instance, while Moroccans love spices and dried fruits. However, one food ingredient unites these culinary traditions: olive oil. Some scientists say it's one reason the people of the Mediterranean are among the healthiest in the world.

Does olive oil prevent heart disease?

YES Scientists have known for decades that people who consume plenty of olive oil have low rates of heart disease. Now they've figured out how it works its magic.

Nutritionists have been lavishing praise upon the Mediterranean diet for so long that it's easy to forget how radical the idea was that certain fats, like olive oil, could be good for the heart. But the evidence was strong: In the mid 1980s, a long-term study comparing rates of cardiovascular disease in seven countries revealed that heart attacks were relatively uncommon in countries where the people consumed lots of olive oil, including Italy and Greece.

Today there is little doubt that olive oil—especially virgin olive oil, which undergoes minimal processing—protects the cardiovascular system. Researchers at the University of Pennsylvania asked 22 people to eat several different meal plans for 24 days at a time, including a low-fat diet and a diet rich in olive oil and other sources of monounsaturated fat. They found that diets high in olive oil lowered cholesterol just as effectively as a low-fat

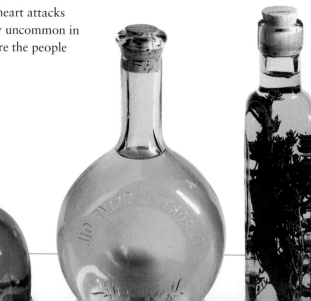

diet. These diets lowered triglycerides, too, while the low-fat diet actually caused levels of these blood fats to rise. Overall, the study showed that the olive oil diet lowered the risk of heart attacks by 25 percent, which made it twice as effective as the low-fat diet.

More recent studies suggest that olive oil does more than lower cholesterol and blood fats. In a study involving 772 volunteer subjects, people who prepared meals with olive oil lowered their risk factors for heart disease more than others who ate a low-fat diet. Their blood pressure improved more, as did their ratio of total cholesterol to HDL cholesterol. Their blood sugar fell slightly, too, lowering the risk of type 2 diabetes, a condition linked with heart disease.

Still other studies show that olive oil acts a bit like aspirin, reducing levels of chronic low-grade inflammation, another culprit behind heart attacks. Finally, olive oil is teeming with antioxidants, which act on cholesterol to make it less likely to stick to artery walls.

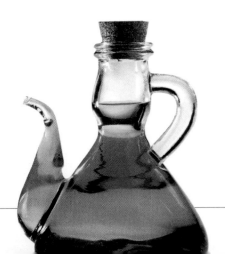

How Fats Stack Up

All fats and oils contain monounsaturated, polyunsaturated, and saturated fatty acids. Monos protect against heart disease and have other benefits, polyunsaturated fatty acids are a mixed bag, and saturated fat is unambiguously bad for you. Olive oil is the best source of monounsaturated fat. Here's how other oils and fats in your kitchen compare. Remember that vegetable shortening and margarine often contain trans fats, perhaps the worst fats of all for your heart. Avoid products with the word *hydrogenated* on the label.

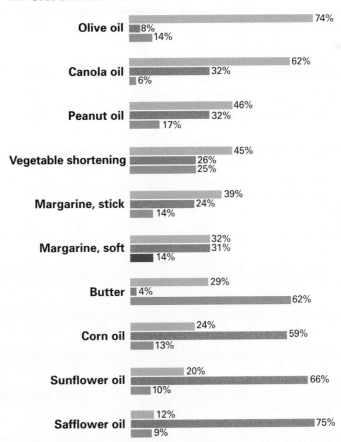

- MONOUNSATURATED FAT
- POLYUNSATURATED FAT
- SATURATED FAT

Oil/Fat	Monounsaturated	Polyunsaturated	Saturated
Olive oil	74%	8%	14%
Canola oil	62%	32%	6%
Peanut oil	46%	32%	17%
Vegetable shortening	45%	26%	25%
Margarine, stick	39%	24%	14%
Margarine, soft	32%	31%	14%
Butter	29%	4%	62%
Corn oil	24%	59%	13%
Sunflower oil	20%	66%	10%
Safflower oil	12%	75%	9%

Source: Adapted from *The American Dietetic Association's Complete Food & Nutrition Guide* (Chronimed Publishing, 1996).

Note: Values do not add up to 100 percent because oils contain components other than fatty acids.

OLIVE OIL

Does olive oil prevent cancer?

MAYBE Some early research suggests that olive oil may do more than protect the heart; it could guard against certain cancers, too.

The same researchers who discovered that heart disease was relatively uncommon in the Mediterranean region made another intriguing observation: Overall cancer rates were lower in that sunny region than in most Western countries. In particular, the women of Greece developed breast cancer about one-third as often as women in the United States. Some scientists suspected that a diet rich in olive oil was the secret.

The olive oil theory didn't make sense to some skeptics. After all, population studies suggest that women who eat a lot of fat increase their risk of breast cancer fivefold. Yet some intriguing evidence suggests that the monounsaturated fat in olive oil is a cancer fighter.

For starters, a 1995 study of nearly 2,400 Greek women found that those who consumed olive oil at least twice a day had a 25 percent reduced risk of breast cancer. A more recent study found that women on the Canary Islands who consumed slightly less than two teaspoons of olive oil daily cut their breast cancer risk by even more—73 percent.

Although it's still not clear whether olive oil protects against breast cancer, scientists have uncovered some compelling evidence to suggest that some women may benefit. One-fifth to one-quarter of breast cancer patients carry too many copies of a gene known as HER2. As a result, they tend to develop

Our BEST ADVICE

When it comes to olive oil, virgin or extra virgin is best. It contains far more antioxidants than other olive oils. To preserve those antioxidants, keep your oil away from heat, light, and air. They not only turn the oil rancid but also lower antioxidant content. Store your oil in a cool, dark place in an airtight opaque container.

aggressive, hard-to-treat tumors. Lab studies by Spanish researchers have shown that the oleic acid in olive oil reduces the expression, or activity, of HER2 by up to 46 percent. It also appears to enhance the effectiveness of trastuzumab (Herceptin), a breast cancer drug that blocks the expression of HER2. ∎

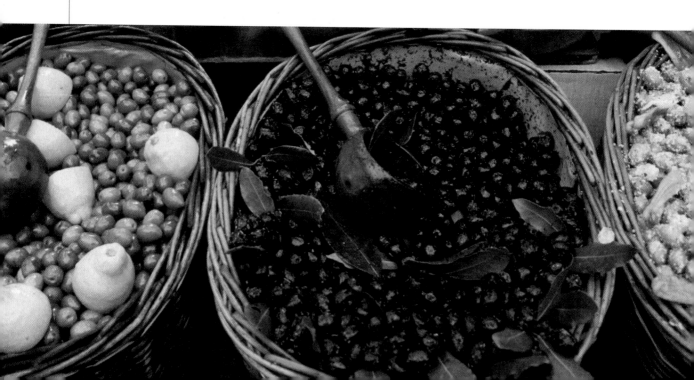

Organic Produce

Once available only at farmer's markets or natural foods stores, organically grown fruit, vegetables, and other goods now have a foothold in most supermarkets. Foods labeled as organic must meet certain standards that prohibit or greatly restrict the use of synthetic fertilizers, pesticides, hormones, antibiotics, and other chemicals. And they almost always cost more.

Is organic produce worth the extra cash?

MAYBE The answer depends on your pocketbook. If you can afford to buy organic and still eat plenty of produce, the answer is yes.

Shoppers who decide it's time to try organic foods may suffer from acute sticker shock at the register: Organic produce almost always costs more, sometimes up to 100 percent more, than its conventionally grown counterparts. If the high price tag means you buy—and eat—fewer fruits and vegetables, it's a devil's bargain. Most experts agree that the health benefits you get from conventionally grown produce far outweigh any risks posed by pesticide residues.

On the other hand, if price is no object, who wouldn't want to eat apples, peaches, and cucumbers grown without bug-killing chemicals?

Here's the bottom line on three aspects of organic produce that may or may not sway you to spend more.

Taste: Some organic food devotees swear that carrots, cucumbers, and other produce free from exposure to agricultural chemicals simply taste better. Taste is subjective, of course, yet some evidence suggests that certain organic foods may have bolder flavors. For example, a recent study in the *European Journal of Clinical Nutrition* found that some species of organically grown apples have higher concentrations of sugar. The organic apples also had a greater concentration of antioxidants called phenols, which could influence flavor, too.

Nutritional value: Surveys show that many consumers believe organic foods are more nutritious than conventional foods. A small amount of scientific research suggests that may be true in some instances, although the case for organics is hardly overwhelming. For example, even skeptics concede that leafy greens and potatoes grown using organic methods tend to have slightly

At the end of the day, it comes down to how worried **pesticide residues** make you.

ORGANIC PRODUCE

higher levels of vitamin C. Given the overall lack of research on this question, however, there's no clear evidence that organic foods are healthier than conventional products.

Safety: In most first world countries, pesticides are strictly regulated; their use is approved only if the levels of residues in resulting crops are a fraction of the level—as little as one one-hundredth—that is safe for lab animals. As new science emerges, however, the risk assessments of these chemicals are refined, and this has led to certain pesticides being banned or severely restricted. To the best of scientists' knowledge, the pesticides in use today have a positive risk-benefit ratio. It's possible, though, that chemicals may have subtle effects that show up only after years of exposure or that the cumulative effect of the many different pesticides in our food today may do more damage than we can know by studying them individually.

We do know that the fruits and vegetables you bring home from the supermarket often retain detectable levels of insect-killing chemicals. In one analysis, the US nonprofit Environmental Working Group found that 97 percent of peaches and 94 percent of

WHEN TO SPEND, WHEN TO SAVE

The Environmental Working Group, a Washington, D.C.–based watchdog organization, analyzes the pesticide content of fruits and vegetables and publishes its list of the "Dirty Dozen" and "Clean 12." Use their findings to spend extra on the fruits and vegetables that retain the most pesticide residue and to save money on those that don't.

THE "DIRTY DOZEN"	THE "CLEAN 12"
Peaches	Onions
Apples	Avocados
Bell peppers	Sweet corn (frozen)
Celery	Pineapples
Nectarines	Mangos
Strawberries	Sweet peas (frozen)
Cherries	Asparagus
Lettuce	Kiwifruit
Grapes	Bananas
Pears	Cabbage
Spinach	Broccoli
Potatoes	Eggplant

apples had pesticide residue. Rinsing produce before you eat it helps, but it doesn't remove all of the agricultural chemicals. Peeling fruit such as apples eliminates some pesticides but strips away important nutrients, too.

At the end of the day, it comes down to how worried

these pesticide residues make you. Note that certain fruits and vegetables tend to contain more residues than others. If you want to spend your money on organic versions of the ones that contain the most, see "When to Spend, When to Save" above. ■

Pasta

For many people, a steaming bowl of spaghetti and meatballs or baked ziti with cheese is the ultimate in comfort food—but is pasta a dietary disaster? At 210 calories per cup, it isn't especially low in calories, and of course, it's high in carbs. So will it kill you, or at least pack on the pounds?

Does pasta make you fat?

NO Pasta's reputation as fattening is undeserved. Eat pasta in moderation, without high-fat sauces, and it won't pad your waistline.

Bread is severely restricted on most low-carb diets on the theory that it makes you fat. There is some truth to the idea that starchy and highly refined carbohydrate foods, such as white bread, white rice, and potatoes, work against weight control by sending blood sugar soaring, only to crash and make you ravenous again in no time. But does pasta fall into the same category?

It doesn't. A system called the glycemic index (GI) ranks foods on a scale of 1 to 100 according to how much they cause blood sugar to rise. Yet while a slice of white bread can have a GI value as high as 80, spaghetti's value is a modest 44, fettuccine checks in at 46, and macaroni's GI is just 47.

How can that be? After all, aren't bread and pasta both made from wheat? Yes—but not the same kind of wheat. Most pasta is made from durum wheat or another type of hard wheat, and that wheat is coarsely ground into what's known as semolina. The enzymes in the digestive system aren't very good at breaking down the starch in semolina and turning it into blood sugar, so when most people eat a reasonable amount of pasta, their blood sugar doesn't soar.

Our BEST ADVICE

To maintain pasta's low GI value, cook it al dente, that is, a noodle should give a little resistance when you bite into it and not be mushy. Overcooked pasta has a high GI because its starch granules expand, which makes it easier for the digestive enzymes in your system to break them down and turn them into blood sugar.

Of course, eating huge portions of pasta, or any food, will make you gain weight. And drowning your pasta with sauces that contain butter, cream, cheese, and other high-fat foods will make the noodles' low GI value irrelevant. ■

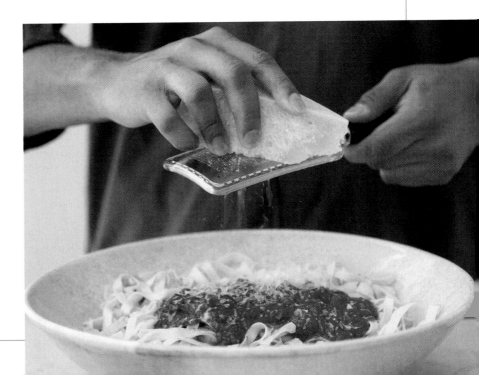

Red Meat

Robert Atkins, MD, the low-carb guru, outraged the scientific community when he proposed that a diet high in meat and low in carbohydrates could protect the heart. After all, he of all people—he was a cardiologist, you may recall—should have known better. But while big, juicy steaks and fast-food cheeseburgers have become symbols of all that's bad about the modern diet, lean meats have proven their rightful place in a healthy diet.

Does red meat raise cholesterol?

NO Solid, well-designed studies show that eating red meat will not raise your cholesterol if you choose lean cuts.

If you switched from whole milk to fat-free to protect your heart, you should know that trading a porterhouse steak for a top sirloin or other lean cut will have a similar effect. While saturated fat has been shown to raise cholesterol, a review of 54 studies determined that eating *lean* red meat that has been trimmed of visible fat—which is surprisingly low in saturated fat—does not raise total cholesterol or artery-clogging LDL ("bad') cholesterol.

In fact, research shows that lean red meat can take its place on the table alongside other heart-friendly protein sources, such as skinless chicken breasts. For example,

in a study by the Chicago Center for Clinical Research, 191 men and women were split into two groups. Researchers instructed one group to eat diets that included chicken and fish as their main sources of protein. The second group got their protein mainly from lean beef, pork, and veal. After nine months, there was no difference between the two groups in total cholesterol, LDL cholesterol, HDL cholesterol, or triglycerides (a form of blood fat linked to heart disease).

Does red meat cause colon cancer?

MAYBE Scientists don't agree. Some say eating red meat probably increases the risk of colon cancer, while others say the evidence is weak.

Eating too much red meat has been blamed for increasing the risk of several types of cancer,

but none more than colon cancer. In one study published in the *Journal of the National Cancer Institute*, researchers followed close to a half million European men and women for 10 years. During that period, people over 50 who ate the most red meat were 35 percent more likely to develop cancer of the colon or rectum than others who ate little or no red meat. Investigations by several other groups of researchers reached similar conclusions.

These alarming studies are in the minority, however—most others have failed to find any link between red meat and colon cancer. According to a review in the *European Journal of Clinical Nutrition*, just 3 out of 15 studies in which scientists studied the

Our BEST ADVICE

To keep an appetite for red meat healthy, follow a few rules: Look for "loin" (such as "sirloin" or "tenderloin"), "round, "or "chuck" in the name of the cut. Choose cuts that are surrounded by a layer of fat no more than 1/8 inch thick and trim off visible fat. Avoid cuts that have lots of marbling, or white streaks of fat, in the meat. And favor low-fat cooking methods, such as grilling, broiling, and roasting, over frying.

dietary habits of large groups of people for extended periods turned up evidence linking red meat to colon cancer. In 30 other studies comparing colon cancer patients with healthy people, 20 failed to identify red meat as a suspect.

If there is a connection between red meat and colon cancer, the risk may be limited to people who eat red meat every day. A committee of medical experts in the United Kingdom concluded that only those who consumed about 5 ounces or more of beef, pork, or lamb a day have an increased cancer risk. Moreover, several studies suggest that processed or cured meats (such as bacon, deli meats, and sausage) may be the real problem, possibly due to their high levels of nitrites and nitrates. A study of nearly 150,000 men and women published in the *Journal of the American Medical Association* found no connection between overall intake of red meat and colon cancer, but a 50 percent increased risk among people who ate the most processed meats over a 10-year period. ■

The Skinny on Beef

All red meat has saturated fat, but lean cuts have so little that eating modest portions has little or no effect on cholesterol levels. Fatty cuts are another story. Skinless chicken is your leanest option of all.

CUT (3 OZ. BROILED)

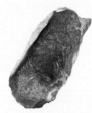

Top Round
Sat. Fat. = 1.6 g
Calories = 157

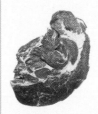

Bottom Round
Sat. Fat. = 1.7 g
Calories = 139

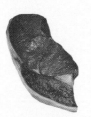

Top Sirloin
Sat. Fat. = 1.9 g
Calories = 150

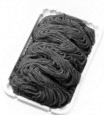

Ground Beef
(97% lean)
Sat. Fat. = 2.5 g
Calories = 145

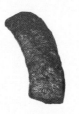

Tenderloin
Sat. Fat. = 2.7 g
Calories = 170

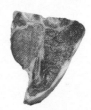

Porterhouse
Sat. Fat. = 3.4 g
Calories = 178

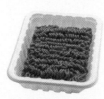

Ground Beef
(75% lean)
Sat. Fat. = 6.2 g
Calories = 236

Chicken Breast
(skinless)
Sat. Fat. = 0.38 g
Calories = 130

Chicken Breast
(with skin)
Sat. Fat. = 3.85 g
Calories = 249

Source: USDA Nutrient Database.

SALT

Salt

You won't hear a chef say bad things about salt. It's the ultimate flavor enhancer, irreplaceable in the kitchen. But you will hear doctors speak plenty ill about it. Your body can't live without salt, since the mineral provides elements that are necessary for human health. But a constant craving for salty foods could be raising your risk of serious medical problems.

Should everyone cut back on salt?

YES Sodium raises blood pressure in some people and not others, but it's hard to tell who's who, so experts advise that everyone eat less of it.

It's inevitable: When a doctor delivers a diagnosis of high blood pressure, he'll also deliver a mandate to eat less salt. The offending ingredient is sodium, which makes up a little more than one-third of every salt crystal. The average adult requires only about 500 milligrams of sodium per day (and you could probably get by on as little as 115 milligrams). Yet most people consume more than 3,000 milligrams of sodium daily.

Most experts agree that eating salty foods causes blood pressure to rise in people who are "salt sensitive." By some estimates, half of all people

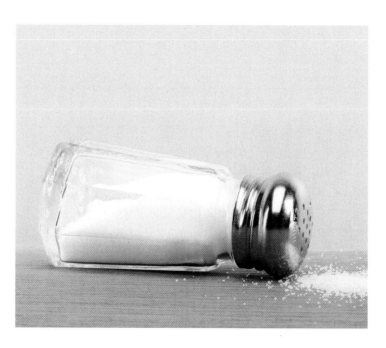

Our BEST ADVICE

Eating fewer salty foods has an even greater impact when you eat *more* foods that are high in potassium, such as fruits and vegetables. Potassium actually promotes healthy blood pressure levels. In one major study, hypertension patients who cut back on salt and ate more produce lowered their systolic blood pressure by 11.5 points. That's a better result than some hypertension drugs can achieve.

who have high blood pressure are salt sensitive. Unfortunately, there's no way to test for salt sensitivity. That's why physicians hedge their bets and instruct patients with high blood pressure to consume less sodium—no more than 1,500 milligrams per day.

A review of 17 long-term studies found that hypertension patients who make modest reductions in their salt intake lower their systolic blood pressure (the top number in a blood pressure reading) by 5 points and their diastolic pressure (the bottom number) by 3 points.

According to the review's authors, if all people with high blood pressure ate fewer salty foods, deaths from heart attacks and strokes would drop by 9 and 14 percent, respectively.

Sodium in Food

Experts say that healthy people should consume no more than 2,300 milligrams of sodium per day. Adopting a light touch with the saltshaker can help, but it's far more important to cut back on processed and packaged foods, which—along with restaurant dishes—provide about 75 percent of the sodium in most diets.

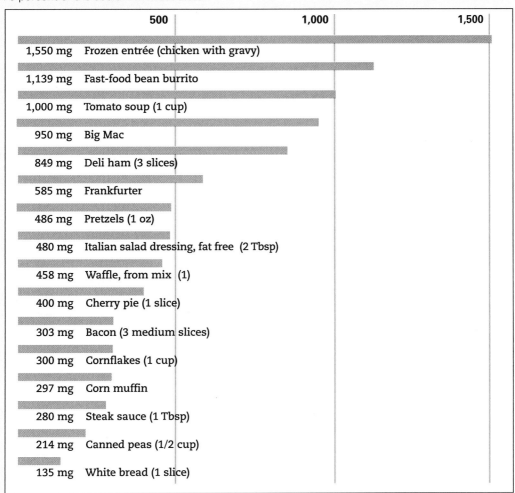

	500	1,000	1,500
1,550 mg	Frozen entrée (chicken with gravy)		
1,139 mg	Fast-food bean burrito		
1,000 mg	Tomato soup (1 cup)		
950 mg	Big Mac		
849 mg	Deli ham (3 slices)		
585 mg	Frankfurter		
486 mg	Pretzels (1 oz)		
480 mg	Italian salad dressing, fat free (2 Tbsp)		
458 mg	Waffle, from mix (1)		
400 mg	Cherry pie (1 slice)		
303 mg	Bacon (3 medium slices)		
300 mg	Cornflakes (1 cup)		
297 mg	Corn muffin		
280 mg	Steak sauce (1 Tbsp)		
214 mg	Canned peas (1/2 cup)		
135 mg	White bread (1 slice)		

Source: *Bowes and Church's Food Values of Portions Commonly Used* (Lippincott, 1998).

What if you don't have high blood pressure? Some scientists argue that telling everyone to cut back on sodium makes no sense since many people can eat large amounts without any effect at all on their blood pressure. But here's one reason to curb your intake anyway: Studies show that about one in four people who don't have hypertension are salt sensitive, and they stand a greater risk of developing high blood pressure as they age.

Most doctors agree that people without high blood pressure should limit their sodium intake to no more than 2,300 milligrams per day, or the amount in one teaspoon of salt. ■

Shrimp

Like all shellfish, shrimp wears a coat of armor to guard its tender flesh, which is sweet and coveted by seafood lovers. However, as they dip a shrimp in cocktail sauce or dig into a plate of shrimp scampi, many people feel a twinge of guilt due to lingering concerns about this crustacean's high cholesterol content. The good news: Shrimp is almost completely devoid of saturated fat.

Is shrimp bad for your cholesterol?

NO Despite shrimp's high cholesterol content, your levels of blood cholesterol actually become healthier when you eat this popular seafood.

As a health food, shrimp has much to recommend it. The curl-shaped crustacean is low in fat and calories and rich in protein, iron, and vitamin B_{12}. It even has a respectable dose of healthy omega-3 fatty acids. Yet ounce for ounce, shrimp has more cholesterol than just about any other common food, including the fattiest meats and richest dairy products. For that reason, people concerned about their arteries often avoid it—but they shouldn't.

A study at Rockefeller University in New York City showed that there's no reason to shun this shellfish. Researchers asked 18 men and women to eat large servings of steamed shrimp every day—more than 10 ounces, or 30 to 40 shrimp, which was enough to give them nearly 600 milligrams of dietary cholesterol. That's twice the daily limit recommended by the American Heart Association. After three weeks, the researchers took blood samples from the volunteers and found that their levels of LDL ("bad") cholesterol had jumped 7.1 percent, on average. That doesn't sound like very good news, but all that shrimp had an important benefit: The volunteers' levels of HDL cholesterol, the kind that keeps your arteries clear, rose 12.1 percent. In other words, eating shrimp actually improved the ratio of good cholesterol to bad cholesterol. Many cardiologists believe that this ratio is a better indicator of cardiovascular health than total cholesterol levels. ∎

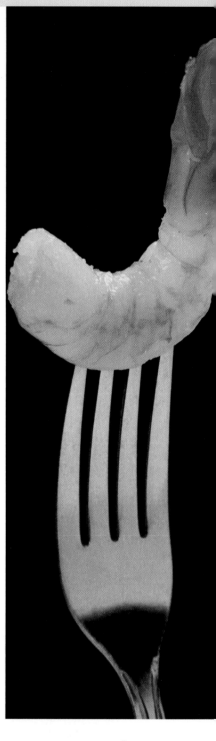

Eating shrimp improved the ratio of good cholesterol to bad cholesterol.

Soft Drinks

Just about everyone loves the refreshing fizz of an icy-cold soft drink. Yet many people cringe when they see someone giving a baby one of these bubbly beverages, and for obvious reasons: The drinks are devoid of nutritional value and full of sugar, usually in the form of high-fructose corn syrup. Are they carbonated killers, or merely innocent indulgences?

Do soft drinks make you fat?

YES Studies show that people who drink lots of soda and other sugary beverages have a high risk of becoming overweight.

People in nations all over the world are getting fatter, and some scientists say it's no coincidence that consumption of soft drinks has been soaring in many of those same countries. Nowhere is this trend more alarming than the United States, where obesity rates have doubled since 1976—a period when consumption of sweetened beverages increased by 135 percent.

Soft drinks don't deserve all the blame for the current obesity crisis, of course, but a large body of research points to soda and other sugary thirst quenchers as one key cause. Recently, researchers at Yale reviewed 88 studies and found convincing evidence that people who consume soft drinks regularly take in a greater number of total calories and weigh more than people who avoid them. A similar review by Harvard scientists a year earlier reached the same conclusion.

One problem with soft drinks is that the body doesn't seem to register the calories in drinks the way it does those in food, explains Marlene B. Schwartz, PhD, one of the study's authors. Normally, when you consume a lot of calories from food, you compensate later in the day by eating less. Many studies show, however, that people fail to compensate for the calories in soda and other sweet beverages. "Soft drinks are probably worse than candy or other solid empty calories," says Dr. Schwartz.

How bad are soft drinks for your waistline? A 2004 study in the *Journal of the American Medical Association (JAMA)* offers a clue. Harvard researchers asked more than 50,000 female nurses to describe their diets in 1991, then again in 1999. They found that women who went from rarely consuming soft drinks to having one or more servings per day during that eight-year period gained more than 17 pounds, on average. Meanwhile, women who cut back on soft drinks maintained a stable weight.

Do soft drinks cause diabetes?

YES Large studies show that people who drink a lot of these beverages have an increased risk of type 2 diabetes.

The *JAMA* study linking soft drinks to weight gain came to another disturbing conclusion: Women who drank one or more sugar-sweetened beverages per day increased their risk of developing type 2 diabetes by an astounding 83 percent. Maybe it's no surprise since soft drinks cause weight gain, and being overweight increases diabetes risk. But the link went beyond weight. In the study, drinking soda, fruit drinks, and other sweetened beverages regularly seemed to increase the threat of diabetes independent of any influence on body weight.

The real problem? Soft drinks (other than diet varieties) contain lots of sugar. A typical 12-ounce can has between 40 and 50 grams, usually in the form of high-fructose corn syrup, which is chemically similar to table sugar. Studies show that downing sugary soft drinks causes a steep increase in blood sugar, which triggers an answering increase in insulin, the hormone responsible for escorting blood sugar into cells. Over time, forcing your body to churn out a lot of insulin makes cells less sensitive to the hormone, causing insulin resistance, a problem at the core of type 2 diabetes.

Another emerging theory holds that high-fructose corn syrup may contribute to insulin resistance not so much by raising blood sugar (in fact, fructose has less of an impact on blood sugar than does glucose, the other component of table sugar) as by its effects on the liver, which metabolizes it.

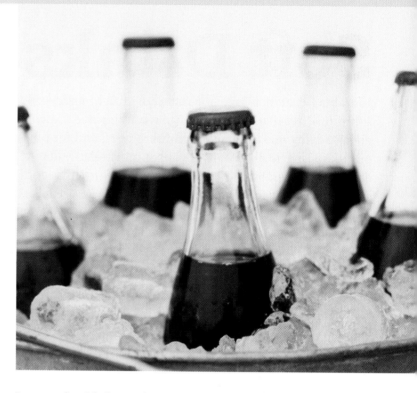

Does cola weaken bones?

YES Emerging evidence suggests that additives in cola drinks interfere with the body's ability to build new bone.

Scientists who study bone health say that carbonated drinks may increase the risk of crippling fractures. And while not all types of soda are guilty, studies suggest that the most popular variety of all—cola—is the culprit.

At first, experts thought soda was bad for bones because people who drink it often do so at the expense of drinking calcium-rich milk. Recent studies suggest, however, that low-calcium diets don't necessarily increase the risk for weak bones. Scientists also posited that the caffeine in colas might diminish bone strength. But other beverages, namely coffee, contain far more caffeine than the typical carbonated drink, and coffee drinking is no longer thought to be associated with osteoporosis.

Now experts have trained their sights on the phosphoric acid added to colas. This acid, which gives colas a sharper flavor, blocks calcium from being absorbed by bone, and studies suggest that it may increase the risk for weak bones.

Scientists at Tufts University asked more than 2,500 men and women about their daily diets, then checked their bone density with x-rays. They discovered that women (but not men) who drank cola beverages every day had weaker bones than those who rarely drank cola. Diet cola appeared to have a similar effect, while non-cola carbonated drinks (which don't contain phosphoric acid) had none at all. In another study of 460 teenage girls, those who were physically active and drank cola regularly were five times more likely than other girls to have had bone fractures.

Skeptics point out that phosphorus is present in many other foods, such as meat, dairy foods, and eggs, so why blame soda? But scientists who study bone health argue that consuming too many cola drinks throws off the balance between phosphorus and calcium in the body, which could make bones fragile. ■

Soy

Remember when the only person you knew who ate soy was your weird college roommate, the one who wore Birkenstocks and always smelled like patchouli? Today more people eat soy foods—now sold in "normal" supermarkets—for their health. But how much bang are they getting for their tofu cubes and edamame beans? Perhaps not quite as much as they think, though there's no harm in eating soy for its taste (yes, taste), versatility, and protein.

Does soy stop hot flashes?

NO Although soy foods and supplements are promoted as a defense against hot flashes, studies show they do little to turn down the heat.

Controlling hot flashes used to be easy and straightforward: A woman simply asked her physician to write a prescription for hormone replacement therapy (HRT), which is capable of reducing hot flash frequency by 60 to 85 percent. In 2002, however, a study of more than 16,000 subjects found that HRT increased the risk of heart disease, stroke, and breast cancer, leading many women to search for alternatives.

Soy foods and supplements seem like a logical choice for several reasons. In Asia, where tofu and other soy dishes are diet staples, only 10 to 20 percent of women develop hot flashes. Soy contains compounds called isoflavones, which are structurally similar to estrogen. Soy supporters claim that these hormone-like compounds fool the body into thinking it's receiving estrogen, thereby reducing hot flashes and other menopause symptoms.

Unfortunately, soy may not quite live up to its billing. A group of doctors and scientists led by Heidi D. Nelson, MD, of Oregon Health and Science University, analyzed a stack of research on nonhormonal approaches to relieving hot flashes. They found 17 well-designed studies on the benefits of soy extract and red clover, an isoflavone-rich herb that's also used to fight off episodes of flushing. Their findings, published in the *Journal of the American Medical Association* in 2006, found no consistent relief from hot flashes among women who took soy extract. (There was even less evidence that red clover helped, according to this review.)

Is soy good for the heart?

YES Eating soy foods produces only a modest drop in cholesterol, but replacing fatty meats with soy brings additional benefits.

Food processors in the United States can claim that products containing at least 6.25 grams of soy protein per serving "may reduce the risk of heart disease." Research shows, however, that soy's benefit to the cardiovascular system is modest, even when you consume a lot of the stuff.

Scientists began to suspect that eating soy foods may protect the cardiovascular system in the 1970s. Once again, the inspiration came from the

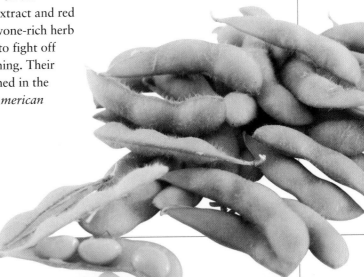

SOY

East, as studies showed that the soy-loving citizens of Japan and other Asian countries had fewer heart attacks and lower cholesterol levels than people in the West. Later, studies in which patients with high cholesterol ate diets high in soy protein showed impressive improvements. Some subjects lowered their LDL ("bad") cholesterol levels by 20 to 30 percent.

In many of these studies, however, subjects were given diets that not only included soy foods but were also low in saturated fat and cholesterol. In many cases, study volunteers lost weight. These other factors make it difficult to sort out what actually produced the improved blood cholesterol levels.

When all other influences are considered, it appears that soy's actual impact on cholesterol is rather small. Recently a panel of experts looked at 22 different studies and determined that consuming 50 grams of soy protein with isoflavones every day lowers LDL cholesterol by about 3 percent, on average. If that doesn't sound like much, then this news will be really hard to swallow: To get 50 grams of soy protein, you need to eat up to 1 1/2 pounds of tofu or drink seven or eight cups of soy milk.

Yet the panel still believes that anyone will benefit from eating more soy. When you swap a T-bone steak for a tofu burger, after all, you avoid lots of saturated fat and cholesterol.

Does soy protect against any cancers?

YES There is modest evidence that soy may help prevent prostate cancer. It appears less useful against breast cancer.

Some common forms of cancer in Western countries are relatively rare throughout Asia. Many scientists believe that diet plays a role. While the typical Westerner eats too much saturated fat, which may promote certain cancers, studies suggest that some elements of Asian cuisine could slow or prevent the dreaded diseases.

Mounting evidence suggests that one staple of Japanese and Chinese cooking—the soy-

Our BEST ADVICE

Don't like tofu? Try frozen green soybeans, or edamame. They make a fun, protein-rich snack when you squeeze them out of their pods (thaw them first), or you can sprinkle shelled soybeans on salads or into soups.

bean—may protect against prostate cancer. For example, a study by Chinese researchers showed that men who ate the most tofu (about an ounce or so daily, on average) cut their risk of prostate cancer by nearly half. A Japanese study came to a similar conclusion, though it found that men who ate natto (made from fermented soybeans) gained even greater protection. If tofu and natto are too exotic for your taste, try soy milk. One study of more than 12,000 men in California found that men who drank soy milk at least once a day reduced their risk of prostate cancer by 70 percent.

Other research offers clues about how soy might protect against prostate cancer. A recent study by University of Minnesota scientists found that men at high risk for the disease who drank soy protein shakes for six months had prostates with fewer receptors for androgens, or male

Some doctors caution **women at risk for breast cancer** to avoid consuming large amounts of soy.

hormones, which fuel the growth of tumors on this gland. That may help to explain why other studies have shown that prostate cancer progresses less aggressively (as measured by levels of prostate-specific antigen, or PSA) in patients who consume frequent servings of soy foods.

Is eating large amounts of soy a smart idea?

NO Some doctors caution women at risk for breast cancer to avoid consuming large amounts of soy, since some studies suggest it may increase their risk for the disease. Likewise, a limited amount of research hints that a soy-rich diet could make men more vulnerable to the most serious forms of prostate cancer. A Japanese study found that eating soy foods appeared to protect against localized prostate cancer, the less dangerous kind that remains contained within the gland. But a hearty diet of tofu and other soy dishes may have *increased* the risk of advanced prostate cancer, which spreads to other organs.

Should you take soy supplements?

NO Soy pills, powders, and other supplements don't offer the same health-promoting qualities as soy foods and

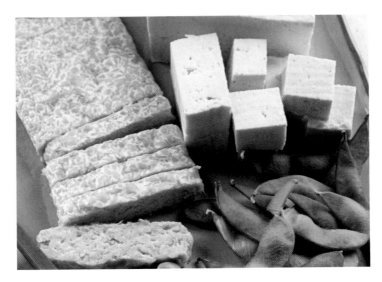

could even pose a health threat.

You've been hearing for years that highly processed refined grains, such as white bread, are less healthy than whole grains, such as whole wheat bread. In a similar way, research suggests that highly processed soy—like the kind found in soy supplements—seems to lose some of its health benefits. It may even be unsafe.

In Asian countries, where soy-rich diets have been linked to lower risk of heart disease and breast cancer, most people eat minimally processed foods made from soybeans and soy flour. In most Western countries, however, many people who want the purported health benefits of this illustrious legume take pills, capsules, and other dietary supplements that contain protein and isoflavones extracted from soybeans. That way, you get all the benefits of soy

without having to retrain your taste buds, right?

Maybe not. Although there is evidence that consuming more soy foods may reduce the risk of heart disease and some forms of cancer, other studies have raised the disturbing possibility that soy supplements may actually raise the risk of certain forms of the disease. Notably, researchers at the University of Illinois found that feeding isoflavones extracted from soy to lab animals actually stimulated the growth of breast tumors. Meanwhile, feeding soy flour (which undergoes minimal processing) to lab animals had no effect on tumor growth.

True, results from animal studies don't always apply to humans. Until scientists demonstrate that supplements containing isoflavone extracts are safe, however, it's best to get your soy in the form of food. ◼

SUGAR

Sugar

Our taste buds adore it, even on our very first exposure; our waistlines, however, seem to despise it. You've heard sugar described as a source of "empty calories" because it provides calories (about 50 per tablespoon) but virtually no nutrients. But is it even worse than that? Does sugar actively ruin our health, or is it relatively harmless as far as guilty pleasures go?

Does eating sugar cause diabetes?

NO But candy and other sugary foods contribute plenty of calories, which can lead to weight gain, and being overweight greatly increases the risk of type 2 diabetes.

Studies have failed to produce consistent evidence that links a sweet tooth with type 2 diabetes. A study of more than 39,000 women, for instance, found that those who ate the most sugar did not have an increased risk for the disease.

Type 2 diabetes occurs when blood levels of glucose, or blood sugar, become chronically elevated. Consuming sugar makes blood sugar levels rise, so it seems logical that eating candy, cakes, and cookies would cause diabetes. But it doesn't—at least not directly.

In recent years, many experts (though not all) have pointed their fingers at diets with a high glycemic index (GI) as a main culprit behind the obesity epidemic as well as an epidemic of insulin resistance, a core problem in type 2 diabetes. The GI is a measure of how much the carbohydrate in a food raises blood sugar (see page 139). When you eat foods that cause a steep rise in blood sugar, your body churns out of lot of insulin to "process" that blood sugar and get it out of the bloodstream and into cells. Over time, repeated floods of insulin make the body less sensitive to the hormone, leading to a condition called insulin resistance—and so the path to diabetes begins.

Refined grains (like white bread) and starches (like potatoes) actually have a higher glycemic index value than sugar does. Still, certain sugar sources may not be entirely off the hook. An emerging theory suggested by a handful of experts holds that fructose, a component of table sugar, may cause insulin resistance. Fructose, in the form of high-fructose corn syrup, is abundant in many sodas and commercially processed foods.

Insulin resistance aside, eating too many sweets—or potatoes, pork chops, or peanut butter sandwiches—can make you gain weight, and well-established science indicates that becoming overweight or obese raises the odds of developing type 2 diabetes.

Does sugar cause hyperactivity?

NO Despite what parents and teachers believe, sugary foods and beverages don't make kids misbehave and run amok.

Mothers and fathers who have seen one too many children's birthday parties erupt into chaos accept this theory as fact: Heavy doses of cake, candy, and soda turn well-behaved little ones into wild things. Scientists seemed to

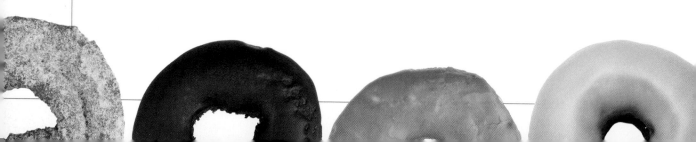

agree—until fairly recently. Contemporary research has largely knocked this age-old belief off its feet. For example, a study conducted by researchers at the University of Iowa and published in the *New England Journal of Medicine* tested whether parents and teachers can tell when children have consumed a large amount of sugar. The families of 58 children under age 10—about half of them identified by their parents as "sensitive to sugar"—were provided with all of their at-home meals for nine weeks. For part of the study, the families ate high-sugar diets; for the remainder, they consumed little sugar. Instead, they were given foods flavored with the artificial sweeteners aspartame and saccharin so they still tasted sweet. All of the food looked alike, and participants weren't told which foods they had been given.

Throughout the study, parents, teachers, and research assistants observed the children and rated their mood and how impulsive, attentive, or aggressive they acted. Their reports showed that the children behaved similarly whether or not they ate lots of sugar.

White bread and potatoes have a greater impact on blood sugar and insulin than sugar does.

A large body of research supports this study's finding. A review of 23 studies published in the *Journal of the American Medical Association* found no evidence that eating sugar affects a child's behavior or thinking ability.

Does sugar hamper your immune system?

NO Although some holistic healers insist that eating sugar makes your body more vulnerable to illness, there is little evidence to support this claim.

A few small studies in animals and humans conducted in the 1970s found that consuming sugar lowered the activity of white blood cells, which the immune system produces to defend the body against germs and infections. However, there has been little research on this matter in the ensuing years, and leading immunologists say there is no current scientific data to confirm the theory that eating too much sugar harms the immune system.

One reason this belief persists may be that people with poorly controlled diabetes—who have elevated blood sugar levels—are at unusually high risk for many types of infections, says immunologist Richard F. Lockey, MD, of the University of South Florida College of Medicine. The high blood sugar levels that can accompany diabetes can damage many organ systems, including the immune system. Simply eating sugary foods, however, does not have this effect.

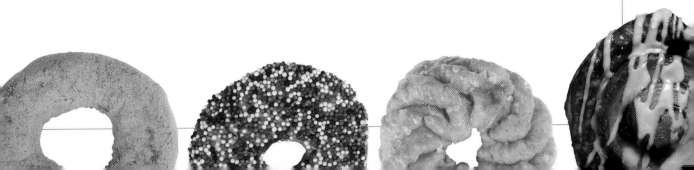

Is sugar addictive?

MAYBE Recent studies suggest that sweets and addictive drugs cause similar changes in the brain that can lead to cravings and dependence.

It's easy to rationalize buying a box of chocolate truffles with the excuse: "I can't help myself—I'm addicted!" Yet there may be a biological explanation for why some people are compelled to gorge on candy, ice cream, and the like. For years, many scientists and physicians denied that sugar addiction exists. But according to mounting research, some people may truly become hooked on the sweet stuff.

For starters, research suggests that eating sugar and other refined carbohydrates creates a vicious cycle in some people, causing them to crave sweets. When you eat refined carbohydrates, the pancreas churns out large amounts of insulin to convert blood sugar into energy. Over time, chronically elevated insulin levels can cause cells to ignore this hormone. This condition, known as insulin resistance, leaves cells low on blood sugar, which triggers a desire to eat more sweet foods.

Furthermore, intriguing evidence suggests that certain foods—sugar in particular— act on the brain in much the same way as addictive drugs. For example, cocaine increases

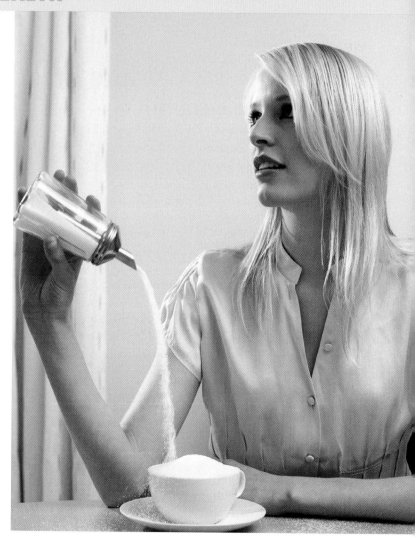

levels of dopamine, a brain chemical that seems to play a role in producing sensations of pleasure. Studies by researchers at Princeton University show that lab rats allowed to binge on sugar-sweetened water produce large amounts of dopamine, too. When the same rats are deprived of sugar, they develop withdrawal symptoms, such as trembling and chattering teeth.

Sugar may mimic other addictive drugs as well. Heroin and morphine, both opiates, produce a sense of well-being or euphoria by locking into opioid receptors in the brain. Studies have shown that humans given medications that block opioid receptors lose their craving for sweet foods.

Finally, early humans probably developed a strong taste for sugar to ensure that they consumed enough calories to survive. Some scientists theorize that walking past the candy aisle may send that primitive desire for sugar into overdrive. ■

Tea

For years, health nuts shunned regular tea in favor of herbal tea. They may have been seriously missing out. An impressive body of research now shows that traditional tea—that is, black, green, and other varieties made from the leaves of the *Camellia sinensis* plant—is one of nature's richest sources of disease-fighting antioxidants.

Does green tea fight cancer?

YES Compounds in green tea block cancer cells, at least in test tubes, but you may need to drink a *lot* of tea or take supplements to get a benefit.

Despite its subtle flavor, green tea packs a wallop against cancer cells. The grassy-tasting brew is brimming with antioxidants called catechins, particularly one known as EGCG, one of the most potent of all antioxidants. Green tea is one of the richest sources of EGCG among all foods and drinks, packing 3 to 10 times more than black tea.

Lab and animal research leaves little question that EGCG has the potential to destroy cancer cells. The antioxidant blocks the growth and spread of cancer by triggering a process within cancer cells that makes them self-destruct. It also starves the cells by cutting off their blood supply and inhibits an enzyme needed for cancer cell growth.

The strongest evidence that tea fights cancer in humans comes from population studies conducted in Japan and China, where most people sip the green variety. In particular, some (but not all) studies show a benefit against colon cancer and other gastrointestinal cancers. A recent review found that green tea drinkers cut their risk of colon cancer by 18 percent, while black tea appeared to have no effect. Also, studies show that Japanese women who drink vast quantities of green tea—10 or more cups a day—are less likely to be diagnosed with breast cancer.

Antioxidants in green tea may have an unusually potent effect on prostate cancer. In one of the first clinical studies to test tea's catechins against cancer in humans, a group of Italian scientists divided 60 men at high risk for developing prostate cancer into two groups. Half the men received tablets containing green tea catechins, and the other half received placebos. A year later, just one of the men who took the green tea extract had been diagnosed with prostate cancer, compared to nine men who took placebos.

Is tea good for the heart?

YES Tea helps keep arteries supple, which lowers the risk of heart attacks and strokes.

Tea is the second most popular beverage in the world, after water. Cardiologists wish it were even more popular—though their business might suffer.

Drinking tea appears to benefit the heart mainly by improving blood vessel function. Tea's massive stash of antioxidants appears to make the blood vessels dilate wider and more efficiently, which promotes good circulation. One study of 50 heart disease

People who sipped tea every day **reduced their heart attack risk** by 44 percent.

TEA

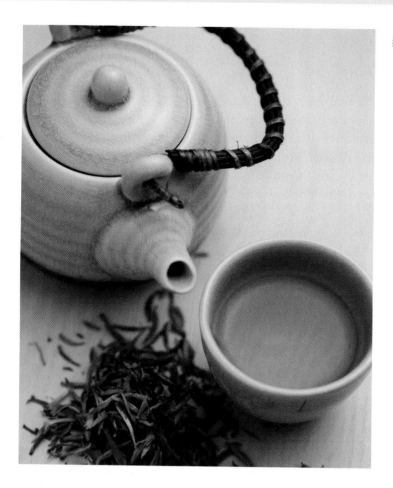

Here's how to get the most antioxidants from tea.

Drink your tea "black." If you sip your tea the British way, with milk or cream, consider lightening up. A 2007 study showed that drinking black tea improved blood flow in 16 female volunteers. When the women drank tea with milk, however, the milk blocked tea's benefit.

Buy a teapot. Studies show that hot brewed tea has a far greater concentration of antioxidants than instant powders or bottled tea.

Try white tea. It's lightly processed, which allows it to retain higher levels of antioxidants than other varieties. Some research shows it may have the highest level of antioxidant activity—higher even than green tea.

patients at hospitals in Massachusetts and Oregon found that drinking three or four cups of tea per day brought impaired blood vessel function—the result of their heart disease—back to near-normal levels according to ultrasound tests that measured blood flow.

Tea's catechins, part of a larger class of antioxidants called flavonoids, probably play a starring role. Dutch scientists evaluated the flavonoid content of the diets of more than 800 men over age 65. They found that tea was the leading source of this important antioxidant and that men who consumed the most flavonoids cut their risk of heart disease by 58 percent.

Another study of more than 700 men and women found that people who sipped one cup or more of tea per day reduced their heart attack risk by 44 percent. And a team of doctors and scientists at several Boston hospitals found that people who drank two or more cups of tea per day were 39 percent more likely to survive heart attacks. ■

Tomatoes

Whether they say to-*may*-to or to-*mah*-to, most people say these juicy fruits (that's right, they aren't vegetables) are delicious. Sliced and eaten with salt and a bit of olive oil, chopped for a salad, or cooked to make a sauce, they are unquestionably good for you, rich in vitamin C and antioxidants. Lately, though, one of their main claims to fame has been called into question.

Do ketchup and tomato sauce prevent prostate cancer?

NO There are plenty of reasons to eat tomatoes, but recent research suggests that they do not prevent prostate cancer as once believed.

Can eating a hamburger with ketchup or a steaming plate of spaghetti with red sauce really fight prostate cancer? That was the message that came from a series of studies dating back to the mid 1990s, when Harvard researchers first reported that men who ate frequent servings of tomatoes, tomato sauce, and other foods made with cooked tomatoes lowered their risk of prostate cancer. One study of more than 47,000 male participants by the Harvard team found that men who ate two or more servings of tomato sauce per week cut their risk of prostate cancer by 23 percent.

Tomatoes appeared to draw their cancer-fighting strength from the antioxidant lycopene. Cooking tomatoes increases their lycopene content and makes the antioxidant more active.

Since foods and beverages made from cooked tomatoes are cheap, tasty, and nontoxic, many doctors began telling their male patients to eat more marinara sauce and drink tomato juice. Sales of supplements containing lycopene took off. But meanwhile, other groups of scientists began to look more closely at lycopene, and its reputation began to rot on the vine.

For example, five out of eight studies in which scientists compared the diets of men who developed cancer with those of healthy men failed to produce any evidence that eating tomatoes prevented the disease.

In 2007, the largest study of its kind cast more doubt. Researchers studied lycopene levels in 137,001 men in eight European countries and found that the antioxidant did not protect against prostate cancer.

Tomatoes are an excellent source of vitamin C and other nutrients, but enthusiasm for the possibility that they prevent prostate cancer seems to have exceeded the science. ■

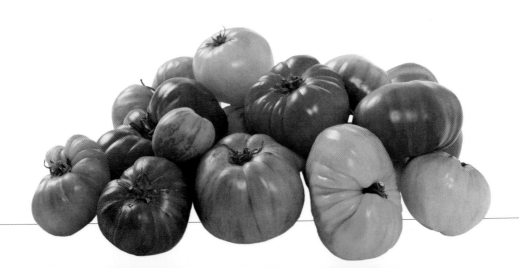

Vegetarian Diets

When your teenager becomes a vegetarian, should you worry or rejoice? Most vegetarians eat fairly healthful diets, although people who subsist mainly on pasta, cheese, and junk food are hardly doing their bodies a favor. Vegetarians get plenty of protein from beans and other foods, though they must take care to get enough of certain nutrients, such as iron and vitamin B_{12}, which come only from animal foods and foods fortified with the vitamin.

Are vegetarians healthier than meat eaters?

YES Several large long-term studies have produced persuasive evidence that people who eat plant-based diets are protected from heart disease and other serious health problems.

Saying so long to bacon and farewell to fried chicken pays off not only with a smaller waistline but also with a longer life. One study found that typical vegetarians live about 3 1/2 years longer than meat eaters. Not only are they unlikely to be overweight, but vegetarians also have healthier hearts. And some evidence suggests that they gain protection from other leading killers as well.

While it's true that vegetarians tend to live healthier lives apart from what they eat—they're unlikely to smoke, for example, and they tend to exercise regularly—studies suggest that a diet dominated by fruits, vegetables, and grains protects against these and other conditions.

Heart disease: Fatty meat is a major source of saturated fat, which raises cholesterol, so it's no surprise that vegetarian diets improve cholesterol levels. (Vegans have even lower cholesterol since they avoid the saturated fat in dairy foods, too.) Vegetarians also tend to have low blood pressure; one large study found that male meat eaters were about

2.5 times more likely than male vegans to develop high blood pressure. It's no wonder, then, that people who eat plant-based diets have relatively few heart attacks. For example, a study of more than 34,000 Californians found that men who eat beef three or more times a week or more are 2.3 times more likely than vegetarians to die of heart disease. Another study of more than 76,000 adults found that vegetarians cut their risk of fatal heart attacks by 24 percent.

Cancer: It's less clear whether shunning meat will cut your risk for cancer. A review of five major studies of vegetarian diets found no consistent evidence that avoiding meat lowers the risk of cancers of the breast, colon, lung, prostate, or stomach. Yet other research shows otherwise. Authors of the Oxford Vegetarian Study, which compared 6,000 vegetarians and 5,000 meat eaters, found that the former cut their risk of developing any form of cancer by up to 39 percent.

In a recent review, 24 out of 26 studies showed that men who are diagnosed with prostate cancer may have a better chance of surviving if

Vegetarians tend to have low blood pressure and weigh less.

they eat a vegetarian-style diet. Also, a British study found that women from India, Pakistan, and Bangladesh who were lifelong vegetarians appeared to be less likely to develop breast cancer, although researchers couldn't determine whether eating no meat or consuming large amounts of vegetables provided the protection.

Diabetes: Vegetarians are less likely to develop diabetes, according to one study of more than 25,000 people who were followed for two decades. Type 2 diabetes, the most common form of the disease, is closely linked to obesity. Vegetarian diets promote healthy weight, which often leads to improved blood sugar control. In one study, researchers asked 652 diabetes patients to adopt a low-fat vegetarian diet and a regimen of regular exercise. After four weeks, 39 percent of the patients who had needed insulin injections to maintain normal blood sugar levels were able to discontinue the medication, and 71 percent who took oral diabetes drugs were able to stop. ■

Yogurt

It's unusual for people to willingly eat food that contains bacteria, but yogurt is one exception. It's made by fermenting milk with certain strains of bacteria, known as "starter culture," causing it to develop a firm texture and tart taste. Like all dairy products, yogurt is a good source of calcium and protein, but the real benefits may come from "good" bacteria added by the manufacturer.

Can yogurt ease digestive problems?

YES Yogurt is an excellent addition to the diets of people with lactose intolerance and other gastrointestinal problems.

When most people hear the word *bacteria*, they think of nasty germs that make people sick. However, the body is home to millions of "good" bacteria that help keep the bad kind in check. One type of these bacteria, known as *Lactobacillus acidophilus*, helps maintain a healthy balance of microorganisms in the digestive tract. Many yogurt makers now add it and other types of bacteria believed to have health benefits, known as probiotics, to their products. Solid research suggests that this enhanced yogurt can help relieve the following gastrointestinal problems.

Lactose intolerance. People who lack a certain enzyme in their gastrointestinal tracts can't digest lactose, or milk sugar, which may cause them to develop gas, bloating, or diarrhea if they consume more than a small amount of milk. While yogurt contains lactose, it also contains the "antidote"—the cultures used to make it produce lactase, the enzyme needed to break down milk sugar. Studies show that when people with lactose intolerance consume yogurt, they

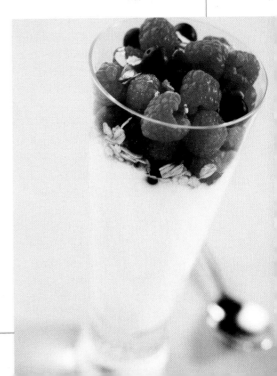

YOGURT

experience fewer gastrointestinal symptoms than when they drink milk.

Diarrhea: If you've ever gotten diarrhea while taking antibiotics, here's the likely reason: Antibiotics kill indiscriminately, wiping out both bad and good bacteria, the kind that keeps your gut healthy. This can lead to diarrhea and other tummy troubles. But taking probiotics, the good bacteria in yogurt, can help. In a recent study of 135 hospital patients receiving antibiotic treatment, just 12 percent who were given probiotic milkshakes developed diarrhea compared to 34 percent who received a placebo drink.

Lactobacillus can also help with diarrhea caused by infections, a common problem in children. A review published in the journal *Pediatrics* found that treating sick children with this healthy bacterium shortens the duration and severity of a bout of diarrhea. Other studies suggest that probiotic therapy may help prevent "traveler's diarrhea," too.

Peptic ulcers: Most stomach and intestinal ulcers are caused by a type of bacteria called *Helicobacter pylori.* Treatment with antibiotics and drugs called proton-pump inhibitors can cure peptic ulcers, but this first-line therapy fails to eliminate *H. pylori* in 10 to 23 percent of patients. Studies in humans show that yogurt

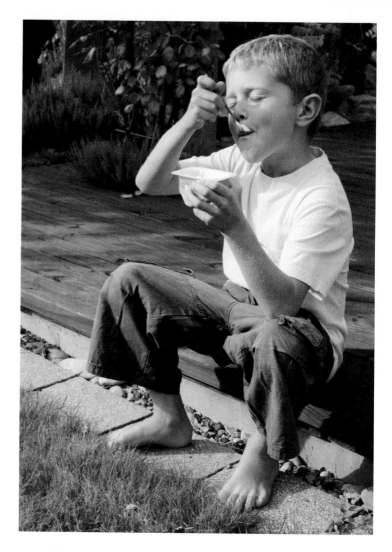

containing live cultures suppresses the activity of the bacteria. Taiwanese researchers asked a group of 69 patients with hard-to-treat ulcers to eat six ounces of yogurt containing live cultures twice a day while undergoing a second round of therapy. After four weeks, 91 percent were cured, versus 77 percent of patients in a comparison group.

Other gastrointestinal problems: Several studies have

shown that the probiotics found in yogurt may relieve some symptoms of irritable bowel syndrome, including abdominal pain and bloating. Less is known about the benefits of yogurt for inflammatory bowel disorders such as ulcerative colitis and Crohn's disease. However, a recent study found that eating yogurt containing probiotics for one month reduced levels of inflammation in a group of patients with these two conditions.

Does yogurt stimulate the immune system?

YES Eating yogurt appears to be a tasty way to bolster your body's defenses against microbes that can make you sick.

Your gastrointestinal tract does much more than process your breakfast, lunch, and dinner. As unlikely as it sounds, it also serves as a vital part of the immune system. That's right, your gut contains a vast preponderance of immune cells, and it seems the probiotics in yogurt can help them function at their peak.

Studies in both animals and humans show that consuming probiotics commonly added to yogurt—*L. acidophilus*, *L. casei*, and *Bifidobacterium bifidus*—increases levels of an important infection-fighting protein called secretory immunoglobulin A in the intestines. White blood cells known as lymphocytes are another critical part of your body's defense system, since they produce antibodies and other proteins that fight infections, and a recent Austrian study found that the cells became more active in young women who consumed either a probiotic supplement or 3.5 to 7 ounces of yogurt a day for a month. Other research suggests that probiotics make germ-eating white blood cells called macrophages more voracious.

What does all of that mean for *your* health? At minimum, regularly eating yogurt with live cultures could keep you out of a sickbed. A study of 262 employees at a Swedish company found that men and women who drank a beverage containing probiotics every day missed work half as often as other workers given a placebo beverage and were 60 percent less likely to develop gastrointestinal distress or the common cold and other respiratory tract conditions.

Yogurt's immune-stimulating properties could have even greater benefits; preliminary evidence suggests that they may help reduce the risk of some cancers, including colon and bladder cancer.

Can yogurt prevent or treat yeast infections?

MAYBE Eating yogurt every day is a popular home remedy for recurrent yeast and urinary tract infections. Some women keep yogurt in the fridge for just this reason. Does it work? There's not enough research to say for sure.

Yeast infections are caused by the overgrowth of a microorganism called *Candida albicans* in the vagina, which can occur when a woman takes antibiotic medications, among other reasons. Naturally occurring healthy bacteria, including *L. acidophilus*, exist in the vagina, too. A few studies have examined whether eating yogurt containing *L. acidophilus* can cure yeast infections by restoring normal bacteria levels in the vagina. In one, women with recurrent vaginitis (itching and irritation) caused by yeast overgrowth who ate eight ounces of yogurt a day experienced a threefold drop in infections. The study was small, though (just 13 women finished), and there were other problems that affected its credibility. There is equally limited scientific support for another folk remedy for yeast infections: inserting yogurt directly into the vagina.

Can yogurt prevent or treat urinary tract infections?

NO Urinary tract infections (UTIs) are caused by bacteria and can arise anywhere in the urinary system, including the bladder, kidneys, and any of the tubes that transport urine. The probiotic *Lactobacillus* shows some promise in the treatment of UTIs, but so far only strains that are not added to yogurt have proven successful. Eating a cup of yogurt offers many health benefits, but to relieve a UTI, you'll need to turn elsewhere (see page 325 for more information). ■

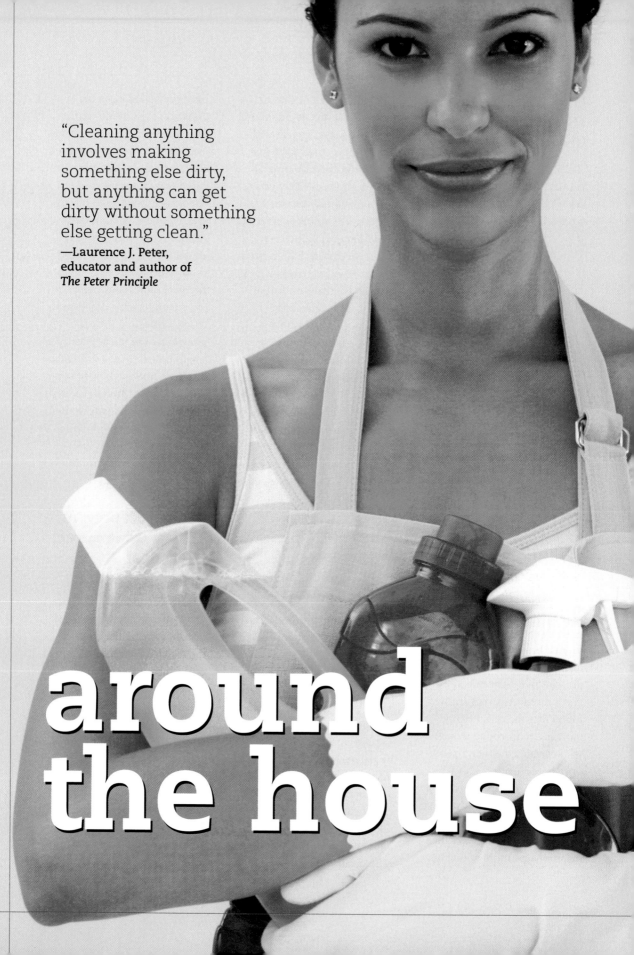

"Cleaning anything involves making something else dirty, but anything can get dirty without something else getting clean."

—Laurence J. Peter, educator and author of *The Peter Principle*

around the house

Air Filters

If microscopic airborne particles of pollen, dust, or pet dander make you sneeze or wheeze, filtering the air you breathe seems like a logical solution. Air filters work best if you also take another smart step: Controlling the irritants that get into your home or your bedroom in the first place.

Do air filters ease allergy and asthma symptoms?

NO Filters do scrub some sneeze- and cough-provoking particles from the air, but often not enough to improve breathing or lessen annoying reactions.

Advertisements proclaim that air filters are "essential" for people with allergies to pollen, dust mites, mold spores, and pet dander, and it seems to make sense that removing these misery-producing bits from the air would bring relief. But here's the odd truth: While plenty of studies show that air filters—especially those with high-efficiency particulate air (HEPA) filters—can reduce the amount of microscopic sneeze makers in the air, there's scant proof that they ease most allergy and asthma symptoms. When Canadian doctors reviewed 10 air filter studies, they concluded that filtered air didn't improve lung function and improved symptoms like coughing, sneezing, watery eyes, and runny noses only a little.

If you're a dog or cat lover with pet-dander allergies, though, and you can't bear to part with your pet, an air filter may help. One study of 30 allergic pet owners found that two-thirds of those who installed HEPA filters in their bedrooms and living rooms needed less allergy medication. The filters worked best when pets were also banned from bedrooms. In a study of dog owners, air filters removed just 75 percent of dander in bedrooms where dogs were allowed to roam free, but 90 percent when they were kept out. Air filters eliminated 50 percent of cat dander in feline-free bedrooms.

Are ion-generating filters safe?

NO These purport to work by attracting and trapping particles with positive or negative electrical charges. The high-voltage wire used to ionize air particles converts oxygen into ozone, a highly reactive molecule. Even in tiny amounts, ozone damages lung tissue and can cause throat irritation, coughing, chest pain, and shortness of breath—something you don't need, especially if you have allergies or asthma. ∎

THE TRUTH ABOUT AIR-DUCT CLEANING

Many duct-cleaning companies would have you believe that the air ducts for your heating or air conditioning system are breeding grounds for the mold spores and dust that aggravate allergies and asthma. The fix: A high-priced clean-out.

The truth? Duct cleaning has never been proven to prevent health problems, according to the EPA. One study even found that, contrary to what duct cleaners claim, most of the ducts tested were virtually free of dust mites. And unless the vacuum equipment used to clean ducts is vented to the outdoors or uses a HEPA filter, the project could actually stir up dust rather than cleaning the air.

Your ducts need repair—not just cleaning—if you find a buildup of mold, dirt, or moisture inside or if insects or rodents have taken up residence there. Keeping air filters clean and fixing leaks are the first steps.

Antibacterial Products

Commercials for antibacterial soaps and sprays would have you believe your home is infested with a horror movie's worth of bacteria, viruses, yeasts, and molds, all waiting to make you and your family sick. But do you really need these products? While it's true that the world faces new germ threats, including antibiotic-resistant bacteria, science is reinforcing old truths about the best ways to fight germs, which old-fashioned homemakers have known for generations.

Does antibacterial soap kill more germs than plain soap?

NO Regular soap is just as effective. Germ-killing soaps don't actually kill more bugs or prevent colds or tummy troubles.

Antibacterial soaps are no better than old-fashioned soap and water for killing disease-causing germs or preventing the illnesses they can cause. When University of Michigan scientists reviewed 27 studies examining purported germ-fighting products containing ingredients like triclosan, they found no evidence that they were superior for battling microbes in the home. These products seem to have little effect on viruses that cause colds, flu, and gastrointestinal woes, researchers say. When

238 families used liquid hand soaps, spray cleaners, and laundry detergents with or without antibacterial ingredients for 48 weeks, scientists found no difference in the number of parents and kids who got runny noses, coughs, fevers, nausea, diarrhea, or skin rashes.

In fact, antibacterial products can be downright risky if you think they're more effective than soap and therefore wash your hands less thoroughly. Washing your hands for 15 to 20 seconds every time you use the bathroom and before handling food or eating is a proven germ stopper that experts say can get rid of 99.9 percent of germs—by washing bacteria and viruses down the drain and by outright killing nasties like the highly contagious rotavirus, which causes

gastrointestinal problems. When 1,445 military recruits were ordered to thoroughly clean their hands five times a day for one year, respiratory tract infections—including colds, flu, and pneumonia—fell by 45 percent, say scientists at the US Naval Health Research Center.

Are antibacterial hand gels worth using?

YES When you can't get to a sink, germ-battling gels can reduce your exposure to bugs that cause respiratory and gastrointestinal illnesses.

When a sink and a bar of soap are out of reach, alcohol-based antibacterial gels and towelettes are a proven alternative for ridding your hands of bacteria and viruses. In a recent study of 292 families with young children, those who used hand sanitizers for five months had 59 percent fewer infections than those who didn't use them. In another study, families who washed up with hand gels about five times a day cut the risk of colds by 20 percent compared to families who scrubbed less often.

ANTIBACTERIAL PRODUCTS

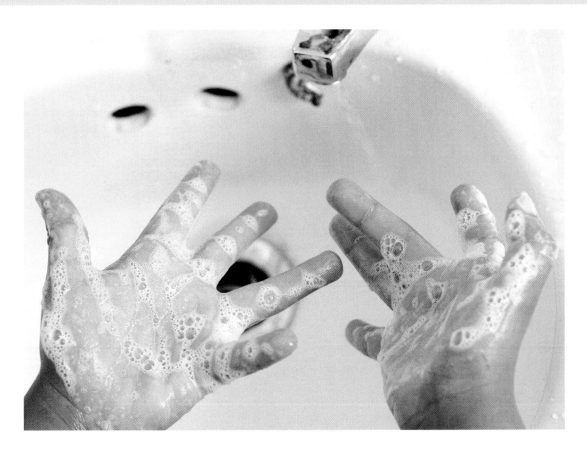

For best results, squeeze out 1/2 teaspoon of gel (about the size of a nickel) or grab a towelette and vigorously rub your hands front and back.

Tuck an antibacterial cleaner into your child's backpack, too. When 420 elementary school kids used hand sanitizer several times a day at school—when coming into the classroom, before eating, and after using the bathroom—for four weeks, they got 29 percent fewer gastrointestinal illnesses and 49 percent fewer colds. Kids who used sanitizers also had 31 percent fewer sick days.

Most antibacterial cleaning products aren't designed to kill viruses.

Do germ-killing cleaning products make my home cleaner?

YES But don't expect them to cut down on viruses within your family. They may, however, cut down slightly on cases of illnesses caused by bacteria.

Kitchen countertops, dining room tables, and bathroom surfaces all can harbor disease-causing bacteria like E. coli, salmonella, staph, and strep. While regular cleaning removes dirt, only sanitizing kills the bacteria that may remain. In a head-to-head study comparing disinfectant

ANTIBACTERIAL PRODUCTS

and antibacterial sprays and cleaning solutions against homemade solutions of baking soda or vinegar, the store-bought products won. They killed 99.9 percent of bugs, including salmonella, *Staphylococcus aureus*, and *Escherichia coli*, while the homemade natural concoctions killed just 90 percent.

In theory, that could mean the difference between staying well and getting sick, the study's authors say, which is especially important if your household includes young babies, older people, or anyone with weakened immunity. But remember that all the bugs listed are bacteria, not viruses. The fact is, most antibacterial cleaning products aren't designed to kill viruses, and they may or may not do so. (Even alcohol kills some viruses and not others, depending on the concentration used.) That may explain why, when researchers studied 292 families, those who used antibacterial cleaning products got just as many colds and other upper respiratory infections as those who didn't use the products. The study didn't rule out the possibility that these products might cut down on illnesses caused by bacteria, however.

Should you go crazy about the prospect of germs living on doorknobs, telephones, and light switches? In general, no. But if someone in your home is ill, it can't hurt to take

ANTIBACTERIAL PRODUCTS YOU DON'T NEED

Can your toothbrush, dish detergent, or cutting board really battle germs all by itself? Food safety experts at the University of Wisconsin-Madison say no. Among the antibacterial products you can skip are toothbrushes, cutting boards, detergents, telephone guards, baby toys, mops, and sponges.

precautions, since germs can survive for 20 minutes to two hours on a hard, dry surface, long enough to be transferred to the next victim unless someone cleans up. Experts recommend a solution of 1 part bleach to 10 parts water, which effectively kills germs and some viruses. Leave the solution on the surface for 10 to 20 seconds before wiping dry.

Are antibacterial sponges superior to regular kitchen sponges?

NO All sponges pick up dirty liquids and food particles that can harbor bacteria. And germ-fighting sponges can't disinfect your countertops.

Wiping your kitchen counter with a dirty sponge leaves a writhing film of bacteria on every surface—yuck! No wonder experts call sponges the number one source of germs in the house. Your best defense: A new cleaning strategy for your kitchen sponge—and for your countertops. Relying on

"antimicrobial" sponges isn't enough because germs can still breed in the warm, wet crevices of a sponge, especially once tiny food particles become lodged in them.

Your best bet? Ditch the sponge entirely and clean countertops and tables with paper towels and a disinfectant spray or the bleach solution we suggest above. If you prefer sponges, clean them daily. How? When researchers compared five methods of cleaning super-dirty, germ-laden kitchen sponges, they found that soaking them in a 10 percent bleach solution, lemon juice, or deionized water eliminated just 37 to 87 percent of bacteria and just 7 to 63 percent of yeasts and molds. In contrast, cleaning sponges in a dishwasher (including the drying cycle) killed 99.998 percent.

While some experts recommend microwaving sponges, this strategy has its flaws. There's no way to be sure how long it will take your microwave to heat a sponge sufficiently to kill germs—and an overheated sponge could catch fire. ∎

Brain-Boosting Software

As fun and fast-paced as a teenager's video game or placid enough for the eyes and ears of a baby, new computer software programs and videos promise to boost brainpower while you have fun. Research shows that older people may get benefits, but barely more than you'd gain from regular exercise, an active social life, and regular mental challenges. Meanwhile, experts warn that computer fun may not be best for babies.

Does brain-training software improve thinking skills and memory?

YES But experts disagree about how much they can help.

As we age, most of us don't mind if some things slow down a bit, like the pace of our daily lives. But our minds aren't one of those things. In fact, dozens of "brain-training" computer games and Web sites are hitting the market with claims that they make the brain younger and ward off memory loss and fuzzy thinking, and some of them may help—a little.

In a recent study at Wake Forest University Baptist Medical Center in North Carolina, researchers scanned the brains of 23 older people and found that those who'd gone through a brain-training program were less distractible and better able to focus. And in a landmark study of 2,832 people, those who used computer brain-training programs for 10 weeks showed improvements in memory, information-processing speed, and reasoning ability five years later.

Still, the notion that working your brain can forestall age-related mental declines is controversial. Plenty of studies have found that people who are involved in more activities, from social groups to hobbies to continuing education, seem to maintain sharper mental skills. But when a University of Virginia neuroscientist analyzed studies purporting to show that mental challenges slow or reverse age-related brain decline, he concluded that there's no hard proof that they do.

At the end of the day, though, there's no harm in keeping your brain active in as many ways as possible.

Will brain-building videos and software make my baby smarter?

NO Despite marketing claims, videos and computer programs that promise to make babies smarter or learn language faster don't work—and can even backfire. When University of Washington researchers surveyed 1,000 parents by phone about their children's vocabularies and time spent watching infant DVDs and videos, they got a shock. Babies and toddlers between the ages of 8 and 16 months understood six to eight fewer words, on average, for every hour per day they spent watching the videos, compared to babies who didn't watch them. (These "educational" programs had no effect of any kind on the vocabularies of toddlers between 17 and 24 months old.) The reason: Babies don't learn through passive listening, but actively—when a parent or caretaker talks, sings, or reads to them. ■

Home Defibrillators

Portable, easy-to-use automatic external defibrillators (AEDs), found in airports, shopping malls, school gyms, and even gambling casinos, are proven lifesavers. In the hands of fast-thinking yet untrained citizens, they've jump-started the hearts of thousands of victims of sudden cardiac arrest. Now you can buy them for your home, although some skeptics aren't sure they belong there.

Can a home AED save your life?

YES AEDs in public places triple the odds of surviving sudden cardiac arrest. Home devices save lives too, but so does CPR, at less cost.

Unlike a heart attack, sudden cardiac arrest happens when the heart's electrical activity is disrupted and the heartbeat becomes perilously rapid or dangerously out of rhythm, so the heart is unable to effectively pump blood. It kills hundreds of thousands of people each year, and most people are home when it strikes.

Your survival odds are nearly 100 percent if an AED delivers lifesaving electrical shocks within 2 minutes but drop by 7 to 10 percent with each passing minute, falling to a dismal 4 percent at 10 minutes. Since emergency medical crews may take 10 minutes or more to reach you, it makes sense in theory to have an AED at home if someone in your household is at risk for cardiac arrest.

Yet in a study of more than 7,000 people at moderate risk for the condition, AEDs didn't save any more lives than CPR. All of the people had someone in the household willing and able to perform CPR (which they'd been well trained in) and use an AED. The researchers split them into two groups: One group was told to call an ambulance and perform CPR if something happened; the other group was given defibrillators and told to use them first, then call for help. People in both groups died at the same rate, though so few people in the study suffered cardiac arrest at home while someone else was present that it's hard to say how conclusive the results are. And of course, if no one in your household knows CPR, an AED can indeed be a lifesaver.

The devices do work; no one argues that point. But they are expensive, and experts argue the money could be better spent elsewhere (on CPR training, for instance).

Can anyone operate an AED?

YES AEDs have easy-to-follow directions. Studies show that sixth graders and senior citizens age 60 and older can successfully use them, though medical groups still recommend that everyone in your household receive training. The machine confirms a victim's cardiac arrest and won't shock someone whose heart is still beating.

You must also remember to call for an ambulance as soon as possible. Your loved one still needs prompt medical care, and experts worry that AED owners may skip this vital step.

If you have an AED at home, it's important to keep up with safety advisories and recalls. Just as crucial is ensuring that your AED has fresh batteries and is accessible—retrieving it from the back of a closet or the depths of the basement wastes precious time. ■

Home Medical Tests

Back in the day, your doctor's office was the only place to have your cholesterol checked, get screened for colon cancer, and find out your HIV status. Today you can walk into a drugstore or order a test online and play doctor at home. But if you plan to use a home medical test, choose it wisely. While a few can give you fast, accurate, useful information, others are useless at best and dangerous at worst.

Are home tests as good as tests in the doctor's office?

NO A few tried-and-true home tests are a good idea, but using home tests to diagnose a medical condition could be dangerous.

We're all for home monitoring of blood pressure if you have hypertension and of blood sugar if you have diabetes. But playing doctor by using home tests to find a cause for troubling symptoms or for screenings usually done in the doctor's office isn't a great idea. For example, if you take a home cholesterol test and the results look normal, you may never discover that your ratios of "good" and "bad" cholesterol are out of balance and that you're in fact at high risk for a heart attack. You may also never find out that you have other significant heart risks, such as high triglycerides.

Experts suggest you don't go it alone. If you think you have a medical problem, see a doctor for a checkup and a careful screening. And think twice about these home checks.

HIV: Tests that promise results in minutes may be inaccurate (those that ask you to send a blood sample to a lab may be as accurate as a clinic test, however). The bigger issue: If

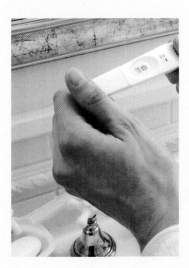

TWO HOME TESTS WORTH TAKING

Trying to get pregnant? Or worried that you might be? These two proven, highly accurate tests deliver the info you need right away.

Ovulation: This urine dipstick checks for luteinizing hormone (LH) and sometimes for estrone-3-glucuronide, both of which rise near ovulation. It's usually 90 percent accurate.

Pregnancy: While it's possible to get a false positive result (if you have traces of blood in your urine) or a false negative result (if you test too soon after a missed period), home pregnancy tests are usually accurate and can give you the news you're looking for, fast. Of course, if you get a positive result or have taken a few tests with mixed results, see your doctor. She can confirm your results with a blood test or pelvic exam.

you test positive, it's imperative to see a doctor immediately to begin treatment. Also, a negative result may not mean you're in the clear: It takes three weeks to six months after HIV exposure for antibodies to appear in your bloodstream.

Cholesterol: Some home tests give only *total* cholesterol—not the details you need about "bad" LDL cholesterol, "good" HDL cholesterol, and potentially dangerous triglycerides (another blood fat). While expensive versions do give you this important breakdown, it's still important to see your doctor so she can evaluate a range of other important factors that affect your heart's health, including your age, weight, activity level, and the presence or absence of other health problems, such as diabetes.

Urinary tract infections: Home dipstick urine tests are considered accurate for revealing UTIs. But then what? You need fast antibiotic treatment to end the pain and clear the infection, so you'll still end up going to the doctor.

Menopause: Hot flashes? Missed periods? This urine check for rising levels of follicle-stimulating hormone (FSH) could reveal whether perimenopause—the years-long process leading to menopause—is under way. They're accurate 90 percent of the time, but test results can be skewed by drinking lots of water or by not using first morning urine for the sample. These tests are fine if you're in your mid to late 40s or older and are curious about your shifting hormones, but you should see a doctor if you're a younger woman who may be going through early menopause.

Is human error a problem?

YES Becoming a do-it-yourself medical technician isn't a simple task. If you don't follow the directions precisely, you could easily skew the results.

Home tests promise to be easy to take, but not all of them live up to that promise. Wondering if you're pregnant? Just urinate on a special stick, wait a few minutes, and check your results. But sometimes matters are more complicated. Pitfalls of home testing range from buying an expired test (check the sell-by date) or one that's been improperly stored (some need to be refrigerated or kept out of humidity) to not following directions. Mistiming a test could throw off results (if you're supposed to time a step carefully, use a watch with a second hand). Ignoring instructions to fast or skip certain foods or medicines may also skew results. A prime example: Having a T-bone steak, broccoli, or vitamin C before some colon cancer risk tests could leave you with a false positive result. So could squeezing blood from a pricked finger instead of collecting droplets as they form (squeezing adds bits of tissue).

Since genetic tests look for only a few genes, their **results are impossible to interpret.**

Do home genetic tests work?

NO More and more home tests promise to reveal whether your genes put your future health at risk. But experts say they aren't ready for primetime.

Expensive new home genetic tests claim to help you see your future health. Just swab the inside of your cheek and send a sample to a lab, and you can find out whether your chromosomes contain risks for everything from heart disease and diabetes to cancer and Alzheimer's. Some companies will even sell you special supplements or diet programs purported to lower your risk.

Experts warn that scientists don't yet know which combinations of genetic glitches really raise your risk for serious medical conditions. Since genetic tests look for only a few genes, their results are impossible to interpret. Another problem: Many labs use their own "homebrewed" formulas for evaluating samples since the science of the personal genome is so new that no standard test procedures exist yet. The results? Murky at best. ∎

Mattresses and Pillows

We spend nearly one-third of our lives sleeping, so shouldn't we be comfortable? Too often, the wrong mattress or pillow can make sleep difficult and morning aches and pains worse. Or an invasion of pollen, dust mites, and pet dander unleashes allergic reactions just when we most need to reach slumberland. Fortunately, science has been hard at work discovering the best bed essentials for ache-free, sneeze-free snoozing.

Is a firm mattress best for a bad back?

NO It's time to rethink conventional wisdom about mattresses for aching backs. A little give, it turns out, is a good thing.

Three out of four orthopedic surgeons—the specialist docs who operate on the spines of people with the most excruciating cases of back pain—think a firm mattress is best for nighttime relief of an aching back, surveys show. But if your doctor suggests that a hard-as-a-rock bed is best, show him this: In a Spanish study of 313 people with back pain, a mattress with a little "give" to it eased aches at night, in the morning, and all day long.

While 77 percent of volunteers had some pain improvement on a hard bed, 85 percent felt better on a medium-firm bed. Medium-firm mattress sleepers also had 40 percent less pain during the day. Why? Some experts suspect that a slightly softer mattress offers better support for people whose muscles and joints are stiff. In contrast, an extra-firm mattress doesn't allow your shoulders and hips to sink in; instead, your spine

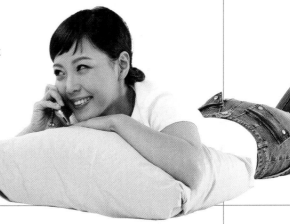

MATTRESSES AND PILLOWS

ends up bending into uncomfortable positions.

Will I sleep better on a high-tech mattress?

MAYBE High-priced mattresses are loaded with gimmicks, from double innersprings to astronaut foam. But get smart: A mid-priced bed may be just as comfortable.

If you've ever walked into a mattress showroom, you may have felt as if you were at a car dealership, complete with salesmen ready to take you for a ride. The fact is, mattresses are big business, and every manufacturer wants you to believe they're offering something special with the unique ability to transform your sleep—for a price, of course. Yet despite the hoopla about layered innersprings, "viscoelastic" polyurethane foams, latex, and air-filled adjustable chambers, the best mattress is still the one that feels right to you. And that's a very individual thing. While some back experts recommend these high-priced new mattresses, especially for people with back pain, no mattress emerged a clear winner in a *Consumer Reports* magazine test.

The choices are tantalizing. Viscoelastic, originally created by the US space program to help absorb the G-forces in astronaut's seats, promises to conform to your personal dimensions and support every "pressure point" on your body. Yet in one test, some users said it didn't cushion or support their bodies. An air-filled mattress that can be adjusted for each bed partner was deemed heavenly by some and not worth the money by others. A mattress with layered innersprings got similarly mixed reviews.

Do neck pillows ease neck pain?

YES The right pillow can help you sleep better and wake up feeling great. The catch? You'll have to try several to find the one best suited to your anatomy.

Up to 80 percent of adults endure neck pain at some point in their lives—the result of muscle injury, arthritis, osteoporosis, or simply the wear and tear associated with bad posture (hunching forward at the computer or in the car) or with aging. The good news? Several studies suggest that neck pillows can relieve the ache, though you may have to try out several types before finding the perfect one for you.

Some neck-support pillows look like standard pillows with an extension for your neck and upper spine; others are rolls or rectangular pillows with indentations for your head and firmer support for your neck. Some are made from foam or

Our BEST ADVICE

To find the best mattress for you, put on loose clothes and shoes you can kick off, then visit a mattress store. Plan to spend 15 to 20 minutes lying on each mattress: 5 minutes on each side and 5 each on your back and your stomach, if you sleep on it.

You may need a new mattress if your current bed is over 10 years old (or just 5 to 7 years if you're over 40—muscle and joint changes with age mean you may need different support) or if it's saggy. Sleep better in a hotel bed? That's another sure sign that your home mattress needs an update.

filled with water, air, buckwheat, or other materials.

In a Johns Hopkins University study of 41 chronic neck pain sufferers who tried out a roll pillow and then a water pillow for two weeks each, researchers found that half preferred the water pillow because it improved their sleep and reduced morning pain. Others preferred the roll pillow or their own standard pillow. When 52 Australians with neck pain tried out four different neck pillows plus a standard pillow, 77 percent said the neck pillows improved their sleep, and 61 percent reported fewer morning headaches. But there

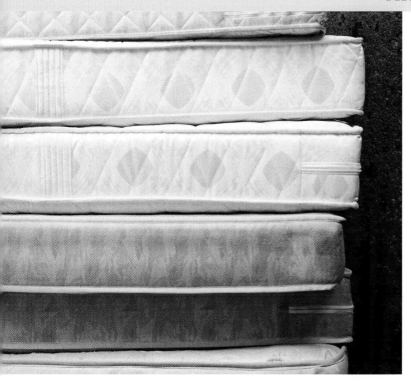

In several studies, these mite-trapping covers did little to ease the sneezing, runny nose, coughing, and watery eyes that come with a dust-mite allergy. In a Swiss study of 30 women and men with asthma, those who used anti-allergy mattress covers had lower levels of some types of dust mites on mattresses, but their lung function didn't improve, and they used "rescue" medicines—usually reserved for relief during an asthma attack—just as often as people whose beds didn't have mattress covers. Two other studies—one of 1,122 people and one of 279 women and men—found similar results: fewer mites, but no reduction in symptoms.

The covers may work better as part of a larger strategy that includes washing bedding weekly in 130°F water, lowering humidity (below 40 percent is optimal) with an air conditioner or dehumidifier, using washable area rugs instead of wall-to-wall carpeting in your bedroom, and using wood, leather, or vinyl chairs instead of mite-friendly upholstered ones. ■

was no clear winner among the pillows: Several types offered relief; volunteers simply said the best were soft and gave good support to the natural curve of the spine at the neck. Researchers suggest testing a variety of pillows for yourself.

Do anti-allergy mattress and pillow covers relieve asthma and allergy symptoms caused by dust?

NO Coverings alone can't beat the critters that provoke respiratory problems. You'll need an overall dust-mite reduction strategy.

Microscopic eight-legged dust mites thrive where there's high humidity and lots of human skin scales—the dead skin cells our bodies slough off around the clock—to eat. Their favorite haunts are pillows and mattresses, making bedtime unbearable for the millions of people allergic to the mites. But allergists' standard mite-control advice—to invest in anti-allergy covers for pillows and mattresses—won't work if it's the only step you take to discourage the critters.

SNORE-STOPPING PILLOW

Bedmates of snorers, rejoice! Someday, a computerized pillow may eliminate night noises—and let both of you sleep more soundly. Developed by a German scientist, the prototype pillow is attached to a computer that analyzes snoring patterns and adjusts air compartments inside the pillow to improve breathing and minimize snoring.

Pain-Relief Gadgets

The search for drug-free pain relief has prompted millions of people with arthritis, lower-back pain, fibromyalgia, and other chronic pain problems to experiment with everything from electricity and magnets to crystals and shoe inserts. Many makers of pain-relieving gadgets use stories of miraculous recovery to lure pain sufferers in. It's tempting, especially if you're among the many whose pain isn't fully relieved by drugs and other medical treatments. But don't be fooled—get the facts first.

Do magnets ease pain?

NO Science suggests that these pieces of metal belong on your refrigerator door, not in your medicine cabinet.

For decades, magnets have been marketed for reducing the pain of foot problems, arthritis, fibromyalgia, and other health problems. But when researchers from the Peninsula Medical School in England analyzed nine well-designed studies on magnets for pain, they found no significant reduction in aches and discomfort. In another study published in the *Journal of the American Medical Association* of 100 people with a painful foot problem called plantar fasciitis, researchers found that those who used magnetic insoles in their shoes got no extra relief.

Magnets have been touted as a pain reliever for hundreds of years. Advocates claim they boost circulation, alter nerve impulses, relax muscles, and increase levels of feel-good endorphins in the body. So far there's no proof any of these claims are true.

Can a TENS unit relieve a backache?

NO Low-voltage electricity may alter pain signals to the brain, but it doesn't seem to help relieve back pain.

For more than a decade, doctors have suggested that people with lower-back pain use a home transcutaneous electrical nerve stimulator (TENS) unit to "scramble" pain signals sent by nerves to the brain. Yet studies consistently show that this low-voltage electrical therapy doesn't really work. When researchers at the University of Ottawa analyzed five randomized controlled medical studies of people with lower-back pain who used TENS units, they found no difference between people who used real units and those who used fake ones. In another study, Canadian researchers tracked 324 people with lower-back pain who received one of three types of TENS therapy or fake TENS. None worked.

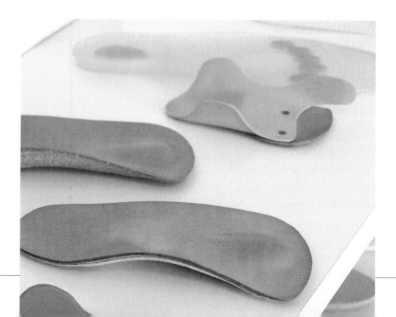

Can orthotic insoles stop knee pain?

YES "Lateral wedge" insoles keep knee joints from twisting when you walk. For some people, these special foot cushions cut knee pain significantly.

If you have medial osteoarthritis of the knee, the most common form of knee arthritis, in which the pain seems to radiate from the part of the knee near the inner thigh, a shoe insert could provide extra, drug-free pain relief. In one two-year-long study of 156 people with knee arthritis, those who wore custom-made lateral wedge insoles in their shoes took 24 percent fewer pain relievers than those who didn't wear the insoles.

These shoe inserts raise the outer edge of the foot slightly—just enough to reduce excess twisting of the bones in the knee joint. One caveat: The insoles won't help people with two other types of knee arthritis: patella femoral osteoarthritis, in which pain comes from underneath the kneecap, and lateral knee arthritis, in which pain seems to radiate from the side of the knee near the outer thigh. ∎

Sunglasses

Nothing says "cool" like a signature pair of sunglasses. But the right sunglasses have more going for them than mere fashion cachet: They protect against common vision-robbing eye conditions caused by the sun's ultraviolet rays. Over time, sunlight can raise your risk of cataracts and age-related macular degeneration, a major cause of blindness.

Are pricey sunglasses better than cheap ones?

NO Many inexpensive sunglasses work as well—or better—than high-priced brands at protecting against ultraviolet rays.

The right spectacles protect your peepers from long-term exposure to the UVA and UVB rays in sunlight—the solar radiation that raises the risk of cataracts and age-related macular degeneration (ARMD).

The proof: When scientists checked the eyes of nearly 900 Chesapeake Bay fishermen, they found that those who spent the most time in the sun were three times more likely to have vision-dimming cataracts than those who spent the least. But wearing sunglasses reduced the risk by two-thirds. Experts suspect that solar radiation alters proteins in the eye's normally crystal-clear lens, causing it to cloud. In another study, people who wore sunglasses and hats just half of the time they were out in the sun had 45 percent fewer early signs of ARMD.

You don't have to spend lots of money to get the best protection. When one Washington, DC, television station had the sun protection power of

Cheap sunglasses were just as good at blocking UVA and UVB rays as those costing 10 times more.

SUNGLASSES

4 SUNGLASS MISTAKES TO AVOID

Get the most from your sunglasses by sidestepping these pitfalls.

Relying only on contact lenses. Most contacts block less sunlight than UVB-protective sunglasses—but they do protect the sides of the eyes better than many sunglasses (except wraparound types). The best plan: contacts plus shades for more complete protection.

Not wearing a hat. A wide-brimmed hat cuts eye exposure to UVB rays by a whopping 50 percent. A hat plus sunglasses reduced risk of age-related macular degeneration by 50 percent in one 10-year-long study of 2,764 people. And in a study of 900 Chesapeake Bay shellfish harvesters, those who wore sunglasses plus brimmed hats cut cataract risk by two-thirds.

Wearing sunglasses only at midday. Japanese researchers say the sun's low angle in the morning and late afternoon is the reason study volunteers' eyes received twice as much damaging UVB radiation at 9 am and 2 pm as they did at noon.

Skipping sunglasses in the winter. Snow reflects 80 percent of sunlight—three times more than water and five times more than beach sand.

various sunglasses analyzed, they found that cheap pairs were just as good at blocking UVA and UVB rays as those costing 10 times more. As long as the label or tag says the lenses protect against 99 percent of UVB and 95 percent of UVA rays—or says "UV absorption up to 400 nm"— you're covered. (Cheaper sunglasses have the major advantage of being easily replaced when you lose them.) Steer clear of "blue-light blocking" lenses, which don't offer UV protection. And don't assume that polarized lenses meet the criteria unless they say they have extra UV-blocking material in or on them.

Are certain lens colors better for your eyes than others?

NO Whether your lenses are tinted gray, brown, or yellow doesn't make a difference in the amount of UVA or UVB light the lens filters. Nor does the darkness of the lens. Lens color might make a difference to your eye comfort, however. Gray and brown lenses distort colors the least. Yellow lenses, popular with skiers, increase contrast and work well in low light or hazy conditions. ■

Toothbrushes

Toothbrush technology has come a long way from the days of brushing with twigs or with hog's hairs attached to a bone handle. But while home dental equipment has never been better, our teeth are in greater peril than ever before thanks to high-sugar diets that "feed" the bugs that promote tooth decay and gum disease. And the stakes are higher than you may think: Gum disease has been linked to heart disease and stroke.

Do electric tooth-brushes clean better than manual toothbrushes?

YES Unless you're utterly devoted to proper brushing, do your teeth a favor and trade in your manual tooth-brush. Powering up means better cleaning for most people.

It's the rare person who faith-fully brushes his pearly whites for a full two minutes at least twice a day, paying equal attention to the fronts, backs, and chewing surfaces of all those choppers. If you're that person, a regular toothbrush is probably all you need to keep your teeth sparkling and plaque-free. But surveys show that half of us brush just once a day, and most of us devote just 46 seconds to the task.

Electric toothbrushes can help by removing more plaque. A definitive review of 42 well-designed studies involving nearly 4,000 women and men has found that an electric toothbrush with bristles that rotate in alternating directions removed 11 percent more plaque and reduced gum disease 6 percent more than manual brushes after one to three months of use. After three months, electric tooth-brush users had 17 percent less gum disease. Worried that a buzzing, whirring power brush will nick or irritate your gums? Don't be. The researchers found that manual and electric types didn't harm gums.

The catch? Only the brushes with bristles that spun in one direction and then the other (called rotation oscillation) were this effective, and these are often the most expensive kind. Ultrasonic brushes and those with brush heads that moved from side to side or rotated in only one direction were no better than a manual toothbrush. Brushes that work by "counter oscillation"—some tufts circle in one direction while others circle the other way—were just a little more effective.

Can I skip flossing if I use mouthwash?

NO Mouthwash helps, but only floss can remove hard-to-reach debris that threatens your teeth and gums.

"Swish instead of flossing!" was the surprising message that emerged just a few years ago from two studies that compared twice-daily rinses with a popular antiseptic mouthwash to once-a-day flossing. Sponsored by a mouthwash manufacturer, these small studies found that their product worked better than traditional flossing. The result: TV ads proclaiming that mouthwash beat out floss at preventing gum disease.

But don't toss that floss. A later study found that a dental-care routine featuring

Our BEST ADVICE

If you'd rather use a quiet, human-powered brush, there's no need to switch. You'll still give your mouth good care if you brush for two minutes at least twice a day, use a fluoride toothpaste, and floss afterward to remove food particles and plaque between teeth and below the gumline.

TOOTHBRUSHES

brushing, flossing, *and* rinsing with an antiseptic mouthwash cut plaque by 50 percent—better than flossing or mouthwash alone. Another reason to keep on flossing at least once a day: It's the only way to dislodge that strand of spinach that got lodged behind your right bicuspid at lunch.

Emerging evidence suggests that flossing every day can cut your risk for some surprising and life-threatening diseases elsewhere in the body. Researchers are discovering that unchecked gum disease raises levels of bacteria in the bloodstream, setting off a chemical chain reaction that increases chronic inflammation. The result is higher risk of developing the following conditions.

CLEAN—OR TOSS—A DIRTY BRUSH

A toothbrush's wet bristles can be a breeding ground for bacteria. These steps can keep brush bugs in check.

- Rinse in cool water, then store your brush in an upright position after each use so the water drains away from the bristles. Don't store a wet toothbrush in a closed case.

- Don't let the bristles of family members' brushes touch.

- After a bout with a cold, the flu, a sore throat, or mouth sores, it's best to simply replace your toothbrush or the brush head of your electric toothbrush.

- Still worried about germs? Consider dunking your brush in antimicrobial mouthwash. Studies show a 20-minute soak can eliminate germs. Don't reuse the disinfection liquid or soak more than one brush in it.

- Replace all toothbrushes every three to four months.

By the way, plenty of Internet sites suggest disinfecting your toothbrush in the microwave or dishwasher, but no well-designed studies have confirmed the benefits, and these methods may damage the bristles.

Atherosclerosis: When scientists at Columbia University Medical Center measured the bacteria levels in the mouths of 657 people, they found that high bacterial counts were directly related to the thickness of the carotids, major arteries in the neck. Thickened carotids raise the risk of heart attack and stroke.

Chronic obstructive pulmonary disease (COPD): When scientists checked the dental records and respiratory health of 13,792 women and men, they found that those with more signs of gum disease were 1 1/2 times more likely to develop COPD—a set of lung problems including

bronchitis and emphysema—and more likely to have breathing problems.

Stroke: In a study of 771 people, researchers found that severe gum disease quadrupled stroke risk. ■

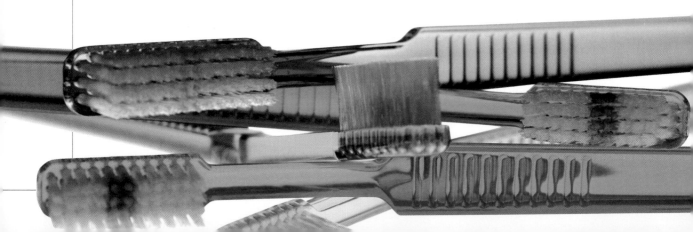

Vacuum Cleaners

Buying a device to suck up dust and dirt (a huge portion of which is made of sloughed-off human skin cells!) has never been so complicated. You can choose one that promises extra suction or allergen filtering. You can even opt for a robotic vacuum that does the work for you. But good luck finding a machine that really gets your floors and carpets clean and keeps the dirt in the vacuum where it belongs.

Do anti-allergy vacuum cleaners keep dust and dander out of the air?

NO Vacuums with allergy filters aren't perfect—and many vacuums spew almost as much dust and dirt as they suck up.

If you're allergic to dust mites, pollen, or pet dander, you've no doubt heard the advertising claims about the wonders of vacuum cleaners equipped with high-tech HEPA (high-efficiency particulate air) filters. These systems are sometimes touted to remove 100 percent of the microscopic nasties that provoke coughing, sneezing, watering eyes, and even full-fledged asthma attacks. But scientific research suggests otherwise.

When British researchers wearing particle-trapping devices in their nostrils tested old vacuum cleaners and new HEPA-equipped models in homes, they found that all types sent clouds of cat dander and dust mites flying into the air—and into their respiratory systems. Even more particles wafted into their noses when they changed the filter bags or emptied the machines.

Floor coverings like wall-to-wall carpet and area rugs are the single largest "reservoirs" of sneeze-producing particles in your home. Studies conflict about whether vacuuming really removes any of these allergens at all. In one, researchers found that vacuuming redistributed dust and dander built up in older rugs. Another found that vacuuming released a whopping 90 percent of small-diameter cat dander particles into the air. But one, conducted in 60 homes over the course of a year, found that regular vacuuming—with a standard machine or a HEPA model—cut levels of cat dander by about 50 percent in carpets and upholstered sofas. Levels fell by 80 percent in mattresses. Dog dander levels fell, too—and standard machines often did a better job. The downside? While vacuuming may have helped with pet dander, it increased levels of dust mites.

Do new high-suction vacuum cleaners do a better job?

NO Real-world tests show that lower-priced machines often work better.

Despite manufacturer's claims, several head-to-head tests of vacuum cleaners have found that expensive, bag-free machines purported to "never lose suction" were outperformed by less expensive models. While these vacs cleaned carpeting well, they left dust and dirt on bare floors and were unexceptional when it came to sucking up pet hair. One model didn't lose suction, but reviewers noted that it had less dirt-removal power to begin with. Another reviewer said that his machine leaked clouds of dust when he tried to empty it. Your best bet: Consult an up-to-date consumer review for the latest ratings before you buy. ∎

Water Filters

Even crystal-clear, odor-free, good-tasting tap water can be hazardous to your health. In one major analysis, 22 of 25 American cities had water quality problems such as high levels of lead, chlorine, or bacteria. Thanks to old pipes, over- or undertreatment, and runoff from farm fields, highways, and industries, your water's vulnerable. Bottled water may be no safer, experts say. The answer? A water filter, but only if you choose the right one.

Will water filters make your water safer?

YES Some are great at removing lead, others at ousting disease-causing microbes. The key is to know which one you need.

Home water filters range from pitchers fitted with activated-carbon "strainers" to whole-house systems. Most are quite effective, studies show. But no filter system is capable of removing every contaminant, off taste, and unpleasant odor from tap water. The key is knowing what's in your water, then choosing a filter that can get it out.

How important is the right filter? Consider this: When the city of Milwaukee experienced a massive outbreak of water-borne cryptosporidium infection in 1993, residents who used extra-fine carbon filters (called submicron filters) had 96 percent less diarrhea than those who sipped unfiltered tap water or

used filters with bigger holes, which let this tiny microorganism slip through. And in a study of people with weakened immune systems, those who purified their water with carbon filters plus ultraviolet light disinfection were three times less likely to have gastrointestinal illnesses than those who drank untreated tap water.

Local water-treatment authorities often make annual reports on water quality available to their customers. But if you have a private well or can't get a free report, you may have to pay for a water

test by a private company. Ask for a basic test that looks for arsenic, bacteria, chlorine, copper, lead, manganese, nitrates and nitrites, and sodium. Recheck for bacteria and nitrates/nitrites (from agricultural runoff) every year and for other compounds every three years. Test for radon and volatile organic compounds from gasoline and industrial solvents every three to five years.

If the results show a problem, find the filter best suited to removing it. If all's well, but you're dissatisfied with your water's taste or smell, an activated-carbon filter may be all you need. If there's chemical contamination, consider reverse osmosis, a type of filter system. For bacteria, a submicron filter or ultraviolet disinfection may be good choices. See the chart at right for more details. ■

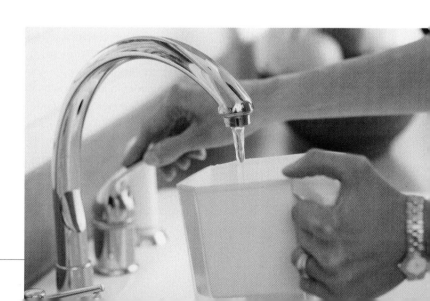

Water Filters

Activated Carbon Filter

How it works: Positively charged, highly absorbent carbon in the filter attracts and traps many impurities.

Type of system: Pitchers, water bottles with filter inserts, faucet attachments, countertop and under-sink units.

What it removes: Bad tastes and odors, including chlorine. Some also reduce contaminantssuch as heavy metals (copper, lead, and mercury), parasites (giardia and cryptosporidium), pesticides, radon, and volatile organic chemicals (methyl-tert-butyl ether, or MTBE, and dichlorobenzene and trichloroethylene, or TCE).

Disadvantage: Bacteria can grow on these filters overnight, even on "bacteriostatic" types that claim to resist bacterial growth. Follow the manufacturer's directions for flushing the filter regularly.

Anion Exchange

How it works: Water passes through a resin bed, which removes certain minerals.

Type of system: Whole-house unit that cleans water before it's sent to faucets throughout your home.

What it removes: Nitrates, nitrites, fluorides, sulfates, and bicarbonates.

Disadvantage: Water may taste salty.

Cation Exchange Softener

How it works: "Softens" hard water by swapping minerals with a strong positive charge for ones with a lower charge.

Type of system: Whole-house unit.

What it removes: Calcium and magnesium, which form deposits in plumbing and fixtures, plus barium.

Disadvantage: Increases sodium in water.

Distiller

How it works: Water is heated to the boiling point and vapor is collected as it condenses.

Type of system: Whole-house unit.

What it removes: Disease-causing microorganisms, heavy metals, and most chemicals (volatile organic chemicals such as gasoline, as well as radon, may remain in drinking water).

Disadvantage: Gives water a bland taste because it removes many minerals.

Ultraviolet Disinfection

How it works: Water is exposed to ultraviolet light from a mercury vapor lamp.

Type of system: Under-sink unit, often combined with a carbon filter.

What it removes: Bacteria and parasites such as cryptosporidium and giardia.

Disadvantage: You'll also need a filter to strain out sediment, heavy metals, pesticides, and volatile organic compounds.

Reverse Osmosis

How it works: A semipermeable membrane separates impurities from water.

Type of system: Under-sink units as well as whole-house system.

What it removes: Pesticides; heavy metals such as cadmium, copper, lead, and mercury; and other pollutants, including arsenic, barium, nitrates/nitrites, perchlorate, and selenium.

Disadvantage: Uses lots of water, and only 10 to 30 percent is released as treated drinkable water; won't remove microbes.

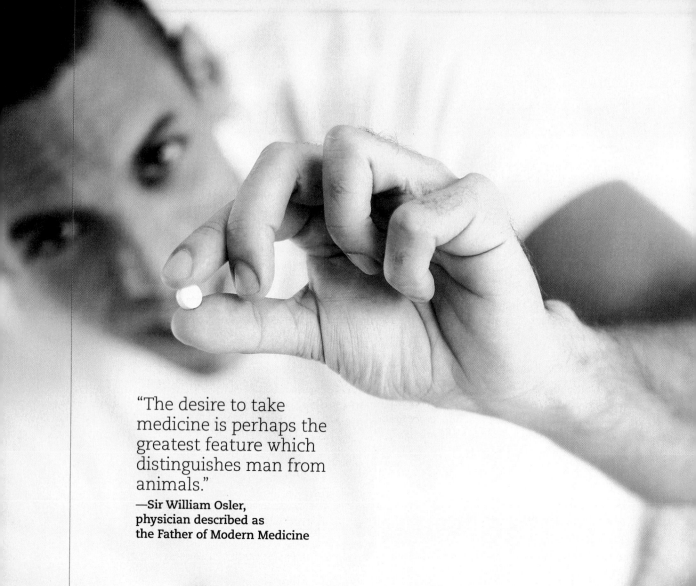

"The desire to take medicine is perhaps the greatest feature which distinguishes man from animals."
—Sir William Osler, physician described as the Father of Modern Medicine

in your
medicine
cabinet

Acetaminophen

If you have a bottle of this stuff in your medicine cabinet, it's likely to be hidden behind the aspirin and ibuprofen. There are instances when it may be the best choice, however. Acetaminophen first became widely available in 1955 with the introduction of Tylenol Elixir, which was sold by prescription and marketed as a children's medication that was gentler on the stomach than aspirin. Within a few years, Tylenol and other acetaminophen-based drugs were on sale over the counter and quickly became popular general-purpose pain relievers.

Is acetaminophen weaker than other over-the-counter pain relievers?

YES Although you may want to keep acetaminophen on hand, NSAIDs have the edge when it comes to relieving most varieties of pain.

Studies show that acetaminophen relieves pain about as well as another old standby, aspirin. Most research, however, shows that NSAIDs, such as ibuprofen, are more powerful than both. For instance, one study of 455 patients with tension headaches found that a single dose of ibuprofen (400 milligrams) produced greater pain relief, faster, than a dose of acetaminophen (1,000 milligrams). Also, a recent review of 15 studies involving nearly 6,000 people with osteoarthritis in the knee or hip found that people who took NSAIDs like ibuprofen (not aspirin) had less pain than others who took acetaminophen. Asked to rate their pain on a scale of 0 to 100, patients using NSAIDs ranked their discomfort six points lower than patients taking acetaminophen. NSAID users had less stiffness and greater mobility, too.

Is acetaminophen sometimes the better choice?

YES It's safest for people with stomach problems and for treating fever in kids and teens.

Acetaminophen may be best for people who can't tolerate NSAIDs (which also include naproxen sodium, ketoprofen, and others), since these drugs can cause a range of gastrointestinal problems, from heartburn to stomach bleeding and even ulcers in some people. Doctors may also advise patients who have poor kidney function to use acetaminophen instead of NSAIDs.

It's also the best choice for lowering fevers in children and teenagers, since aspirin may trigger a rare but potentially fatal disorder called Reyes' syndrome.

It's worth noting that some doctors think it's a mistake to treat fever in the first place. After all, the toasty internal temperature produced when you have a fever helps your body kill off germs that cause infections. However, treating fever usually makes patients feel better. If you take acetaminophen or give a dose to a child to treat fever associated with a virus, keep in mind that some cold remedies contain the drug, too, and be careful not to overdose. ■

Acetaminophen may be best for people who can't tolerate NSAIDs like ibuprofen.

Antibiotic Ointments

It used to be that when we got a cut or scrape, we'd wash it and stick on a bandage. Today people are likely to add a third step to that process, applying an antibiotic ointment to the wound. But are we going overboard, or do these ointments really provide a benefit?

Does antibiotic cream make wounds heal faster?

YES But it may be the cream, not the antibiotics, that does the trick.

Applying antibiotic cream to a cut or wound appears to speed the healing process. One study of 48 people with infected skin blisters found that a commonly used ointment (Neosporin) healed the wounds faster than an antiseptic treatment containing hydrogen peroxide. In the same study, however, a nonantibiotic first aid cream worked better than the peroxide, too.

"It's not entirely clear whether antibiotics actually help with wound healing," explains Stanford University dermatologist Hayes Gladstone, MD. Instead, the protective cover the cream or ointment provides may encourage cells to build "bridges" to one another, the process by which skin repairs itself.

Our BEST ADVICE

All out of antibiotic ointment? Try honey. Traditional doctors have long recommended the sweet, sticky stuff for treating skin injuries. Lab research shows that honey does indeed block the growth of bacteria. A 2001 review found that six out of seven studies showed honey to be an effective treatment for healing wounds and eradicating infections.

Do the creams reduce scarring?

MAYBE Makers of some antibiotic ointments claim that their products minimize scarring. While no over-the-counter salve can *prevent* scars, Dr. Gladstone says applying an antibiotic cream may help smooth them over somewhat. Once again, however, the effect probably isn't due to the antibiotics. Instead, the cream keeps the wound moist, which may have the added benefit of softening a scar's appearance.

Should you use the creams?

YES With concerns about the rising problem of antibiotic resistance, why use one of these ointments at all? The answer: To prevent the number one complication that may occur when you have a cut or wound—infection. No matter how commendable your personal hygiene may be, everyone has bacteria on their skin. A cut or wound is an open door for these germs, so applying antibiotic cream makes sense. One study found that only about 5 percent of skin wounds treated with antibiotic therapy became infected compared with nearly 18 percent treated with petroleum jelly. ■

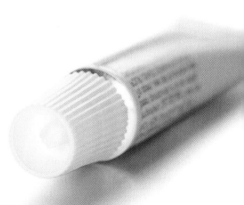

Antifungals

You may think that diabetes and heart disease are the epidemics of our day, but just as many people will fall prey to a highly annoying, albeit less dangerous, plague sometime in their lives: fungus. The kind that infects our skin and nails has seemingly driven us to desperation.

Do over-the-counter products for athlete's foot and jock itch work?

YES Some studies show that over-the-counter products work just as well as prescription creams.

You don't need to be a gym rat to develop athlete's foot or jock itch, though the fungi that cause these conditions do thrive in warm, damp environments, such as gyms, locker rooms, and swimming pools. Sweat and friction (from the straps of an athletic supporter rubbing against the skin, for example) are contributors, too.

Athlete's foot and jock itch are caused by fungi known collectively as tinea. Although its appearance and symptoms vary depending on which body part it afflicts, tinea generally causes skin to become red, itchy, scaly, and cracked. Athlete's foot usually affects the skin between the toes but can spread and infect the nails. Jock itch arises in the groin.

Over-the-counter antifungal creams, gels, and sprays such as clotrimazole (Lotrimin), miconazole (Desenex), and terbinafine (Lamisil AT) can be effective treatments, though they aren't necessarily cure-alls. In some studies, antifungals have eliminated symptoms and signs of tinea infections in 80 to 90 percent of users, though in other studies, the products seemed to work about half the time. A recent review determined that terbinafine may be the most effective choice for athlete's foot.

Can over-the-counter creams and ointments eliminate nail infections?

NO These treatments don't penetrate the surface of the nail, so they have little or no effect.

The same family of fungi that causes athlete's foot is the culprit behind the stubborn nail disorder known as onychomycosis, which leaves fingernails and toenails yellowed, thickened, and brittle. So if you can clear up athlete's foot with antifungal cream, getting rid of a nail infection should be a snap, right?

Wrong. Unfortunately, fungus infects nails beneath the hard exterior, which creams can't penetrate. Most dermatologists agree that fungus treatments have no effect on nail infections. (Truth-in-advertising alert: Some fungus treatments that have the word *nail* in their names state in small print on their labels that they are *not* effective for nail infections.)

What does work? The prescription antifungal ciclopirox (Penlac), a lacquer that's painted onto the nail and seems to penetrate the surface, may provide short-term relief if applied daily. But you must be persistent—it may take months before you see any improvement. And ciclopirox doesn't prevent nail infections from returning, which they often do.

Prescription pills containing fungus-fighting medication are more effective, eliminating about 50 percent of nail infections. However, these drugs can cause unpleasant side effects, such as headaches, nausea, and insomnia, and can even harm the liver. Antifungal medications can interact with several drugs, too, including blood thinners and birth control pills. To prevent nail infections, keep your hands and feet clean and dry. ∎

Antihistamines

If your nose runs, your eyes itch, or you break out in hives because of pollen, dust, or any other allergen, you can blame histamine. Your immune system produces this chemical to help combat allergy-causing substances that enter the body, but it can also trigger unpleasant symptoms. Antihistamines were discovered by accident and first went on sale in the 1940s. Recently a new generation of these histamine blockers, with fewer side effects, has flooded the market.

Do newer, "nondrowsy" antihistamines work as well as older formulas?

NO They are safer, however, because you're less likely to doze off at the wheel.

For decades, the only antihistamines on the market were strong—and sedating—drugs such as brompheniramine (Dimetapp and others) and diphenhydramine (Benadryl). But now there are "second-generation" antihistamines such as loratadine (Claritin), which is available over the counter in some countries; fexofenadine (Allegra); and cetirizine (Zyrtec).

Doctors and pharmacists, as well as many of their patients, generally agree that the older drugs do a better job of erasing allergy symptoms. The few head-to-head comparisons that have been conducted tend to support that impression. A 1998 study found that the active ingredient in Dimetapp dried up runny noses and prevented sneezing more effectively than the active ingredient in Claritin, for example. A more recent study of 610 patients with moderate to severe allergies found that the active ingredient in Benadryl reduced nasal symptoms by 78 percent, compared to 21 percent for desloratadine (Clarinex).

However, these studies also underscored a well-known downside to the older drugs: They were far more likely to make people sleepy. These medications are made up of small molecules that pass easily through the blood-brain barrier, the layer of tightly packed blood vessels that controls which substances enter the brain. As a result, the older antihistamines cause drowsiness and poor concentration in 20 to 35 percent of users (though in some users, the sedating effects subside over time).

Second-generation antihistamines are made up of larger molecules that are less likely to cross the blood-brain barrier and cause drowsiness. In simulated driving tests, some people given first-generation antihistamines drive as though they have had a few cocktails, while subjects given the newer medications show little or no sign of impairment.

For some consumers, the older antihistamines remain attractive since they are cheaper and don't require a prescription. Most allergists, however, recommend trying the newer antihistamines first and using the older drugs only if all other treatments fail or if you won't endanger yourself and others by being drowsy.

Our BEST ADVICE

Take an antihistamine *before* you are exposed to an allergen instead of waiting until the sneezing fits and watery eyes begin. For example, if you're allergic to ragweed, start taking antihistamines before pollen season begins. If you're allergic to animal dander, take an antihistamine a few hours before visiting your friend the cat lover.

ANTIHISTAMINES

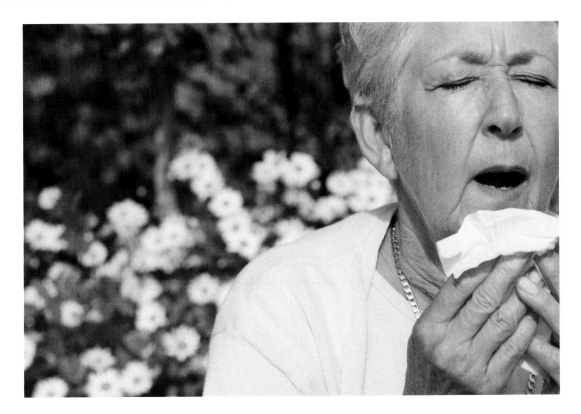

Some doctors and pharmacists recommend using loratadine or some other new-style antihistamine during the day and one of the older types at night. (Be careful, though: Taking a first-generation antihistamine at bedtime may leave you feeling sleepy the next day.)

Are allergy medications and cold remedies useful as sleep aids?

YES If you choose an older antihistamine like Benadryl, that is. But beware: These drugs actually keep some people awake.

Most over-the-counter sleep aids are actually antihistamines, usually either diphenhydramine, the stuff in Benadryl, or doxylamine, the drug in Vicks Nyquil and other "nighttime" cold remedies and pain relievers that makes you drowsy.

So, if you can't sleep some night, is it okay to pop an allergy pill or knock back some nighttime cold medicine? The latter is a bad idea, since the product is likely to contain other medicines you don't need. The allergy pill may help—but only certain people. For others, it may backfire. These drugs tend not to have a sedative effect on Asians, for instance. Oddly enough, some people (especially children and the elderly) respond to a dose of Benadryl as though they just gulped down a triple espresso, leaving them very much awake.

Antihistamines can worsen symptoms of glaucoma, chronic bronchitis, and difficulty urinating due to an enlarged prostate gland. If you have chronic insomnia, you're better off finding out what's causing it and addressing the root problem. ∎

Aspirin

Aspirin may have been the only pain reliever your parents kept in their medicine chest. It's no longer the first choice against aches, pains, and fever, however. Most people today turn to ibuprofen and other newer pain pills. Nonetheless, aspirin is still a top seller, thanks to the discovery that it lowers the risk of heart attacks.

Should everyone take aspirin to prevent heart attacks?

NO Doctors recommend daily aspirin only for people who have an increased risk of heart attacks and strokes, and women may not benefit as much as men.

When you have a headache or sore muscles from gardening, aspirin relieves the misery by blocking production of hormone-like substances called prostaglandins. In addition to sending pain signals to the brain, prostaglandins cause blood platelets to bunch together and form clots. Because aspirin blocks the formation of clots in arteries, doctors have been recommending daily aspirin as preventive therapy to patients at high risk for heart attacks since the 1970s.

Since then, aspirin has saved many lives. A 2002 analysis of 287 studies found that aspirin reduces the risk of heart attacks, strokes, and death by about 25 percent. However, doctors don't tell all of their patients to pop an aspirin with their morning juice because the little white tablets are not entirely benign. Aspirin blocks prostaglandins that protect the stomach lining, so some people who take it regularly develop ulcers and stomach bleeding.

Furthermore, certain people—especially women—may not gain as much heart protection from aspirin as doctors once thought. In one major study of 40,000 women 45 and older, there was no overall difference in the number of heart attacks or the risk of dying of any form of cardiovascular disease between those who took 100 milligrams of aspirin every other day for 10 years and those who took a placebo for 10 years.

Aspirin users did have 17 percent fewer ischemic strokes, the most common type, which are caused by blocked arteries in the brain. However, they had slightly *more* hemorrhagic strokes, which are caused by bleeding

in the brain. Furthermore, women in the aspirin group were 40 percent more likely to develop stomach bleeding.

Could I be "resistant" to aspirin?

YES Aspirin does not protect everyone who takes the pills from having heart attacks. Some people have a condition called aspirin resistance.

Imagine two groups of people who have high cholesterol, high blood pressure, and other risk factors for heart attacks. The people in one group take aspirin every day, while the others do not. Over time, there will be about 25 percent fewer heart attacks among members of the aspirin group. While that's valuable protection, it's far from a guarantee. Aspirin prevents clots in the arteries—the culprit behind most heart attacks—so why isn't this drug even more powerful?

There are a number of reasons why aspirin may fail to prevent heart attacks. For example, taking ibuprofen or other anti-inflammatory drugs at the same time blocks aspirin's effect on blood platelets. What's more, some people are born resistant to aspirin's anti-clotting effects. A recent review estimated that about one person in four is aspirin resistant. (The true number could be higher or lower, since there is not yet an agreed-upon definition of the phenomenon.) Even if you have aspirin resistance, though, the drug will still work as a pain reliever.

Some doctors have begun using new aspirin-resistance tests to determine whether heart patients will benefit from taking the drug or if they might be better off taking a more powerful anti-clotting medication such as clopidogrel (Plavix). However, other doctors say it's too soon to know whether the tests are accurate or if enough people have aspirin resistance to warrant routine testing. ■

KEEP YOUR MEDICINE HEALTHY

Don't let the name fool you: The medicine chest in your bathroom is a great place to store toothpaste and moisturizer—but *not* medicine. Medications are formulated to be stored at room temperature in a dry place. Most bathrooms are warm and damp, which can cause some drugs to break down and lose potency. In most homes, the bedroom is a better choice.

Always check the expiration date on the label before you take any drug or supplement, and throw out any that are outdated. But keep in mind that the expiration date represents the manufacturer's estimate of how long the medication or supplement will maintain its potency under *ideal circumstances*—that is, stored in the original container at room temperature in a dry place. No matter what the expiration date is, toss the medicine if:

- Its color has changed.

- Its texture or consistency has changed (tablets may start to crumble or crystallize, for example).

- It has a strong odor (for instance, outdated aspirin smells like vinegar).

- Any other change in appearance has occurred (such as a liquid developing floating particles).

If you take medicine and discover later that it had expired, don't panic. Outdated medicine is very unlikely to make you sick unless it's long past its expiration date, and even then, you probably won't have any problems.

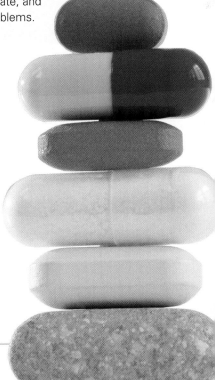

CALCIUM SUPPLEMENTS

Calcium Supplements

Bones are complex structures, and keeping them sturdy and strong requires a diet that provides adequate levels of several key nutrients. For preventing osteoporosis, though, it's calcium that's gotten the most attention. As a result, many people now take calcium supplements to prevent bone fractures. But who should take them, and how, remains a bit of a mystery.

Should everyone take calcium supplements?

NO Doctors often recommend calcium supplements to build stronger bones. But the benefits appear to be modest, so think twice before adding the pills to your daily regimen.

Providing your body with a steady supply of calcium is essential for healthy bones. Yet debate persists over the benefits of taking supplements to strengthen bones and prevent fractures, largely because the results of studies have been inconsistent.

Recently, a team of Australian researchers attempted to clear the air by analyzing 29 studies on calcium and bones. They determined that people over 50 who took calcium supplements, either alone or in combination with vitamin D, reduced the risk of broken bones, but only by 12 percent. However, it's well known that people who volunteer for studies often neglect to take their pills every day. In studies where compliance was high, the reduction in fractures was 24 percent.

Some people appear to gain more benefit than others. As the study authors note, those who gained the most bone protection were people whose diets were low in calcium to begin with, people over 80, and people who lived in nursing homes or other institutions. More modest reductions in the risk of fractures occurred in people under 70 (3 percent reduced risk), people whose diets included a normal amount of calcium (5 percent reduced risk), and people who did not live in institutions (6 percent).

Whether you should take calcium supplements is a decision for you and your doctor. It's important to consider that they are not necessarily harmless. They may cause constipation and increase the risk of kidney stones. And several disturbing—if inconclusive—studies have shown that men who consume high amounts of calcium have an increased risk of prostate cancer.

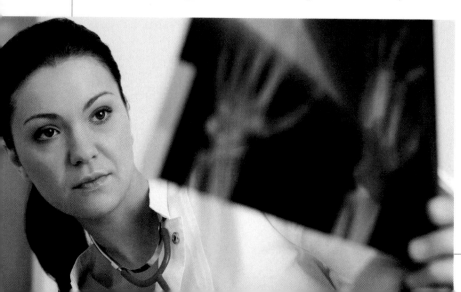

CALCIUM SUPPLEMENTS

Is it okay to take calcium-based antacids instead of calcium supplements?

YES For most people, common antacids can be a cheaper alternative to calcium supplements, though some may benefit by spending the extra money.

Among its many roles in the human body, calcium builds bones and neutralizes stomach acid, which can help to cool heartburn. In fact, the active ingredient in many popular antacid tablets (including Tums and Rolaids) is calcium carbonate—the same ingredient as in some calcium supplements, which cost more. But not everyone who needs extra calcium can take advantage of the bargain, because calcium carbonate can cause gastrointestinal side effects in some people, such as gas, bloating, and constipation. They may be better off using supplements that contain calcium citrate, which do not cause GI symptoms. Because the body absorbs it more readily, calcium citrate may also be a better choice for older people, whose stomachs produce less acid, which is necessary to absorb calcium. Or they can overcome the problem by taking calcium carbonate with a meal.

Should you buy a calcium supplement with added vitamin D and magnesium?

MAYBE Calcium isn't the only nutrient that's essential to sturdy bones. However, it's not clear whether everyone will benefit from high doses of vitamin D and magnesium.

No matter what form of calcium pill you take, it won't do much good if you're low on vitamin D, which stimulates the intestines to absorb calcium. It has become increasingly evident that adequate vitamin D is essential for preventing osteoporosis—not to mention various cancers.

Does that mean that vitamin D supplements prevent fractures? That's still not clear. A review in the *Journal of the American Medical Association* found that people who took high daily doses (700 to 800 IU) reduced their risk of hip fractures by 26 percent and fractures of bones other than vertebrae by 23 percent. But the authors of another study, which reviewed the best research available, noted that the strongest evidence of D's power to prevent broken bones comes from studies involving institutionalized patients, who presumably remain indoors much of the time and aren't exposed to the sunlight that helps the body make vitamin D.

Our BEST ADVICE

Get the most from your calcium supplements by following these rules.

- Take calcium carbonate with a meal to ensure that it is well absorbed. (You can take calcium citrate anytime.)
- Don't take more than 500 milligrams of calcium at a time, since the body can't absorb more than that.
- When possible, avoid taking calcium supplements after eating a high-fiber meal, which may interfere with how well they are absorbed.
- Talk to your doctor if you take any drug that suppresses production of stomach acid, such as the H2 blocker ranitidine (Zantac) or the proton-pump inhibitor omeprazole (Prilosec). They may prevent your body from adequately absorbing calcium.

People who get even a little sunlight, according to the researchers, probably get enough D to absorb their calcium. Still, some experts think that supplementing with D is a smart move.

What about magnesium? Some studies suggest that women with osteoporosis have low levels of the mineral. But a normal diet provides an adequate supply. ■

Cold Medicines

They were staples of medicine chests around the world for decades, but cold remedies have suddenly become controversial. In recent years, various products have made headlines, usually the kind the pharmaceutical industry would prefer to avoid. As a result, consumers are left wondering whether the old standbys they have long relied on to relieve a stuffed-up nose or quell a cough are safe—or if they even work.

Do cold medicines that don't contain pseudoephedrine still work?

NO Alternatives to products containing pseudoephedrine just aren't very effective.

For years, congested consumers have turned to cold medicines containing pseudoephedrine to relieve blocked nasal passages. But this highly effective ingredient has a dark side: It can be used to manufacture the illegal stimulant drug methamphetamine. Because drug dealers were purchasing or stealing large amounts of pseudoephedrine from pharmacies and other retailers, some countries now limit the sale of products containing it. In the United States, stores must keep pseudoephedrine products behind the counter. Consumers can purchase only small amounts at a time and must show identification.

In response to these restrictions, drug companies reformulated many cold remedies by replacing pseudoephedrine with another decongestant, phenylephrine. Consumers can easily find them on store shelves—but maybe they shouldn't bother.

Doctors and pharmacists say that legions of people have come forward complaining that these cold remedies don't work—and studies suggest they're right. One review of

eight studies found that the legally allowed dose of phenylephrine in the United States (10 milligrams) does nothing to unblock clogged nasal passages.

The pseudoephedrine controversy may have a silver lining. "You're probably better off not using an oral decongestant anyway," says University of Florida professor of pharmacy Randy C. Hatton, author of the review of eight studies. Decongestants work by causing blood vessels to

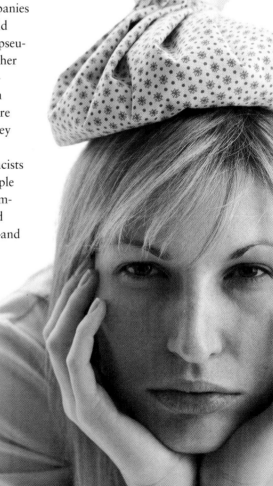

constrict. Taken in pill form, they have this effect throughout the body, which can slow circulation and raise blood pressure. To clear a stuffy nose, Dr. Hatton recommends nasal sprays containing phenylephrine or oxymetazoline (which is longer lasting), since they act directly on the blood vessels in the nasal passages. As you will read in the Nasal Sprays entry (page 212), however, these products should be used only for short-term relief.

When choosing a cold or flu remedy, do more ingredients mean faster, stronger relief?

NO Many cold and flu remedies include several different drugs, each intended to treat different symptoms. But if you don't have *all* of those symptoms, more isn't better.

When it comes to battling a nasty case of the sniffles or a raging bout with the flu, mercy is not an option—you want to clobber the bug with all the ammo you can get your hands on. But before you reach for a pill that contains every symptom buster under the sun, make sure you actually have all those symptoms. These pills and elixirs often contain a pain reliever such as acetaminophen for

aches and fever, an antihistamine for a runny nose, a decongestant for a stuffy nose, and a cough suppressant and/or expectorant. Taking one at night should help you get some rest, if nothing else— if the antihistamine doesn't knock you out, just reading the ingredient list will probably put you to sleep.

If your main problem is congestion, however, does it make sense to use a multisymptom product? "If you don't have fever or pain, why are you taking acetaminophen?" asks Katherine Hillblom, PharmD, a spokesperson for the American Pharmacists Association. Dr. Hillblom rarely recommends multisymptom remedies, since they may expose the user to drugs that won't help and, in some cases, could harm. People who take more than one medication when they have a cold or the flu may be getting acetaminophen or other drugs from more than one source and neglect to add up their daily dose, she notes.

Does cough syrup work?

NO If you have always kept your medicine chest stocked with these syrups, you may have coughed up a lot of money for nothing.

When the leaves are off the trees and the air turns nippy, that means the sound of coughing probably isn't far off in many households. To relieve

If you choose to try cough medicine, don't buy combination products that contain a cough suppressant *and* an expectorant. There is no evidence that either one relieves a cough, but that's only part of the problem. Expectorants are supposed to increase the amount of mucus in your airways, making it easier to cough up, yet a suppressant blunts the impulse to cough, which could cause the airways to become obstructed.

the hacking, many people rely on bottles of colorful—and often vile-tasting—cough syrup. However, many doctors now say that most cough remedies aren't worth using.

One of the first blows against the reputation of these widely used medicines came in 1997, when the American Academy of Pediatrics warned parents that there is no evidence that cough suppressants such as codeine and dextromethorphan work for children. A few years later, in 2001, a review of 15 studies published in the *British Medical Journal* cast doubt on whether *any* form of cough medicine is effective for children or adults. Then, in 2006, the American College of Chest Physicians discouraged the use of cough remedies containing suppressants and expectorants on the grounds that there's no proof they do anything.

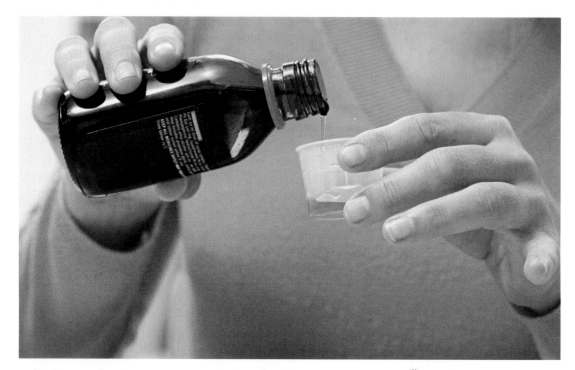

What does help? The only over-the-counter treatments the ACCP recommends for coughs caused by the common cold are antihistamine-decongestant combinations. However, only older antihistamines, such as brompheniramine (Dimetapp), seem to help, and these medications may cause drowsiness. (If the label says "nonsedating," the product won't relieve coughing.) Inhaling steam from a vaporizer and drinking plenty of fluids may help loosen mucus in the lungs, making it easier to cough up.

Do cold medicines work for small children?

NO Although parents have relied on these remedies, there is no evidence that they relieve cold symptoms in small children, and they aren't without risks.

The news stunned parents: In 2007, a panel of experts appointed by the FDA declared that children under age six should not be given cold or cough medicines. The reason: Very few scientific studies have shown that these remedies relieve cold symptoms in small children; in fact, they have proven no more effective than placebos.

This knowledge isn't new. But as evidence that these products pose a threat emerged, health officials began to take notice. A report by the Centers for Disease Control and Prevention found that more than 1,500 children under age two in the United States required emergency treatment for

Our**BEST**
...**ADVICE**

What's a parent of a sniffling, hacking child to do? Make sure the child drinks plenty of fluids and consider putting a humidifier in her bedroom. Give acetaminophen or ibuprofen (not aspirin) for a fever. And sit tight—a cold or cough usually lasts only a few days.

illnesses caused by cough and cold medicines during 2004 and 2005. Three of the children died. Many of these cases involved accidental overdose, which doctors say often occurs because parents administer more than one cold remedy that contains the same drug.

Some parents may wonder: Who cares if there's no

Cabinet Shakeup: Do You Need These?

Here are five over-the-counter products found in many medicine cabinets
that doctors say should be used sparingly, if at all.

1

Hydrocortisone Cream
Used to treat skin inflammation and itchiness from poison ivy, hemorrhoids, and other problems.

The problem: Although it's safe for occasional use, applying hydrocortisone regularly over long periods may thin the skin. Also, the cream won't help a persistent rash.

The alternative: Ordinary moisturizing cream may help relieve mild skin discomfort. If you have a serious skin rash, see a doctor, who can prescribe stronger medication.

2

Hydrogen Peroxide
Used for many purposes, including as a disinfectant for cuts and wounds.

The problem: Hydrogen peroxide actually slows wound healing by preventing inflammatory cells from repairing damaged tissue.

The alternative: Rinsing a cut with water is often all that's necessary. Applying an antibiotic ointment can help. Doctors may recommend using small amounts of hydrogen peroxide solution to treat surgical wounds.

3

Ipecac Syrup
Induces vomiting; once widely recommended for treating accidental poisoning.

The problem: There is no evidence that giving ipecac syrup to victims of poisoning saves lives. Some swallowed toxins may actually be more damaging if vomited. In 2003, the American Academy of Pediatrics recommended against its use.

The alternative: Call your local poison control center (keep the number near the telephone). If someone you believe has been poisoned has convulsions, stops breathing, or loses consciousness, call your local emergency responder.

4

Laxatives
A variety of products designed to make stools easier to pass.

The problem: Frequent use of laxatives can lead to dependence. A strong laxative may empty the intestines, resulting in no need for a bowel movement the next day. Some people interpret this as a sign of constipation, so they take more.

The alternative: Eat a high-fiber diet. Don't use a laxative just because you haven't had a bowel movement for a day—that's normal. See a doctor if you have chronic constipation.

5

Over-the-Counter Sleep Aids
Most of these products contain antihistamines, which cause drowsiness.

The problem: Sleep aids increase shuteye time by minutes, at most, and may lose effectiveness with repeated use. Side effects include dry mouth, dizziness, and fatigue when you awake. Antihistamines make some people jittery and anxious.

The alternative: Improve your "sleep hygiene." Go to bed and wake up at the same hour every day. Avoid daytime naps. Exercise regularly, but not before bedtime. Instead, take a warm bath or listen to soft music.

Cold Medicines
(continued)

evidence that cold remedies ease my kid's colds? At least they help them sleep. To be sure, some cold medicines contain antihistamines that act as sedatives, which may allow the sick child—and everyone else in the house—to get some rest. But at what risk?

"Sedatives are designed to depress your consciousness," says Michael Shannon, MD, professor and chair of emergency medicine at Children's Hospital in Boston and one of several pediatricians who sent a petition to the FDA asking it to reconsider its approval of children's cold remedies. Children, explains Dr. Shannon, are unusually vulnerable to problems linked to excess sedation, such as sleep apnea. Furthermore, a heavily sedated child who develops stomach problems in the night may not awaken and could choke on his own vomit. Other doctors note that the decongestant pseudoephedrine could worsen undiagnosed heart problems in a young child. ■

Diarrhea Medicines

Diarrhea has many causes. Viral infections and contaminated food are two common triggers, but certain medications, various gastrointestinal disorders (such as inflammatory bowel disease), and even stress can roil your insides, sending you on emergency trips to the loo. But be careful what you take to remedy the condition—if you take anything at all.

Do diarrhea meds work?

YES Over-the-counter diarrhea medicine may help if you choose right.

When the FDA studied the safety and effectiveness of OTC diarrhea drugs, they determined that just two—loperamide (Imodium) and bismuth subsalicylate (Pepto-Bismol)—are safe and effective. Imodium slows down the movement of food through the digestive tract, which makes bowel movements less frequent. The pink stuff appears to relieve loose and frequent stools by decreasing fluid in the bowel, easing inflammation, and binding to and killing bacteria.

In one study, diarrhea cleared up about a day sooner in patients who took Imodium than in others who took placebo pills. Pepto-Bismol seems to be a weaker treatment than Imodium but offers some relief for mild diarrhea. One study found that it reduced the typical length of time a person had loose stools, but only by seven hours.

Do you need medicine for most cases of diarrhea?

NO Diarrhea medicine is not the most important therapy and may even be counterproductive.

Because diarrhea usually lasts only a few days at most, you may not need any medicine. In some cases, doctors say, it's best to let diarrhea run its course to allow the body to eliminate the food, virus, or other problem that's making you sick in the first place. Furthermore, these drugs can cause side effects. Imodium, for example, makes some users constipated.

Pepto-Bismol seems to be a weaker treatment than Imodium but **offers some relief for mild diarrhea.**

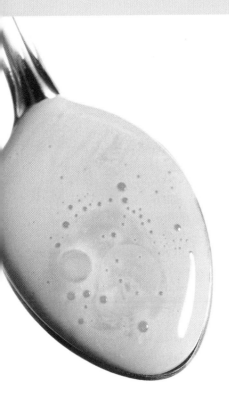

Don't attempt to self-treat diarrhea with any OTC medications if you have a fever and/or blood or mucus in your stools. These are signs of infection, which requires a doctor's care. Finally, the FDA requires manufacturers to recommend that parents ask their doctor before giving Pepto-Bismol to kids under 12. Parents should also check with their doctor before giving Imodium to a child who is younger than 6 or weighs less than 47 pounds.

What *should* you take for diarrhea? Lots of liquids. Diarrhea causes dehydration, so the first and most important step is restoring healthy levels of fluids and important minerals known as electrolytes. Most doctors recommend sipping nonalcoholic,

caffeine-free beverages. (Note that milk and other dairy products may worsen diarrhea in some people.) Soup and broth can help, too. If diarrhea is severe or lasts more than a few days, see your doctor.

Does Pepto-Bismol protect against traveler's diarrhea?

YES Pepto-Bismol and other bismuth subsalicylate products reduce, but don't eliminate, the risk of traveler's diarrhea.

About half of all people who travel to Africa, Southeast Asia, Latin America, the Middle East, and certain other parts of the world develop traveler's diarrhea, usually by consuming food or water contaminated with bacteria. Many frequent international tourists swear by Pepto-Bismol and other medications containing bismuth subsalicylate, insisting that daily doses of the pink drink or tablets protect them against diarrhea. Research suggests that the chalky-tasting cocktail and pills may help, though they

are no guarantee against gastrointestinal turmoil.

In a 1987 study published in the *Journal of the American Medical Association*, students from the United States started taking two 262-milligram tablets of bismuth subsalicylate four times a day within 48 hours of arriving in Mexico. Just 7 of 51 students developed diarrhea. In contrast, 23 of 58 students given placebo pills soon experienced Montezuma's revenge. Overall, this study and others suggest that taking high doses of bismuth subsalicylate reduces the threat of traveler's diarrhea by about 60 percent. So pack Pepto-Bismol when you visit developing nations, but use some common sense, too. Don't drink tap water (or brush your teeth with it), eat only foods that are "peelable, packaged, purified, or piping hot," and follow other precautions.

Talk to your doctor before using Pepto-Bismol if you are allergic to aspirin or take a daily aspirin, or if you currently take blood-thinning medication or drugs to treat gout, arthritis, or diabetes. ■

EYEDROPS

Eyedrops

Not so long ago, the local pharmacy carried just a few bottles of eyedrops, which were used mostly to brighten up tired, "bloodshot" orbs after a late night. You can still find drops that "get the red out," but shelves now drip with products designed to relieve itchy eyes and the seeming epidemic of dry eyes, too. Do you really need them?

Can you overuse eyedrops?

YES Eyedrops can "get the red out," as an old ad campaign used to claim, but using them too often can backfire and actually worsen irritation and redness.

The eyes are sensitive organs and can become irritated when exposed to smoke, polluted air, the chlorine in a swimming pool, or even a late night in front of the TV. Your eyes are filled with tiny blood vessels called capillaries. Irritants cause these capillaries to dilate, which can turn the whites of your eyes into red-streaked road maps.

Eyedrops that promise to erase redness contain decongestant medicine that constricts blood vessels. Narrowing blood-filled capillaries makes them less visible, so the redness fades. But decongestant drops are weak, and their effects wear off quickly. Also, if you use them too many times in a row, you may experience a rebound effect, in which the capillaries become even more dilated, leading to a vicious cycle.

To avoid the rebound effect, don't use decongestant eyedrops for more than a few days at a time. Some eye doctors discourage patients from using them at all. Instead, find out what's causing your eye irritation and try to eliminate the problem. Eye redness that can't be explained may be a sign of infection or other serious condition, so if the problem becomes chronic, talk to a doctor.

Do all eyedrops relieve itchy, watery eyes?

NO Many of the most popular drops lack the critical ingredient that relieves eye symptoms caused by allergies.

If you have hay fever, you probably know that sneezing and sniffling is only half the nuisance of seasonal allergies. Inhaling pollen causes the body to release histamine, a chemical that produces inflammation not only in the nasal passages but in the eyes, too. The more inflamed the eyes become, the more they itch, water, and swell. Decongestant eyedrops that "take the red out" do nothing to battle histamine.

If you take an antihistamine in pill form, such as loratadine (Claritin), your teary, tormented eyes may feel better eventually. But some studies suggest that antihistamine-based eyedrops, which are available over the counter, provide faster relief. Read ingredient lists and look for pheniramine or antazoline, two antihistamines commonly used in allergy eyedrops. But there's a catch: The antihistamines in these products are often paired with a decongestant. As you read earlier, frequently application of

Our BEST ADVICE

Label instructions on eye care products often recommend applying "one or two drops." Yet one drop is enough, according to the *Medical Letter on Drugs and Therapeutics*. One drop of a typical product contains 35 to 50 microliters of fluid, though it may be as much as 75 microliters. An eye can only handle about 30 microliters of fluid. A second drop could wash away the first, wasting money.

EYEDROPS

decongestants to the eyes can worsen redness over time, so these combination drops should be used for only short periods—no more than a few days—if at all.

An exception to this rule is ketotifen (Alaway and Zatidor), which is available over the counter in the United States and some other countries and isn't combined with a decongestant. Ketotifen is a triple threat against allergy eyes: It acts as an antihistamine, stabilizes mast cells (which produce chemicals that cause allergy symptoms), and reduces inflammation. If you have allergy eyes, ask your doctor or pharmacist if ketotifen is right for you and worth the expense; it costs twice as much as other antihistamine eyedrops.

Do "artificial tears" and eye lubricants work?

YES But if you use these eye moisturizers more than a few times a day, you may have a condition that requires medical attention.

You should have tears in your eyes all day, even if you aren't sad. Special glands produce tears to provide a protective film over the eyes to keep them moist and clean and to wash away germs. Some people produce too little tear film, however, or their tears evaporate too quickly. If you are

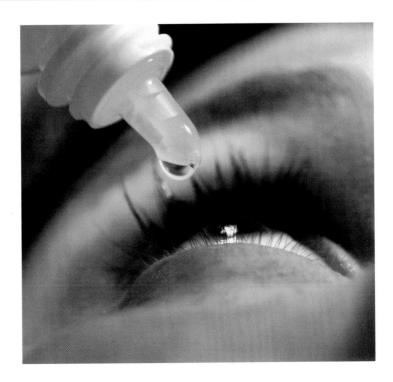

bothered by dry eyes on occasion, eyedrops designed for dry eyes can help, though be braced for some hefty prices and somewhat limited relief.

These products contain chemicals called hydrogels that make the drops linger on the surface of the eye. Even with hydrogels, however, the drops remain on the eye surface for a short time, says University of Illinois ophthalmologist Sandeep Jain, MD. Even if you have a mild case of dry eyes, you may need to reapply drops several times a day.

Higher-viscosity artificial tears, which include Systane, Celluvisc, and Liquigel, offer longer protection (and tend to cost more). But Celluvisc, which has the highest viscosity, can blur vision for up to 20 to 30 minutes, according to

Dr. Jain. Eye gels and ointments are even gooier (some contain petroleum jelly and mineral oil), so they blur vision even longer; that's why they are designed to soothe the eyes while you sleep.

Preservatives are another concern. Some eyedrops contain benzalkonium, which prolongs shelf life but can irritate eyes that are very dry. Try products that contain the preservatives sodium perborate or polyquaternium-1 instead. Better yet, spend a little more and use preservative-free drops, which are sold in single-use vials.

If you use eyedrops more than four times a day, talk to your doctor. Chronic dry eyes can be a sign of a more serious condition, such as rosacea or Sjögren's syndrome. ∎

Fiber Supplements

If dietitians ruled the world, everyone would eat bran flakes for breakfast, lentils for lunch, and brussels sprouts for supper. In short, we would all fill up on fiber at every meal and be healthier for our troubles. Yet most of us fall well short of the recommended 25 to 35 grams of fiber per day. To fill the gap and gain the well-known benefits of roughage, some people turn to fiber supplements. But can pills and powders really replace peaches and peas?

Are fiber supplements always the best treatment for constipation?

NO Some people who take fiber supplements to relieve constipation end up feeling worse. For hard-to-treat cases, other medications may be a better choice.

Your body can't absorb the fiber in food or supplements. Instead, this indigestible stuff helps to form bigger, softer stools that are easier to pass (fiber supplements are sometimes called bulk-forming laxatives). Doctors often recommend supplements for treating constipation, especially for patients who can't or won't add more fiber to their diets. Studies show, however, that about half of all patients who start taking fiber supplements eventually quit. The main reason seems to be that increasing fiber intake makes some people feel bloated, as though their stomachs were stretching and about to burst.

Some patients may give up on fiber supplements because they aren't helping much. One review found that people who take a daily fiber supplement increase their number of bowel movements by only about one per week. A task force for the American College of Gastroenterology found that only fiber supplements containing psyllium are effective for chronic constipation.

If you decide to try fiber supplements to treat a case of constipation, start out with small amounts at first and be sure to drink plenty of fluids. For persistent constipation, see a doctor.

Are fiber supplements an adequate substitute for high-fiber foods?

NO Fiber supplements lack the vitamins, minerals, and other valuable nutrients in high-fiber foods.

If your diet contains too little fiber, supplements can seem like the ideal quick fix. In fact, taking fiber supplements is easier than ever these days.

You'll gain greater disease protection by getting roughage from your daily (whole-grain) bread.

FIBER SUPPLEMENTS

Gulping down gritty cocktails made with powdered psyllium used to be how most people supplemented their diets with fiber, but now you can choose from capsules, tablets, and even crispy wafers as more palatable alternatives.

However, quick fixes rarely work as long-term solutions, and fiber supplements aren't any different. They don't provide your body with the vitamins, minerals, and other disease-fighting benefits that you get from eating high-fiber foods. A pear, for instance, contains about five grams of fiber, but it's also a terrific source of vitamins C and E as well as potassium. Eat a cup of peas with dinner, and not only will you add nearly nine grams of fiber to your daily total, you'll also get a healthy dose of the antioxidants lutein and zeaxanthin, which some studies suggest may help prevent vision loss.

The National Cancer Institute looked at the diets of nearly a half million men and women and found that people who ate the most whole-grain foods, which are rich in fiber,

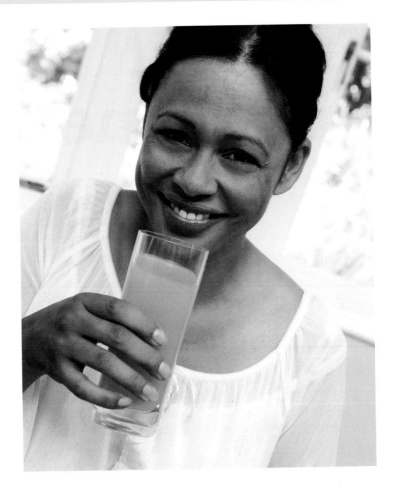

cut their risk of colorectal cancer by 21 percent. You won't get that benefit from a fiber supplement. In fact, the study showed that the fiber in these foods had no effect on a person's cancer risk; something else was doing the trick.

Your doctor may recommend fiber supplements (to lower cholesterol, for instance), and they may help ease occasional constipation. But you'll gain greater disease protection by getting roughage from your daily (whole-grain) bread. ∎

FISH-OIL SUPPLEMENTS

Fish-Oil Supplements

To many people, sitting down to a fish dinner is not a pleasure but a chore to be avoided, along with cleaning the gutters and dusting the blinds. Yet research shows that the omega-3 fatty acids in fish oil have powerful health benefits. That's why a growing number of once-skeptical doctors now recommend fish-oil supplements to patients at risk for heart disease and other conditions.

Our BEST ADVICE

Keep fish-oil supplements in the refrigerator. The cool temperature keeps the capsules fresh and prevents spoiling. Also, many users swear that refrigerating the supplements helps eliminate one of their most common and bothersome side effects, eructation—which you know better as burping.

Are fish-oil supplements a good alternative for people who hate fish?

YES Fish-oil supplements are the next best thing to eating fin food.

Research shows that people who take fish-oil supplements cut their risk of developing cardiovascular disease. For example, a study involving 11,324 recent heart attack survivors found that patients who took one gram of fish oil every day cut their risk of sudden cardiac death (a type of heart attack) by 45 percent. Fish oil, whether from seafood or supplement, stabilizes heart rhythm, lowers levels of artery-clogging blood fats called triglycerides, makes blood less likely to clot, reduces inflammation, and may even reduce blood pressure.

Fish-oil capsules may even have an edge over fish. Although the benefits of eating fish outweigh the risks posed by any toxins in fish, most seafood nonetheless contains at least traces of mercury, PCBs, and other contaminants. Some species have dangerously high levels. Fish-oil supplements seem to be more pure. Consumerlab.com researchers tested the purity of 43 different brands of fish-oil supplements and failed to find a single contaminated capsule.

There are a number of possible reasons why fish-oil supplements are purer than the salmon or tuna on your dinner plate, says consumerlab.com president Tod Cooperman, MD. First, some of the most worrisome contaminants, including mercury, accumulate in fish muscle, not in the oil. Second, many varieties of fish-oil supplements are produced from small fish species, such as menhaden, which are much less likely to be contaminated than larger species like swordfish and shark. Finally, the distillation process used to produce fish-oil supplements removes toxins.

Should you pay more for "pharmaceutical-grade" fish oil?

NO First, most over-the-counter fish oils contain few if any contaminants. And if you choose to pay extra for oil labeled "pharmaceutical grade," you may not get anything different, since this phrase has no legal meaning. If you want to ensure you're getting true pharmaceutical-grade oil, ask your doctor for a prescription for the fish oil Lovaza. Since it's sold by prescription, Lovaza must meet high standards of purity, unlike over-the-counter supplements, which are not closely regulated. Also, the makers of

Lovaza claim that their distillation process removes cholesterol, saturated fat, and oxidized lipids—all stuff you can do without.

Should you avoid cod-liver oil as a source of omega-3 fatty acids?

MAYBE Your grandmother had the right idea—fish oil truly is good for you—but if you take cod-liver oil, you may be overdosing on vitamin A.

People of a certain age may recall the days when taking a daily dose of cod-liver oil was as common as popping a multivitamin is today. Today it seems cod-liver oil is back. Encouraged by claims touted on the Internet, many people now turn to the fishy-tasting liquid (now also available in capsules) to protect their hearts, ward off cancer, strengthen bones, relieve joint pain, promote healthy digestion, and improve mood.

While growing evidence suggests that fish oil has a range of health benefits, it's not clear that there is anything special

about cod-liver oil in particular. Scientists do know this much, however: Cod-liver oil is a very rich source of certain nutrients, including vitamin A. In fact, just a teaspoon contains far more than the recommended daily intake of the vitamin. (Other fish-oil capsules contain somewhat less vitamin A but are still rich sources of the nutrient.) Your body is particularly adept at using the form of vitamin A that comes from animal foods—so-called preformed vitamin A—including cod-liver oil. And emerging evidence indicates that vitamin A toxicity may occur at lower levels than previously believed. For example, osteoporosis and hip fractures have been linked to an intake of preformed vitamin A that's just twice as high as the recommended amount. Liver problems and birth defects have been associated with high vitamin A levels, too. If you choose to include cod-liver oil supplements in your daily regimen, find a product that has 2,000 IU or less of vitamin A per teaspoon. ■

Garlic Pills

We know garlic is good for the heart. It may even help prevent some cancers. But some people *hate* the stuff and never eat it. Others, who may love recipes like Chicken with 40 Cloves of Garlic and are mad for Italian cuisine, probably don't eat the odoriferous bulbs every day. For these reasons, many people take garlic supplements to bolster their health—and avoid garlic breath.

Can garlic pills fight infections?

MAYBE Emerging research suggests that compounds in garlic may fight infections, so these supplements could help prevent colds and more serious conditions.

Traditional healers and mainstream doctors have used garlic to fight infections throughout history. Garlic preparations were used to treat battlefield wounds in World War II, for example. And garlic does kill germs—at least in a test tube. In the lab, garlic extract can block the growth of bacteria, viruses, and fungi. There's little proof that popping a daily garlic tablet will keep you infection free—but it just might help.

One study found that garlic supplements may block the rhinovirus, which causes the common cold. In one study, a British researcher recruited 146 volunteers at the start of winter. Half took daily capsules containing allicin, which appears to be the active element in garlic (it's produced when a clove is chewed, chopped, or crushed). The other half of the volunteers took placebos. By winter's end, the garlic users had caught only 24 colds compared to 65 among the placebo group. What's more, when a member of the garlic group got a cold, the symptoms lasted only a day and a half on average, compared to the typical five-day cold among the people given placebos. Unfortunately, these results need to be reproduced in other studies before anyone can say that garlic supplements stave off the sniffles.

Some scientists also believe that garlic supplements could eventually have a role in combating antibiotic resistance, a serious problem in healthcare in which germs become "resistant" to antibiotics. For example, many of the most widely used antibiotics are worthless against methicillin-resistant *Staphylococcus aureus* bacteria, better known as MRSA, which often infect hospital patients. A study by Taiwanese researchers showed that garlic extract fed to lab mice destroyed MRSA. Here again, however, further study is necessary to confirm whether "nature's penicillin" lives up to its billing.

Do odorless garlic pills work?

MAYBE Removing the smelly stuff in garlic strips away some of its medicinal compounds. Enteric-coated pills are the best bet.

As any garlic lover knows, a meal spiced with chopped fresh cloves can leave you desperate for an industrial-strength after-dinner mint. Taking garlic supplements can make your breath reek, too, or

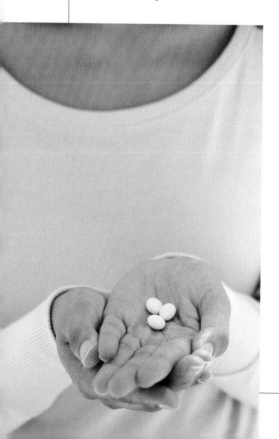

even give you body odor. Most companies that sell garlic supplements claim their products are "odorless," but scientists who study the cloves smell a potential problem with these pills.

Some products are made odorless by "aging" garlic cloves in alcohol for months. This process removes the offending compounds that cause bad breath—but these are the same compounds that provide garlic's health benefits. Aged garlic supplements won't give you bad breath, but they may not do much else either (besides empty your wallet).

A better bet: Enteric-coated garlic tablets. These are designed to dissolve in the small intestine, not in the stomach, so they're less likely to cause bad breath. But do they dissolve at all? Chemist and garlic researcher Larry D. Lawson, PhD, tested one garlic supplement that failed to disintegrate after 66 hours, when he gave up on it. Some garlic pills may be "impotent" for another reason: Dr. Lawson has studied the leading brands and found evidence that some do not produce significant amounts of the all-important sulfur compound allicin, because they either contain too little alliinase (which converts to allicin) or fail to dissolve before passing from the small intestine. He found that only one enteric-coated tablet, Garlicin, produced a significant amount of allicin. ■

Heartburn Remedies

Judging from the number of heartburn remedies advertised on TV, a whole lot of us have burning bellies. Heartburn used to be regarded as a nuisance. Today some doctors believe that frequent bouts can damage the esophagus (though this phenomenon may have been overblown by the drug companies that make heartburn drugs). In recent years, chronic heartburn even acquired a fancy new name—gastroesophageal reflux disease, or GERD—and new drugs to treat it. (See the Heartburn entry on page 288 to read about how well these drugs work.)

Are heartburn drugs harmless?

NO They contain serious medicine and may cause side effects, especially if you don't follow label instructions.

These various pills and liquids can cause mild side effects, such as headaches, nausea, and diarrhea. However, heartburn treatments have also been linked to several other, more serious disorders, particularly among people who take large doses for extended periods.

Dementia: A large recent study in people over 65 found that those who used H2 blockers—common drugs that reduce stomach acid—were 2.4 times more likely than nonusers to develop dementia or some other form of mental impairment. H2 blockers include nizatidine (Axid), famotidine (Pepcid), cimetidine (Tagamet), and ranitidine (Zantac). This report conflicted with the findings of several earlier studies. H2 blockers work by interfering with histamine, which is known to play some role in brain function.

Erectile dysfunction: There have been reports in the medical literature of men developing erectile dysfunction and loss of libido after taking certain heartburn and ulcer medications, particularly Tagamet, Axid, and Zantac. However, these problems are rare and reversible once a man stops using the drugs.

Gynecomastia: Tagamet has also been linked to an embarrassing problem for men. Compared to nonusers, males

HEARTBURN REMEDIES

who take 1,000 milligrams or more every day for an extended period are at least 40 times more likely to develop enlarged breast tissue, known as gynecomastia, according to a study in the *British Medical Journal*. But since the overall risk for gynecomastia is small, that means fewer than 1 percent of male Tagamet users develop this condition.

Soft bones and kidney stones: Some heartburn remedies contain aluminum or magnesium, both of which neutralize stomach acid. These minerals also increase the amount of calcium lost in the urine. There are many case reports in the medical literature of patients who consumed large amounts of aluminum-based antacids and developed osteomalacia, or soft bones, as well as kidney stones and other conditions caused by excessive loss of calcium. High doses of aluminum also appear to deplete other important minerals, including fluoride and phosphorus.

Vitamin B_{12} deficiency: A 2004 study found that people over 65 who are current, long-term users of acid-reducing drugs

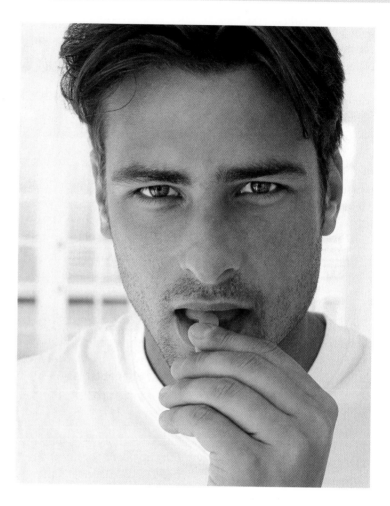

are nearly 4.5 times more likely to have vitamin B_{12} deficiencies than nonusers. Acid-reducing medications include H2 blockers and proton-pump inhibitors, such as omeprazole (Prilosec, which is available over the counter) and several prescription drugs. These medications may pose problems for

some older people, who often have too little stomach acid, which the body needs to help absorb vitamin B_{12}. A deficiency of this vitamin can lead to a drop in red blood cells and result in pernicious anemia, a condition that causes fatigue, weakness, rapid heartbeat, and other symptoms. ■

Ibuprofen and other NSAIDs

For all-purpose pain relief, much of the world turns to ibuprofen (Advil and Motrin are popular brands), a very effective nonsteroidal anti-inflammatory drug (NSAID). Another NSAID, naproxen (Aleve, Naprosyn), is also available without a prescription. Ibuprofen first became available in the 1970s as a safer alternative to aspirin. As some patients discover, however, heavy use of NSAIDs can offset their value as pain fighters.

Do most people who take NSAIDs develop stomach problems?

NO The risk is relatively small, especially if you take them only occasionally. But since the drugs are so widely used, gastrointestinal side effects send many people to hospitals each year.

NSAIDs relieve pain by blocking production of hormone-like chemicals called prostaglandins, which also help to protect the stomach lining. Blocking prostaglandins exposes the inner walls of your belly to damage from acid, bile salts, alcohol, and other irritating substances. Studies of people who take NSAIDs regularly show that about half have erosions in the stomach lining, while 20 percent have ulcers. But NSAID users who have these injuries don't necessarily develop any stomach pain or other symptoms as a result. The most common complaints are heartburn and upset stomach, which occur in about 10 to 20 percent of people who take NSAIDs. (Studies have shown the figure may be as low as 5 percent and as high as 50 percent.)

Stomach bleeding and perforation (literally, a hole in the stomach) are the more worrisome concerns linked to NSAIDs. However, only about 1 to 3 percent of people who use the drugs regularly develop these serious complications. And they *are* serious: 5 to 10 percent of patients hospitalized with stomach bleeding caused by NSAIDs die. The risk is greatest if you are elderly, take high doses of NSAIDs, take more than one NSAID at a time, have a history of peptic ulcers or other GI problems, or take blood-thinning drugs or corticosteroids.

While it's a good idea to discuss which pain relievers you use with your family doctor, most physicians agree that NSAIDs are generally safe for occasional use.

Do ibuprofen and other NSAIDs increase the risk of heart attacks?

MAYBE The evidence is mostly circumstantial, but some studies show that people who take NSAIDs may have a higher risk of heart disease.

Remember Vioxx (rofecoxib)? People who relied on it for their arthritis pain got a shock when it was found to increase

Most physicians agree that NSAIDs are generally safe for occasional use.

IBUPROFEN AND OTHER NSAIDS

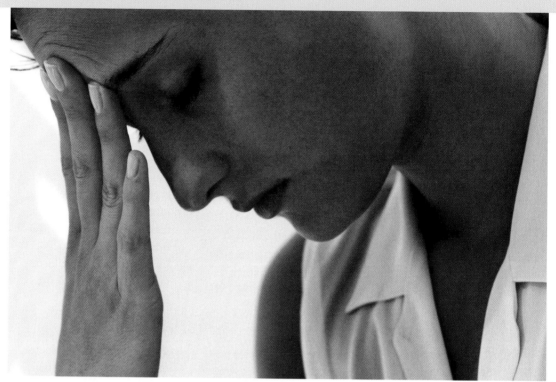

the risk of heart attacks and strokes. When it was taken off the market, many people switched to ibuprofen or naproxen. But are *those* drugs safe for the heart?

That depends. Some studies suggest they may not be, especially if you already have heart problems and take large doses (though other studies have failed to show that NSAID users have more heart attacks or die younger than people who don't take them). A 2005 study led by Danish researchers found that people who had used naproxen and other NSAIDs within the previous month were at least 50 percent more likely than nonusers to have heart attacks. A year later, a second group of Danish scientists showed that heart attack survivors who took large doses of ibuprofen for an extended period— 1,800 milligrams per day for 37 days, on average— increased their risk of death or a second heart attack by 50 percent. (The usual recommended maximum dose is 1,200 milligrams for no more than 10 days.) Use of other over-the-counter NSAIDs was linked to a 29 percent increased risk. These studies did not show any threat to people who use over-the-counter NSAIDs only occasionally.

It's not clear why NSAIDs may imperil the heart. Population studies have shown that regular NSAID users seem to increase their risk of developing high blood pressure. But some preliminary research suggests that acetaminophen, which is not an NSAID, may raise blood pressure, too.

NSAIDs such as ibuprofen and naproxen do appear to interfere with aspirin's ability to prevent blood clots. If you take a daily aspirin for heart protection, ask your doctor whether it's okay to use ibuprofen for pain. The FDA says it's safe to take 400 milligrams of ibuprofen at least 30 minutes before or eight hours after taking an aspirin. ∎

Mouthwash

As you'll read on page 258, while almost all mouthwashes temporarily erase bad breath, germ-killing rinses provide results that last a little longer. But other questions about mouthwash abound, from their safety to their "extra" health benefits. We wash away the myths here.

Can mouthwash cause oral cancer?

NO The long-lingering fear that the alcohol in mouthwash causes cancer of the mouth and pharynx turns out to be unfounded. According to a review in the *Journal of the American Dental Association*, most studies have found no link between mouthwash and cancer.

Can mouthwash irritate your mouth?

MAYBE Some people say that mouthwash containing alcohol stings and causes their mouths to become dry. If you have a condition that causes dry mouth, such as Sjögren's syndrome, swishing with an alcohol-based mouthwash will make it worse (though rinsing with water several times a day is a good idea). However, the alcohol in mouthwash doesn't appear to be a serious health threat for most people. In one study, researchers examined the mouths of people who rinsed with popular brands of mouthwash three times a day for two weeks and found no evidence of inflammation, skin ulcers, or other damage.

Can mouthwash turn your tongue black?

YES Using antiseptic mouthwash too often can cause an unsightly condition with a name right out of a horror movie. Black hairy tongue occurs when the tongue turns dark and the tiny bumps that line its surface become overgrown.

Does mouthwash kill germs that cause colds?

NO Oral rinses that contain antiseptics do indeed kill germs that live in your mouth, but they don't protect against or treat the common cold. In 1978, the U.S. Federal Trade Commission ordered the maker of one popular brand of mouthwash to stop claiming that it prevented colds.

Is using mouthwash as good as flossing?

NO In 2005, a court ordered the maker of that same popular mouthwash to stop claiming that its product cleaned teeth as effectively as dental floss, since the scientific evidence suggested otherwise. ■

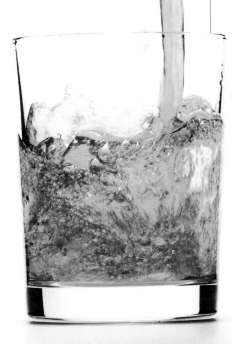

MULTIVITAMINS

Multivitamins

They are your diet's backup plan, a defense against those days when you really meant to have a salad at lunch, but the pastrami sandwich won out. Multivitamins have long been promoted as a modest investment with a big pay-off—a daily guarantee that you'll get all the nutrients your body needs to keep running and ward off disease. Choosing a multivitamin can be hard enough, given the variety of products—but some experts have questioned whether you should use one at all.

Are multivitamins worth taking?

MAYBE Multivitamins are hugely popular, but if you eat a varied, nutrient-rich diet, you probably don't need them.

If you are healthy and eat plenty of fruit, vegetables, and whole grains, then "you are probably not going to benefit from a multivitamin," says Iowa State University nutritionist Diane F. Birt, PhD. Granted, most people's diets aren't ideal. A recent survey of the American diet, for instance, found that most adults and children don't get enough vitamin E, calcium, magnesium, or potassium. The typical adult was low on vitamins A and C, too.

Even if you don't eat a well-balanced diet, though, there is surprisingly little evidence that taking a multi will do you much good. Dr. Birt was on a panel appointed by the U.S. National Institutes of Health to study the scientific literature on the health benefits of multivitamins. The panel determined that there is currently no reason to either recommend or discourage their use.

Few studies have directly examined whether multis reduce the risk for any disease.

Most vitamin studies have examined specific combinations of vitamins and minerals, and these offer some evidence that multivitamins may help certain people, though they are burdened by caveats.

For example, a study involving nearly 30,000 people from small villages in China determined that supplements containing beta-carotene, vitamin E, and selenium reduced the risk of stomach cancer and the overall risk of dying from any cancer. However, many of the people were malnourished, so the study's findings don't apply to everyone.

CHOOSING A MULTI

If you decide to take a multivitamin/mineral, keep three rules in mind.

Don't take "high-potency" supplements. They probably won't make you any healthier, but they may expose you to dangerously high levels of some nutrients, especially if you eat a well-balanced diet. As a general rule, don't take multivitamin/mineral supplements that provide more than 100 percent of the Daily Value for any nutrient unless instructed to do so by a physician. A recent study found that 10 to 15 percent of multivitamin users consume too much vitamin A, iron, and zinc.

Don't take multivitamins containing herbs. There is too little evidence that any confer health benefits, nor is there adequate information about the proper dosage.

Don't worry about form. Multivitamins are available as traditional tablets as well as chewable tablets and liquids. All work just fine, so pick the form that makes you most comfortable.

MULTIVITAMINS

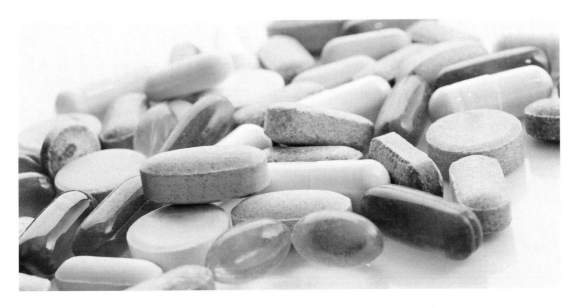

A French study found a 31 percent drop in cancer risk among men who took vitamin C, vitamin E, beta-carotene, selenium, and zinc for eight years. In particular, men who had normal levels of prostate-specific antigen, or PSA (a cancer marker), had a 48 percent reduced risk of prostate cancer. However, prostate cancer risk *increased* in some men. And women gained no cancer protection.

Dr. Birt and her colleagues found no proof that high-dose combinations of vitamins and minerals prevent heart disease or any other major condition, with one exception: One study found that people with the eye disease macular degeneration had slower vision loss if they took vitamin C, vitamin E, beta-carotene, and zinc.

Are "special formula" multivitamins for men, women, and seniors a good idea?

MAYBE Multivitamins designed for specific populations seem to make sense. In reality, though, these specialty supplements probably offer only modest advantages over a basic multivitamin.

The differences between men and women run deep, right down to the way our bodies use vitamins and minerals. What's more, some of our nutrient needs shift as we age. Does that mean a one-size-fits-all multi doesn't fit all? Yes and no. All multis contain similar (though not always identical) core vitamins and minerals. But products geared for men, women, or seniors contain slightly different amounts of certain nutrients to reflect the differences in recommended daily allowances between the sexes and generations. For instance, a men's multivitamin may contain 90 milligrams of vitamin C compared to 60 milligrams in a women's multi.

There are only a few instances where all of this tailoring offers any real benefit, says registered dietitian Roberta Anding, RD, a spokeswoman for the American Dietetic Association. For one, men may be better off with a men's multi since they usually don't include iron (men need less iron than women, and too much iron, found in meat and fortified grains, can be dangerous). Many seniors need extra vitamin B_{12}, since it becomes harder for the body to absorb this nutrient after age 50. Multivitamins marketed to seniors usually contain high amounts of B_{12}, which may help prevent deficiency of this vitamin. ■

MULTIVITAMINS

Vitamin Supplements: Hope or Hype?

Vitamins and minerals are essential to health, but that doesn't mean that megadoses will keep you out of the hospital or make you live longer. Some may be harmful. In most cases, it's preferable to get these nutrients from a balanced diet. Here's the lowdown on eight common supplements—most of which you probably don't need.

High doses of certain vitamins and minerals may be appropriate for certain people, though. Talk to your doctor about supplements if you are a woman of childbearing age, are a vegetarian or vegan, have limited exposure to the sun, are an athlete in training, or suspect for any reason you may be malnourished.

1 BETA-CAROTENE

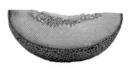

BEST FOOD SOURCES

Carrots, spinach, kale, cantaloupe

RDA*

3,000 IU (in the form of vitamin A) for males, 2,130 IU for females

WHY YOU MAY BE TAKING IT

As an antioxidant, especially to prevent cancer.

WHAT YOU SHOULD KNOW

Beta-carotene supplements *increase* the risk of lung cancer in smokers. There is no evidence that they prevent any other form of cancer.

BOTTOM LINE

Don't take it.

2 FOLIC ACID

BEST FOOD SOURCES

Fortified bread and breakfast cereal, legumes, asparagus

RDA*

400 micrograms

WHY YOU MAY BE TAKING IT

To prevent birth defects.

WHAT YOU SHOULD KNOW

Supplements reduce the risk of neural tube defects in newborns. However, some doctors say supplementation of food with folic acid could be fueling rising rates of colon cancer.

BOTTOM LINE

Only women who are pregnant or may become pregnant are advised to take it.

3 SELENIUM

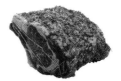

BEST FOOD SOURCES

Brazil nuts, tuna, beef

RDA*

55 micrograms

WHY YOU MAY BE TAKING IT

To prevent cancer, especially prostate cancer.

WHAT YOU SHOULD KNOW

One 2007 study found a 50% increased risk of type 2 diabetes in people who took 200 micrograms a day. A major study will determine whether selenium supplements prevent prostate cancer, but it won't be completed until 2013.

BOTTOM LINE

Don't take it.

4 VITAMIN B_6

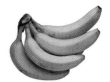

BEST FOOD SOURCES

Baked potatoes, bananas, chickpeas

RDA*

Males/females 19–50: 1.3 milligrams; males over 50: 1.7 milligrams; females over 50: 1.5 milligrams

WHY YOU MAY BE TAKING IT

To prevent mental decline and lower homocysteine levels.

WHAT YOU SHOULD KNOW

Two studies failed to show cognitive benefits. B_6 does reduce homocysteine, but it's not clear whether this prevents heart attacks.

BOTTOM LINE

Take it only if your doctor recommends it.

MULTIVITAMINS

5

VITAMIN B$_{12}$

BEST FOOD SOURCES

Fish and shellfish, lean beef, fortified breakfast cereal

RDA*

2.4 micrograms

**WHY YOU
MAY BE TAKING IT**

To prevent age-related mental decline and boost energy.

**WHAT YOU
SHOULD KNOW**

Vitamin B$_{12}$ deficiency, which can cause anemia and dementia, is a problem for some seniors, so supplements can help. However, high doses of B$_{12}$ have not been proven to prevent cognitive loss, nor do they boost energy.

BOTTOM LINE

Take it only if your doctor recommends it.

6

VITAMIN C

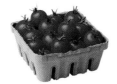

BEST FOOD SOURCES

Citrus fruits, melons, tomatoes

RDA*

90 milligrams for adult males, 75 milligrams for females

**WHY YOU
MAY BE TAKING IT**

To prevent the common cold. Also as an antioxidant to help fight cancer or heart disease.

**WHAT YOU
SHOULD KNOW**

A review of 30 clinical trials found no evidence that vitamin C prevents colds. Exceptions: It may reduce the risk in people who live in cold climates or experience extreme physical stress, such as running marathons. Smokers may need extra vitamin C. High doses of vitamin C do not seem to prevent cancer or heart disease.

BOTTOM LINE

Most people don't need C supplements.

7

VITAMIN E

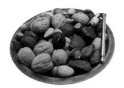

BEST FOOD SOURCES

Vegetable oil, nuts, leafy green vegetables

RDA*

15 milligrams

**WHY YOU
MAY BE TAKING IT**

To help prevent heart disease, cancer, and Alzheimer's disease.

**WHAT YOU
SHOULD KNOW**

Not only have studies failed to show that vitamin E supplements prevent heart attacks or cancer, but high doses may increase the risk of strokes. One study found that vitamin E from food—but not supplements—helps prevent Alzheimer's disease.

BOTTOM LINE

Don't take it.

8

ZINC

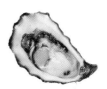

BEST FOOD SOURCES

Oysters, lean beef, breakfast cereal

RDA*

11 milligrams for males; 8 milligrams for females

**WHY YOU
MAY BE TAKING IT**

To prevent and treat symptoms of the common cold.

**WHAT YOU
SHOULD KNOW**

A few studies suggest that cold symptoms are less severe and resolve sooner in zinc users, but others show no benefit. High doses can weaken the immune system.

BOTTOM LINE

Don't take it except for occasional use of zinc lozenges or sprays for colds.

*Recommended dietary allowances for healthy adults are listed; they may be lower or higher for children, women who are pregnant or nursing, the elderly, and other groups.

Nasal Sprays

When you have a stuffy nose from a cold or an allergy, decongestant nasal sprays deliver medicine directly to the problem, unlike pills, which work throughout the whole body and can slow circulation and raise blood pressure. As a result, the sprays work fast—but use them too often, and you may regret it.

Are decongestant nasal sprays addictive?

YES The sprays offer fast relief for a stuffed-up nose, but if you don't use them as directed, your nasal problems may worsen.

Colds and allergies can make breathing through the nose all but impossible because they cause blood vessels in the nasal passages to dilate. The quickest way to unblock a stuffed-up nose is to inhale a few sniffs of nasal spray containing decongestant medicine.

Use one too long, though, and you may find that its effects wear off sooner than expected and that you need increasingly larger and more frequent doses to keep your nasal passages clear. Before you know it, you may end up dependent on nasal spray for months or even years. Doctors call this phenomenon rebound congestion. To avoid this fate, don't use a nasal decongestant spray for longer than three days at a time.

Is nasal spray safe?

MAYBE Most varieties of nasal spray contain a preservative that could cause unwanted side effects.

The preservative is called benzalkonium chloride (BAC) and is used to extend the shelf life of many pharmaceutical products, including decongestant nasal sprays as well as saline nasal sprays. Some doctors steer patients away from sprays that contain BAC—which, it turns out, is most of them. People sometimes complain that sprays containing the preservative irritate their nasal passages. Research also suggests that BAC may worsen the threat of rebound congestion. A few studies suggest that this bacteria fighter may make the nasal passages more prone to sinusitis. Other studies show no short- or long-term risk.

No one should use decongestant nasal spray for more than a few days. If you use saline nasal spray, it may be worth searching for a brand that doesn't contain BAC. As an

ADDICTED TO NASAL SPRAY?

If you become dependent on these products and can't kick the habit on your own, see a doctor. Some physicians recommend gradually weaning yourself from nasal spray by using it only on the side that's most clogged, letting the "good" side go "cold turkey." Over time, the good side should clear up on its own, at which point you should stop using the spray altogether. Other steps that may help include taking oral decongestants and/or an antihistamine to help you sleep and using saline nasal spray. Doctors may also prescribe stronger medicine (such as nasal steroids) to treat this maddening problem.

alternative, you can make your own at home. Mix 1/2 teaspoon of salt and a pinch of baking soda with eight ounces of warm water in a glass jar. Pour the solution into an empty spray bottle or squirt it into your nose using an ear syringe or similar device. Make a fresh batch every day. ■

Supplements and Herbs

Should you stock your medicine cabinet (or more appropriately, the cool, dry place you keep your medicines) with garlic pills, echinacea, or other supplements?

That depends. Here, courtesy of the international research collaboration Natural Standard, we list 26 common herbs and supplements and some of the conditions they're often used to treat. For each use of the supplement, you'll find a letter grade indicating how strongly the available scientific evidence supports it. See the Key to Grades to learn what the grades mean. Important to keep in mind: Some supplements that haven't been thoroughly studied (these usually earn a "C" grade) may still work—we just don't know for sure.

Like drugs, most herbs and other supplements carry a risk of side effects, and some may interfere with prescription drugs. We haven't listed the cautions associated with these products here, so be sure to check with your doctor before taking any of them. Many of these health conditions are potentially serious and require a doctor's care; don't try to self-treat.

More herbs and supplements are covered in Part 3 under the ailments they're most often used for.

KEY TO GRADES:

A Strong scientific evidence for this use

B Good scientific evidence for this use

C Unclear scientific evidence for this use

D Fair scientific evidence against this use (it may not work)

F Strong scientific evidence against this use (it probably does not work)

SUPPLEMENT	USE	GRADE
Acidophilus (*Lactobacillus acidophilus*)	Bacterial vaginosis	B
	Diarrhea prevention	C
	Irritable bowel syndrome	C
	Vaginal candidiasis (yeast infection)	C
Aloe	Constipation	B
	Genital herpes	B
	Psoriasis	B
	Seborrheic dermatitis (dandruff)	B
	Skin burns	C
Arginine	Coronary artery disease/angina	B
	Heart failure	B
	Peripheral vascular disease/intermittent claudication	B
	High blood pressure	C
Beta-glucan	High cholesterol	A
	Diabetes	B
Butterbur	Migraine prevention	B

(continued on page 214)

SUPPLEMENTS AND HERBS

(continued from page 213)

SUPPLEMENT	USE	GRADE
Chamomile	Eczema	C
	Sleep aid/sedation	C
	Upset stomach and other gastrointestinal disorders	C
Chromium	Hypoglycemia (low blood sugar)	B
	Glucose tolerance in women with polycystic ovary syndrome	B
	Obesity/weight loss	F
Coenzyme Q10	High blood pressure	B
	Angina (chest pain from clogged heart arteries)	C
Devil's claw (*Harpagophytum procumbens* DC)	Lower-back pain	B
	Osteoarthritis	B
Echinacea (*E. angustifolia* DC, *E. pallida, E. purpurea*)	Prevention of upper respiratory tract infections	C
	Treatment of upper respiratory tract infections	C
Evening primrose oil (*Oenothera biennis* L.)	Atopic dermatitis (eczema) (taken by mouth)	B
	Menopause (hot flashes)	D
	Premenstrual syndrome (PMS)	D
	Psoriasis	D
Garlic	High cholesterol	B
	Anti-platelet effects (blood thinning)	C
	High blood pressure	C
Ginger	Nausea and vomiting during pregnancy	B
	Motion sickness/seasickness	C
	Nausea due to chemotherapy	C
	Rheumatoid arthritis/osteoarthritis/joint and muscle pain	C
Ginkgo (*Ginkgo biloba*)	Claudication (painful legs from clogged arteries)	A
	Dementia (multi-infarct and Alzheimer's type)	A
	Memory enhancement in healthy people	C
Ginseng	Heart conditions	B
	Mental performance (thinking or learning)	B
	High blood sugar/glucose intolerance	B
	Cancer prevention	C
	Congestive heart failure	C
	Exercise performance	C
	Fatigue	C

SUPPLEMENT	USE	GRADE
Grape seed (*Vitis vinifera, V. coignetiae*)	Chronic venous insufficiency (poor circulation in leg veins causing symptoms such as itching, heaviness, and burning)	A
	Edema (swelling)	A
	Diabetic retinopathy	B
	Vascular fragility (causing a tendency of small blood vessels to leak)	B
Horse chestnut	Chronic venous insufficiency (poor circulation in leg veins causing symptoms such as itching, heaviness, and burning)	A
Kava	Anxiety	A
Lemon balm	Herpes simplex infections	B
Melatonin	Sleep enhancement in healthy people	B
	Insomnia in the elderly	B
Milk thistle (*Silybum marianum*)	Chronic hepatitis (liver inflammation)	B
	Cirrhosis	B
	Liver damage from drugs or toxins	C
Psyllium	High cholesterol	A
	Constipation	B
St. John's wort	Depression (mild to moderate)	A
Selenium	Prostate cancer prevention	B
Willow bark (*Salix* spp.)	Osteoarthritis	A
	Lower-back pain	B
	Headache	C

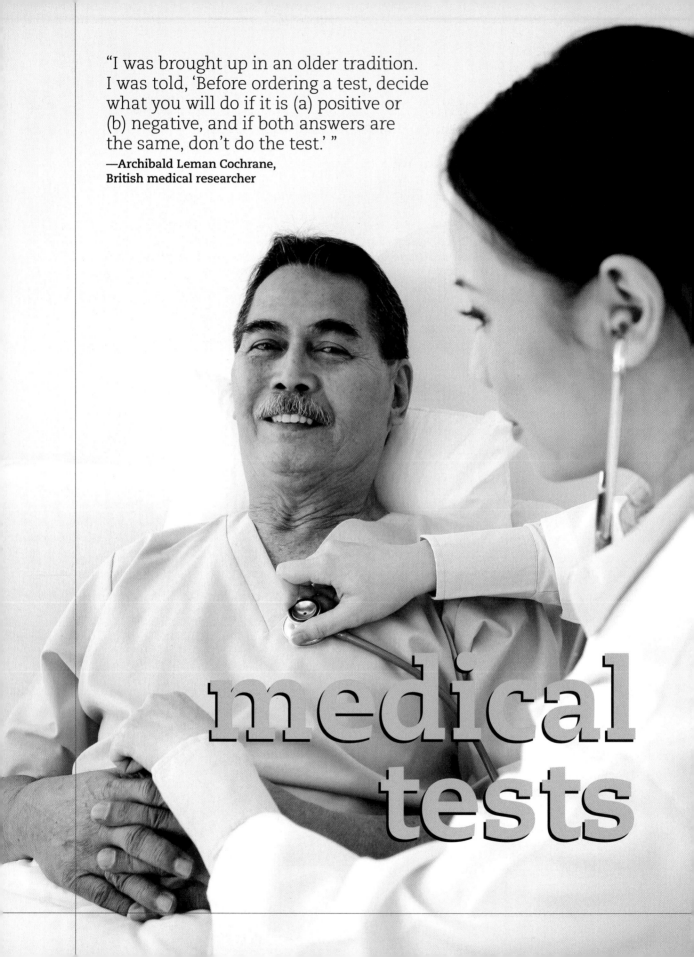

"I was brought up in an older tradition. I was told, 'Before ordering a test, decide what you will do if it is (a) positive or (b) negative, and if both answers are the same, don't do the test.'"
—Archibald Leman Cochrane,
British medical researcher

medical tests

Annual Physical

Your family doctor may be a brilliant, compassionate healer who listens to your concerns and doesn't rush through appointments. But do you really need to see him once a year, even if you feel fine? Many people—and their docs—believe that annual checkups are *de rigueur*. But major medical groups say it just isn't so.

Does everyone need an annual physical?

Despite what your doctor may say, a yearly office visit simply isn't necessary for most people.

During an annual physical exam, doctors measure height, weight, blood pressure, pulse, and much more. They draw blood. They ask questions and take notes. In short, they gather lots of information. Sure, it's nice to know what's going on inside your body. (Want to know your percentage of body fat? A simple test can tell you.) But does all that poking and prodding yield information that actually *changes* anything about your healthcare? In most cases, no. And in fact, a number of studies found that people who saw general practitioners for physicals every year were no healthier than others who saw their doctors less frequently.

The American Medical Association recommends that people under 40 have a complete physical exam every five years; for everyone else, they recommend a checkup every one to three years, at your doctor's discretion. No other major medical organization recommends annual physical exams for everyone.

Many doctors, though, are attached to annual physicals. In fact, a recent survey found that two-thirds of physicians in the United States usually advised their patients to schedule yearly checkups. If you are in good health and your doctor insists that you have an annual physical, ask why. ■

TESTING FOR NOTHING?

Chances are, if you visit your doctor for a physical, he'll draw blood and have you pee in a cup. You may sigh with relief when the doctor calls later to say your test results were normal—but the odds of hearing bad news were tiny to begin with.

In 1996, Mayo Clinic researchers looked at the routine lab results of 531 patients and found that fewer than 1 percent of complete blood count (CBC), urinalysis, and thyroid tests led to a diagnosis that called for a new treatment or a change in therapy. The chemistry panel, which measures total cholesterol, glucose, and many other blood elements, was only a bit more worthwhile, resulting in a new treatment recommendation less than 3 percent of the time. Several groups of medical experts have advised against the routine use of these tests, with one exception: lipid tests, which analyze all blood fats, including LDL cholesterol, HDL cholesterol, and triglycerides. The Mayo Clinic study showed that one out of six lipid tests detected treatable problems. The bottom line: Have your cholesterol checked regularly (see page 220).

Bone Density Tests

Further proof that aging isn't fair: You can drink fat-free milk every day, pop calcium pills religiously, get plenty of weight-bearing exercise—and *still* develop osteoporosis. Medication can slow this disease, which increases the risk of potentially devastating hip fractures and other broken bones. That makes early detection through bone density testing crucial.

Who needs one?

All women should begin having bone density tests by age 65. But some women should start earlier.

Prime candidates for earlier testing include women who have reached menopause *and* have one or more risk factors, such as a family history of osteoporosis or a fractured bone. Doctors also use bone density tests to track how well a patient responds to treatments for osteoporosis and other bone disorders.

There are no established testing guidelines for men, nor are there hard rules about how often anyone should have their bones tested. Women who are several years past menopause may lose only about 1 percent of bone mineral density per year. Such a small change would not be detected, so experts agree that waiting at least two years between exams is probably adequate.

Which type of test is best?

Dual-energy x-ray absorptiometry (DXA or DEXA for short) is the gold standard.

DXA uses a low-dose x-ray to scan the hips and spine. The procedure is painless and takes about 15 minutes.

All bone density tests produce a T score, which reflects the sturdiness of your skeleton compared to that of a healthy young adult. A T score between −1 and −2.5 means you have osteopenia, or low bone mass. A score of −2.5 or lower means you have osteoporosis. Each drop of −1 in your T score indicates that you are 2 to 2.5 times more likely than a healthy young adult to fracture a hip. It also means that your risk of all other bone fractures is increased 1.5 to 2 times.

Keep in mind that fragile bones are just one cause of hip fractures and other broken bones, so acing your DXA test or any other bone exam won't necessarily keep you out of a cast. In a study of more than 8,000 postmenopausal women, more than half the participants who suffered broken hips had received a normal DXA test result within the previous five years. Doctors will soon start using a new scoring system created by the World Health Organization that uses bone density and other factors—such as patient's age and whether she engages in activities such as walking or jogging, which protect against osteoporosis—to determine who's at risk for broken bones.

Is a heel ultrasound as good as DXA?

No. If a heel ultrasound or a similar test suggests osteoporosis, have a DXA test to confirm the diagnosis.

Many small hospitals and clinics don't offer DXA

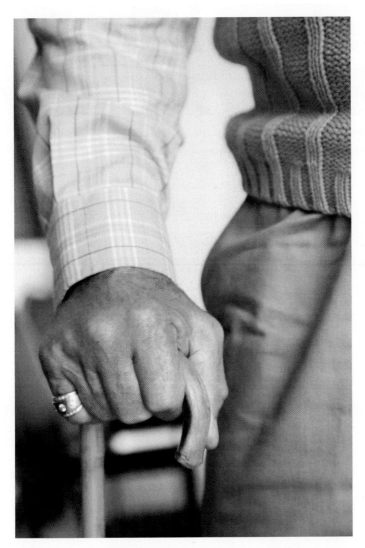

CALCULATE YOUR RISK OF BREAKING A HIP

Even if you don't have your bones scanned, you can get a good idea of how likely you are to break a hip in the next five years by taking an easy online questionnaire at hipcalculator.fhcrc.org. The quiz is designed for post-menopausal women and asks questions such as whether you smoke, have diabetes, or have a parent who broke a hip after age 40. If your risk is high, talk to your doctor about taking calcium supplements, getting more weight-bearing exercise, improving your balance, and fall-proofing your home.

because they don't have the large, expensive machines. The most common alternative is heel ultrasound, which uses a small portable device to measure bone density in the heel. Heel ultrasound assumes that bone density in the foot is a good indicator of a person's overall risk of bone fracture. However, studies show that heel ultrasound misses osteoporosis in the hip about 30 percent of the time. Other alternatives to DXA include pDXA, which measures bone density in the finger, wrist, or other "peripheral" site. Like heel ultrasound, pDXA is not as accurate as DXA but is a reasonable alternative if DXA is not available. However, if one of these tests produces a low T score indicating that you may have osteopenia or osteoporosis, seek out a DXA test to confirm the diagnosis. ■

Cholesterol Tests

Does cholesterol still matter? The answer is a resounding yes, even though recent research suggests that this waxy stuff is just one of several factors that conspire to cause heart attacks and strokes. Experts say that by identifying people who need cholesterol-lowering medication, the tests save lives.

Who needs one?

Everyone 20 and older should have a cholesterol test at least every five years. If you have a family history of heart disease or other risk factors, your doctor may test you more often.

A cholesterol test, also known as a lipid panel or lipid profile, measures how many milligrams of this fat-like substance are contained in one deciliter of blood, which is slightly less than a half cup. The standard test checks your level of total cholesterol as well as LDL ("bad") and HDL ("good") cholesterol levels. It also measures triglycerides, another type of potentially dangerous blood fat. For accurate results, you should fast for 9 to 12 hours before a cholesterol test. Failure to do so is the most common cause of skewed results. (If your test shows that you have elevated cholesterol and triglycerides, your doctor will probably repeat it.)

Patients whose cholesterol levels place them in the danger zone (over 240 mg/dl) usually receive a prescription for a statin or other cholesterol-lowering drug. Studies show that these medications prevent 25 to 50 percent of heart attacks and strokes in high-risk patients.

If my LDL is high but so is my HDL, am I protected?

Somewhat. Having high "good" cholesterol may offset some of the damage caused by "bad" cholesterol.

By now you may know that "bad" LDL cholesterol contributes to plaque in the arteries while "good" HDL sweeps bad cholesterol out of the body. Some doctors believe that a patient's ratio of bad to good cholesterol offers a better indication of their heart disease risk than their LDL or total cholesterol levels.

Most labs determine cholesterol ratio by dividing the total cholesterol number by the HDL number. For example, if your total cholesterol is 195 and your HDL is 50, your ratio is 3:9. A ratio higher than 5:1 increases the risk of heart attacks, while 3.5:1 or lower protects the heart.

The American Heart Association insists that absolute cholesterol numbers are a

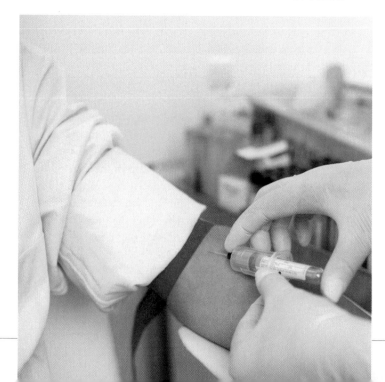

better predictor of heart attack risk, but new studies suggest that cholesterol ratio shouldn't be overlooked. A 2007 review of 61 studies involving nearly 800,000 participants found that cholesterol ratio was twice as accurate as total cholesterol for identifying people at risk for fatal heart attacks.

If my cholesterol numbers are good, can I still have a heart attack?

Absolutely. High cholesterol is just one threat to your heart.

Studies show that one-third to one-half of all heart attacks occur in people who do *not* have high cholesterol. There are at least two morals to this story. First, maybe the bar for "high" cholesterol should be lowered; some doctors argue that putting even more people on cholesterol-lowering drugs would prevent many heart attacks and deaths. Second, your cholesterol numbers don't tell the whole story of your risk for heart attacks and strokes. They say nothing, for instance, about how inflamed the linings of your arteries are. Many cardiologists now believe that most heart attacks occur when inflammation causes cholesterol-filled "plaques" that form along the inner walls of arteries to break apart and form blockages that starve the heart of blood. In

response, some doctors now test the blood for C-reactive protein (CRP), a marker of inflammation. In some cases, doctors may also check the blood for other potential signs of trouble, including elevated fibrinogen (which causes blood to clot), homocysteine (an amino acid linked to heart disease), and Lp(a), a particularly dangerous cholesterol particle.

Should I get a CRP test?

Not necessarily. This test can reveal whether your arteries are inflamed, but many doctors say that doesn't tell them much.

If inflammation triggers heart attacks, as many cardiologists

believe, wouldn't it help to know whether your arteries are overheated? Your doctor can order a simple test to measure CRP, an indicator of inflammation, which can be performed by the same lab that measures your cholesterol. Studies show that people with high CRP (3 milligrams per liter or more) are twice as likely to have heart attacks as people with low CRP (1 mg/L or less). They are also less likely to survive heart attacks, and they have more strokes as well. In fact, people with elevated CRP have a high risk of heart attacks and strokes even if they have normal cholesterol levels.

It sounds like a no-brainer, then, to have your CRP tested—but it isn't. Many doctors shrug and roll their eyes

HEART SCANS—OR SCAMS?

Doctors have many ways of judging your risk of having a heart attack—and deciding how aggressively to lower it with medication. The cholesterol test is one. Another is a fancy x-ray called electron-beam computed tomography, or EBCT (also called Ultrafast CT), which reveals calcium in the arteries. Large deposits of this mineral increase the risk of heart attack by two or three times.

Some research suggests that EBCT offers a more accurate picture of a patient's heart attack risk than older tests, such as the cardiac stress test (which uses an electrocardiogram to measure heart activity while a patient exercises). However, EBCT is expensive and exposes patients to radiation. It can produce false-positive results—and a negative result doesn't necessarily mean you're not at risk for a heart attack.

Do you need the scan? The answer for most people is no, though there are exceptions. A recent study found that women who seemed to have a low risk of cardiovascular disease yet had high calcium scores were six times more likely to have heart attacks than women with no calcium in their arteries.

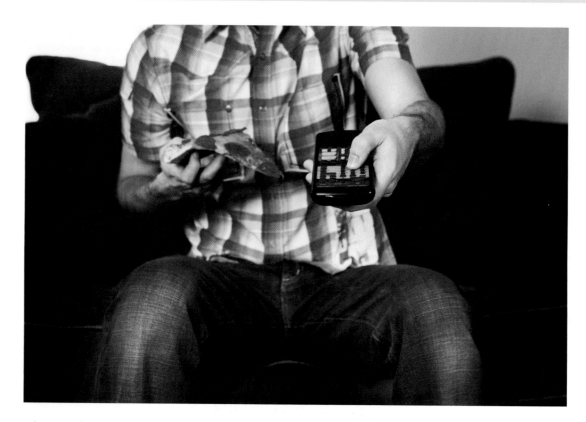

when you bring up CRP. That's because people with elevated CRP almost always have other, more obvious risk factors for heart attacks: They smoke, they're overweight, they have high blood pressure and high blood sugar. In other words, a doctor can tell without a CRP test that the patient is at risk. What's more, a high CRP level may simply be a sign of one of these conditions or, for that matter, an indicator of entirely unrelated inflammation. Perhaps you sprained your ankle recently, for example, or you have rheumatoid arthritis.

Scientists are still studying whether measuring CRP can help prevent heart attacks. The American Heart Association says the test is best reserved for patients who have a borderline risk of heart disease as a way to help doctors decide which treatment to recommend. For example, knowing that a patient with moderately elevated cholesterol also has high CRP may help a doctor decide to prescribe a statin drug (which, by the way, lowers cholesterol *and* CRP). ■

One-third to half of all heart attacks occur in people who do *not* have high cholesterol.

Colon Cancer Screening

As rites of passage go, having a colonoscopy when you turn 50 is a lot less fun than, say, having your first legal glass of beer at age 21. But you'd be a fool to skip it, despite the inconvenience and discomfort, since colorectal cancer is the second most common cause of cancer deaths in the United States. Should you go "virtual"? It's true that new, less invasive methods make screening a relative breeze, but they sacrifice accuracy.

Can I get away with a sigmoidoscopy instead of a colonoscopy?

You can, but you may not want to. Colonoscopy is the gold standard for a reason.

The colonoscopy, which allows a doctor to view the entire large intestine, is the best method for detecting colon tumors and polyps, small wart-like growths on the lining of the intestine that may turn cancerous. Studies show that colonoscopies detect about 90 percent of large polyps and 75 percent of smaller ones. (Doctors can usually remove polyps during a colonoscopy.) The detection rate for full-blown colon cancer is higher still.

A sigmoidoscopy examines only the lower portion of the large intestine, known as the sigmoid or descending colon, and the rectum. The test is cheaper and faster than colonoscopy, doesn't require sedation, and carries a lower risk of complications. The downside? It can't see tumors and polyps in approximately half of the colon. If a doctor finds a polyp, however, she will usually order a colonoscopy in order to view the rest of the colon. For that reason, sigmoidoscopies help to identify up to 70 to 80 percent of the most dangerous polyps and malignant colon tumors. Also bridging the gap between the two tests is the fact that sigmoidoscopy is performed more often (typically every 5 years instead of every

Our BEST ADVICE

If your doctor suggests a barium enema, say "no thanks" and opt for a different test instead. In a double-contrast barium enema (DCBE), a technician x-rays the intestines after they have been filled with the chemical barium and air through a tube inserted in the anus. But DCBE is far less sensitive than a colonoscopy; it may miss more than half of large polyps in a colon. If you do have a DCBE, and it detects signs of trouble, the American College of Gastroenterology recommends having a follow-up colonoscopy.

10) and is often used in conjunction with annual fecal occult blood tests.

The bottom line: A colonoscopy is considered by most doctors to be the first line of defense against colon cancer. But if you can't afford one, don't have access to a doctor who is qualified to perform one, or refuse to have one, a sigmoidoscopy with annual fecal occult blood testing is your next best bet.

One study of 37,702 men and women found that people who had undergone either a colonoscopy or sigmoidoscopy cut their risk of dying from colon cancer by 50 percent. According to another estimate, if all adults eligible for screening were actually tested, deaths from colon cancer would drop by 42 percent.

Is a "virtual" colon-oscopy as accurate as traditional colonoscopy?

We don't know yet. Virtual colonoscopy is a tempting alternative, but more research is needed before experts can recommend it in place of tra-ditional colonoscopy.

Who wouldn't want to forgo having a long tube inserted into all five feet of their colon and instead lie on a table and pass painlessly through a CT (computed tomography) or MRI scanner to have their colon scrutinized "virtually"? Virtual colonoscopy produces three-dimensional images of your colon, no sedation required. The procedure is over in about 10 minutes, which is much faster than conventional colonoscopy.

It sounds great, but there are drawbacks. Virtual colonoscopy doesn't excuse you from the pretest bowel-

WHEN A HOME TEST IS BEST

Many doctors continue to do fecal occult blood tests (FOBTs) based on stool samples obtained during a digital rectal exam, despite clear evidence that tests you perform yourself at home by obtaining samples from three consecutive bowel movements work better.

Colorectal tumors bleed on and off, so a single sample may miss evidence of bleeding. One study found that the single-sample FOBT helped to detect just *5 percent* of tumors. Not surprisingly, no major medical organization recommends this test. Yet a survey by the U.S. Centers for Disease Control and Prevention (CDC) found that about one-third of primary care physicians in the United States screen for colorectal cancer by using it. The CDC researchers speculated that doctors assume that many patients won't complete the at-home test. If your doctor performs an in-office FOBT, ask him to give you a home kit, too.

A new version of the home test kit called the immunochem-ical fecal occult blood test may be more accurate than older tests and eliminate a key reason many people don't like per-forming the FOBT: Having to avoid certain foods (including red meat) and taking certain medications (including ibuprofen and naproxen) for three days to a week before testing. In one study of 5,841 people, the immunochemical test detected 82 percent of existing colon tumors, while the older test identified only 64 percent.

cleansing ritual that no one enjoys—consuming a diet of clear liquids, taking laxatives, and performing an enema. And if the test finds a polyp, you'll need to follow up with a traditional colonoscopy—and repeat the bowel-cleansing ritual—to have the polyp removed.

How accurate a virtual colonoscopy is may depend on who's performing the test and how big your polyps are, if you have any. Some studies, including a 2003 analysis of more than 1,200 patients pub-lished in the *New England*

Journal of Medicine, give a slight edge to virtual colonoscopy. However, the doctors in that study had extensive experience with this new tool. But virtual colonoscopy is still a new screening test, and several other reports suggest that many doctors haven't quite mastered it. For instance, a 2004 study in the *Journal of the American Medical Associa-tion* comparing conventional and virtual colonoscopy at nine major hospitals in the United States showed that the latter detected just 39 percent of small polyps, while the standard test spotted 99 percent. The accuracy of virtual colonoscopy was better for larger polyps—55 percent versus 100 percent for old-style colonoscopy—but still far from perfect. The study's authors blamed lack of experience with the new device for the disparity.

Virtual colonoscopy may one day be a reliable alternative to traditional colonoscopies, but at present, major medical organizations such as the American College of Gastroenterology do not recommend it.

Is a fecal occult blood test worthwhile?

It may be worthwhile between sigmoidoscopies or as a bare-minimum screening method if you can't or won't have a sigmoidoscopy or colonoscopy.

The fecal occult blood test, or FOBT, is a relatively simple test that can detect traces of blood in the stool—often the only symptom of colorectal cancer. A single FOBT isn't as accurate as a colonoscopy, though having one annually increases its effectiveness.

Many doctors perform this test in the office despite evidence that the home version is actually far superior. Blood in the stool may be a sign of cancer, or it may be evidence that you have polyps, small growths that can turn into tumors. However, a positive test doesn't necessarily mean that you have colorectal cancer. A number of gastrointestinal problems can produce blood in the stool, including colitis, hemorrhoids, Crohn's disease, and others. If an FOBT finds blood in your stool, your doctor will order further tests to determine the cause.

Having an annual FOBT is an inexpensive option for colon cancer screening, though doctors recommend having a sigmoidoscopy every five years as insurance. If you have a colonoscopy when you turn 50 and it's negative, you don't need an FOBT or any other form of colon cancer screening for another 10 years.

Persistence appears to pay off with this test: One 13-year study found that people who had annual FOBTs cut their risk of dying from colorectal cancer by 33 percent. ∎

WHEN TO GET TESTED

The risk of colon cancer begins to rise after you turn 40 but remains small until age 50, the point at which most medical groups recommend that all adults begin colon cancer screening. (Your doctor may want you to start earlier and get checked more often if you're at high risk for the disease due to a personal or family history of colon cancer or polyps or you have chronic inflammatory bowel disease, such as ulcerative colitis or Crohn's disease.) Which test is best for you? That's a question to discuss with your doctor. The answer may depend in part on what you're willing to do—and what your insurance will pay for. The American Cancer Society recommends choosing one of the following five screening schedules.

- A fecal occult blood test (FOBT) once a year

- A sigmoidoscopy every 5 years

- An FOBT plus sigmoidoscopy every 5 years (this combination is better than having either test alone)

- A double-contrast barium enema every 5 years (see "Our Best Advice" on page 223 for our take on this exam)

- A colonoscopy every 10 years

If any of the first four tests is positive, you should have a follow-up colonoscopy. If a colonoscopy is negative, your doctor may decide there's no reason for further colon cancer screening of any kind for the next 10 years.

ELECTROCARDIOGRAM

Electrocardiogram

When you think of electricity, you probably think of the juice flowing from wall outlets that powers the TV. But a similar kind of electrical activity allows the heart to pump blood. An electrocardiogram (ECG) checks to see whether the heart's wiring is up to code by measuring the rhythm of its contractions. An ECG is an indispensable tool—if you have reason to have the test. But many people don't.

Who needs one?

If you feel fine and don't have a high risk of heart disease, you probably don't need this test.

The ECG, which records heart activity through electrodes that are attached to the skin, helps diagnose heart disease in patients who have chest pain or other symptoms. Some doctors, however, give all patients ECGs as part of routine physical exams starting at age 50, 40, or even earlier. Yet no major medical organization recommends routine ECGs for healthy people with a normal risk of heart attack.

The American Heart Association and American College of Cardiology say that ECGs may be worthwhile in men over 45 and women over 55 who have a family history of cardiovascular disease or other factors that increase the risk of a heart attack, are about to start rigorous exercise plans, or have jobs that affect public safety (such as airline pilots). But if you don't fall into one of these categories, you probably don't need an ECG. The test can identify some people at risk for heart disease, but it misses many others and causes a large number of false alarms.

An ECG can spot abnormalities such as arrhythmias, which may someday cause serious heart problems. It can also detect evidence that a person already has heart disease, a diagnosis that is typically confirmed with more tests. Unfortunately, there is little evidence that an ECG is a reliable method for spotting potential heart trouble in people who have no symptoms or major risk factors. False-positive results are common when ECGs are used as a routine screening test for heart disease. One study found that 71 percent of people who had abnormal test results on screening ECGs turned out *not* to have heart disease. A false-positive ECG could result in needless additional procedures, such as coronary angiography, which requires having a catheter inserted into a blood vessel. What's more, a resting ECG that turns up no signs of trouble is no cause for celebration; about 50 percent of people with heart disease have normal ECG results.

Stress tests—ECGs conducted during vigorous exercise—are more accurate but still predict whether a person will have a heart attack only 40 to 62 percent of the time.

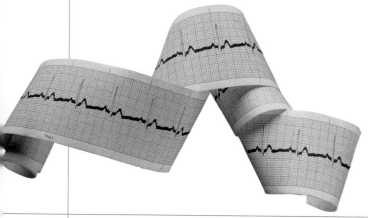

ELECTROCARDIOGRAM

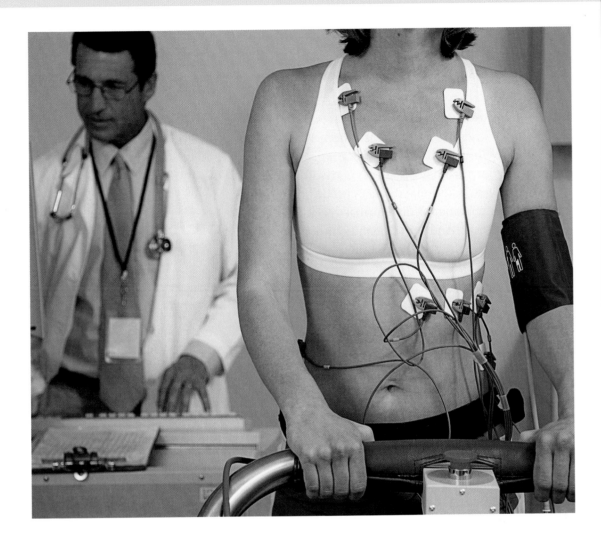

Are ECGs less accurate in women?

Yes. Although the ECG was invented a century ago, this test still does not adequately account for differences in the male and female heartbeat.

Among the countless differences between the sexes, here's one you may not know about:

A woman's heartbeat "looks" different from a man's on an ECG. For instance, on average, a woman's heart beats slightly faster than a man's does. And certain phases of the female heartbeat last longer; they are depicted by greater intervals between the jagged peaks and valleys on an ECG.

Many studies, dating back to 1920, have confirmed these sex-related differences in ECGs, yet doctors typically evaluate an ECG using criteria based on studies of men. As a result, ECGs may produce false-positive results in women 25 to 50 percent of the time. Fortunately, recent studies are providing doctors with new and better criteria for judging women's ECG results. ■

MAMMOGRAMS

Mammograms

It seems hard to argue with a screening test that can cut a woman's risk of dying from breast cancer. But mammograms aren't without controversy, especially in women under 50. Women who get them regularly are more likely to end up having additional medical procedures that can be painful, frightening, or disfiguring—even if they don't have breast cancer. And traditional mammograms spot breast cancer less effectively in younger women.

Who should have routine mammograms?

Many medical authorities say that women should begin at age 40, but research suggests that women over 50 are most likely to benefit.

Women aged 50 to 69 who have routine mammograms reduce their risk of dying from breast cancer by 20 to 35 percent. Mammograms benefit women 70 and older, too, in whom breast cancer risk is even greater. However, doctors may discourage routine screening for breast cancer in patients who are very old or have some other life-threatening condition.

Mammograms offer less benefit to women under 50, for several reasons. Breast cancer is less common in younger women, and younger women tend to have dense breast tissue, which makes tumors more difficult to detect with mammography.

How accurate are mammograms?

They detect about 75 percent of tumors. But false positives are not uncommon, and a negative mammogram does not guarantee you're in the clear.

Mammograms are more accurate in older women and women whose breasts are mostly fat tissue, which is not dense and which x-rays can easily "see" through. Mammograms are less effective in women with dense breasts and those under 50. One study found that when women with very dense breasts have mammograms, tumors are not visible or are not detected 37 percent of the time. (By the way, roughly half of all breast cancers are detected by women themselves.)

About 6 to 10 percent of mammograms produce false-positive results—that is, images that show what look like tumors but prove to be cysts and other harmless masses. Some studies suggest that estimate may be higher, particularly in younger women. Determining whether a suspicious spot is cancer can require additional imaging and in some cases a painful needle biopsy followed by an anxious period of days or weeks waiting for the results. A study published in the *New England Journal of Medicine* found that among 1,000 women who had annual mammograms for 10 years, half received at least one false-positive result. The authors estimated that about one in five women without breast cancer who has regular mammograms undergoes a needle biopsy.

One review estimated that 2,000 women would need to have annual mammograms for 10 years to save one life. Meanwhile, 10 of those women would be diagnosed with DCIS, or ductal carcinoma in situ, a harmless form of cancer that will never spread—and would undergo unnecessary treatment, which may mean surgery and radiation.

MAMMOGRAMS

Are digital mammograms more accurate?

A growing number of clinics now offer digital mammograms, but studies suggest they may not be worth the extra expense for most women.

While the traditional mammogram is little more than an x-ray, digital mammography adds computers and special software to enhance images of breast tissue. But this technology upgrade hasn't necessarily led to better breast cancer detection. A large study involving more than 222,000 women published in the *New England Journal of Medicine* found that switching from traditional mammograms to computer-aided mammograms didn't improve radiologists' ability to detect breast tumors. Women who had computer-aided mammograms *were* more likely to receive false-positive test results and to require needle biopsies.

Some women may benefit from having digital mammograms, however. One study found that the technology spotted more tumors than film mammography in women with dense breasts. It may be worth asking your physician about digital mammograms if you have dense breasts, you're under 50, or you haven't hit menopause yet. Just keep in mind that greater accuracy may come with a higher risk of unnecessary procedures.

Do some women need an MRI in addition to a mammogram?

Yes, but only a small number of women will benefit from this additional imaging.

If you have a very high risk of breast cancer, a doctor may recommend that you undergo magnetic resonance imaging (MRI) in addition to having mammograms. You may be a candidate for an MRI if you have already had breast cancer, you have a strong family history (such as several blood relatives who had the disease at a young age), you carry certain genetic markers for breast cancer, you had chest radiation between the ages of 10 and 30, or you or a close relative have certain rare conditions that increase breast cancer risk.

Studies show that MRI detects far more breast tumors in high-risk women than traditional mammograms do. However, it is also considerably less discriminating. A Dutch study of 1,909 women comparing mammograms to MRI found that the latter led to twice as many unneeded examinations and three times as many unneeded biopsies. ■

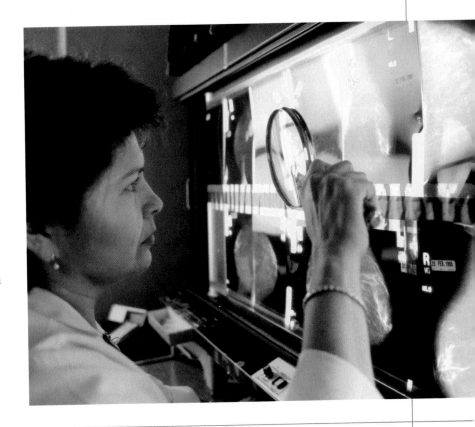

Pap Smear

The Pap smear is a medical success story, largely credited with cutting the rate of cervical cancer by 70 to 90 percent in many countries over the past half century. Named for its inventor, George N. Papanicolaou, MD, the Pap smear (also called the Pap test) detects cancer cells and abnormal cells that may become malignant. Although the Pap smear has near-sacred status in women's healthcare, new approaches to screening for cervical cancer are on the horizon.

Who needs one?

All women, though some may not require annual exams, and older women may not need Pap tests anymore.

The major cause of cervical cancer is human papillomavirus (HPV), which is typically transmitted through sexual intercourse. Most guidelines recommend that women begin having annual Pap smears within three years of their first sexual activity or by age 21. Some physicians believe that women over 30 who have had three consecutive negative Pap smears need to be screened only every two or three years. Some doctors worry, however, that women who don't have annual Pap smears may end up skipping other important screening exams that gynecologists perform. "For most women, getting a Pap smear is synonymous with going to the gynecologist," says Lauren Streicher, MD, of Northwestern Memorial Hospital in Chicago. Regardless of your schedule for Pap smears, you should still plan on having other routine screening tests, including pelvic exams, clinical breast exams, and blood tests for sexually transmitted diseases.

Women aged 65 to 70 may stop having Pap smears if they have had three consecutive negative tests in a 10-year period. A woman who has had her cervix removed doesn't need to have a Pap smear unless the surgery was performed because she had cervical or uterine cancer. (Keep in mind that the cervix is not always removed as part of a hysterectomy; in such cases, regular Pap smears are still recommended.)

How accurate is the Pap smear?

The Pap smear is only modestly sensitive, which is why routine testing is necessary to guard against cervical cancer.

A Pap smear will detect cervical cancer or abnormal cells that could become cancerous about 50 to 75 percent of the time. The test is even less likely to spot cells that are only mildly abnormal. To perform a Pap smear, a doctor, nurse, or other trained healthcare professional removes cells from the cervix with a special scraper (sometimes called a spatula) and/or brush. The cells are smeared on a glass slide and analyzed in a lab. Problems with preparing or reading the slide may affect the test's accuracy. However, cervical cancer develops over many years, so regularly scheduled Pap smears usually detect the disease while it's still treatable.

As with many screening tests, the Pap smear produces a significant number of false-positive results. The risk that a Pap smear will cause a false alarm rises as a woman ages. In one four-year study, 2,500 postmenopausal women had annual Pap smears, which produced 110 abnormal results and led to 231 additional tests, including biopsies. Yet none of the women had cervical cancer, and just one required

PAP SMEAR

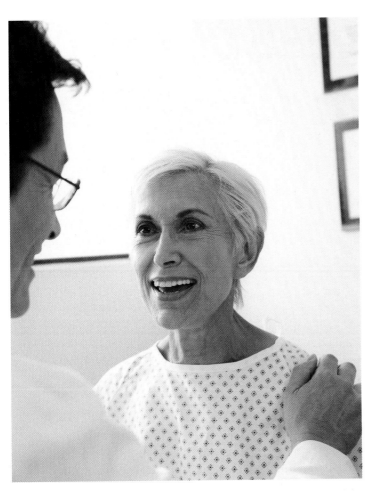

request—and many doctors automatically administer—both tests. Unfortunately, the HPV test is expensive and may not be covered by insurance.

Do young women who have had the HPV vaccine still need Pap smears?

Yes. Although the HPV vaccine is very effective, it doesn't offer 100 percent protection against cervical cancer.

A vaccine called Gardasil that prevents HPV infection and genital warts is now available in the United States and a number of other countries. Other vaccines are on the way. Gardasil is most effective if a person is not already infected with HPV and is currently approved for girls and women aged 9 to 26. Gardasil guards against only four strains of HPV. Two of these strains are responsible for 70 percent of cervical cancer cases, while the other two are responsible for 90 percent of genital warts. Although Gardasil is a powerful defense against cancer, women who have been vaccinated remain vulnerable to other HPV infections. What's more, women who were sexually active before being vaccinated may have already been exposed to HPV. For these reasons, women who have been vaccinated still need Pap smears. ■

additional treatment for precancerous cell growth.

On the other hand, if your Pap smear is negative, you can breathe easy; the chances are 95 percent or better that you do not have cervical cancer.

Should you have an HPV test?

It's a good idea. Recent studies suggest that testing for HPV, the virus that causes cervical cancer, may be more sensitive than the Pap test, though it also produces more false alarms.

Some doctors believe that a test for HPV, which was introduced in 2000, could someday replace the Pap smear. In a study published in the *New England Journal of Medicine*, the HPV test detected 94.6 percent of abnormal growths, far outpacing the Pap smear, which detected only 55.4 percent. The HPV test had a slightly greater chance of producing a false-positive result. Having both tests may be the best bet: In the study, combining the tests was 100 percent effective in detecting precancerous growths. Some women now

Prostate-Specific Antigen (PSA) Test

Deciding to have a blood test that detects cancer when it's still treatable sounds like the ultimate no-brainer. Yet the prostate-specific antigen (PSA) test, which can identify men who have early-stage prostate cancer, has been controversial since its introduction in the late 1980s. There is no doubt that the test can detect prostate cancer in men who otherwise appear healthy. But critics say the test produces too many false alarms and often leads to needless surgery, radiation, and other medical procedures.

Who needs one?

It's tough to find a definitive answer. Most medical groups recommend only that men discuss the PSA test with their doctors.

Millions of men around the world who have reached middle age wouldn't think of letting a year pass without having a PSA test. Yet doctors still disagree—often heatedly— as to whether the test should be used to screen for prostate cancer in healthy men.

Many doctors are firm believers in the PSA test, pointing to a decrease in deaths from prostate cancer since the test was introduced in the 1980s (though it's not clear what actually caused the drop). The American Urological Association encourages men to begin having annual PSA tests when they turn 50, or 40 if they have a high risk of prostate cancer because of their race (African-American males are at increased risk) or a family history of the disease. Doctors generally don't recommend the PSA test for men with a life expectancy of less than 10 years.

Meanwhile, other physicians point out that up to 30 percent of tumors detected by PSA tests and other forms of prostate cancer screening grow very slowly, won't spread, and would never kill a man. Unfortunately, there is no reliable way of telling whether a tumor will remain dormant, so most men diagnosed with early-stage prostate cancer undergo some form of treatment, such as surgery to remove the gland or radiation therapy to destroy cancer cells. These treatments are usually successful but can cause erectile dysfunction, diarrhea, and incontinence.

The case for PSA testing would be strengthened by solid evidence that it saves lives. Two large studies involving more than 50,000 participants failed to show that men who have PSA tests are less likely to die of prostate cancer. Unfortunately, these trials were seriously flawed, so the true benefit of this common test remains unknown.

How accurate is the PSA test?

Elevated PSA may mean a man has prostate cancer. Then again, PSA can rise for other reasons, so a positive test may be no cause for concern.

If a man has prostate cancer, there is a 63 to 83 percent chance his PSA will be higher than 4.0 ng/ml (nanograms per milliliter of blood serum), which doctors have long used as a threshold to decide whether a man should undergo further testing to determine whether he actually has prostate cancer. If his cancer is aggressive, he is even more likely to have a high PSA number. However, many doctors now use lower thresholds, which identify even more men with prostate cancer—and create more false alarms.

Most men who have positive PSA tests—regardless of which threshold a doctor uses—do *not* have prostate cancer. In fact, just 18 to 30 percent of men whose PSA falls between 4.0 and 10.0 ng/ml have the disease. Certain conditions, such as an enlarged prostate and prostatitis, elevate PSA. Some activities, including sex, can raise PSA levels, too. Yet men who have positive PSA tests usually end up having needle biopsies of their prostates to find out whether or not they have cancer, which can cause soreness, bleeding, and anxiety while awaiting results.

Are "new, improved" PSA tests more accurate?

Maybe. By tracking how fast PSA rises and testing "free PSA," doctors may be better able to predict which men are truly at risk.

Many doctors today carefully track PSA velocity—that is, how much a man's PSA rises over time. PSA naturally goes up as a man ages, but a rapid increase may be cause for concern. One study published in

the *Journal of the American Medical Association* found that a man whose PSA climbs 2.0 ng/ml or more in a year is far more likely to have aggressive prostate cancer than a man whose PSA is relatively stable.

Your doctor may mention one of several variations on the PSA test that have been introduced in recent years and are designed to make it more sensitive. One of the more widely used new exams compares a man's level of PSA that's bound to other proteins in the blood with his unbound, or "free," PSA. Men with high levels of free PSA (more than 25 percent) have a low risk of prostate cancer. One study suggests that measuring free PSA in men with borderline-high total PSA could eliminate up to 20 percent of unnecessary biopsies.

If you have a PSA test, do you still need a digital rectal exam?

You do. It's far from perfect (and even less popular), but the exam may improve cancer detection.

Doctors perform the test by inserting a gloved finger into a man's rectum and feeling the prostate for abnormal growths. It's not as accurate as a PSA test. For starters, a physician can touch only the

Our BEST ADVICE

Need another reason to lose that beer belly? Your PSA tests will be more accurate. Research shows that obese men tend to have lower PSA levels than men of normal weight, which means the test could fail to detect prostate cancer. No one is sure why obese men have low PSA. However, a Duke University study of more than 14,000 men with prostate cancer showed that men who carried the most fat also had the largest volume of plasma, the watery portion of blood. That probably means that they only seem to have less PSA because their blood is more diluted.

back and sides of the prostate. In addition, doctors don't agree on what an abnormal prostate feels like. One review found that the test detects fewer than 60 percent of prostate tumors. But having a PSA test *and* a digital rectal exam may turn up more cases of prostate cancer. A study of 6,630 men found that having both exams detected 26 percent more tumors than the PSA test alone. One caveat: Having both tests also increases the risk of a false-positive test result. ■

WHOLE-BODY SCANS

Whole-Body Scans

Skeptical doctors sometimes refer to these screening exams as "whole-body *scams*." The high-priced scans use computed tomography (CT) to examine a person from head to toe, searching for early signs of disease. They sound like the stuff of science fiction novels—and many doctors say that's where these tests belong.

Who needs one?

No one.

No major medical organization recommends whole-body scans that are offered by clinics as one-stop screening for cancer, heart disease, and other conditions. A CT scan produces cross-sectional images of internal organs by passing x-rays through tissue at hundreds of different angles. These high-tech scanners have an important role in medicine. However, most doctors say there is no way to justify the heavy dose of radiation a patient receives during a whole-body scan, given the test's questionable value. The American College of Radiology calls whole-body scans a waste of money that could lead to many unnecessary follow-up procedures.

If you have a whole-body scan, you will probably receive scary news: "We found a suspicious mass." A study published in the journal *Radiology* estimated that nearly

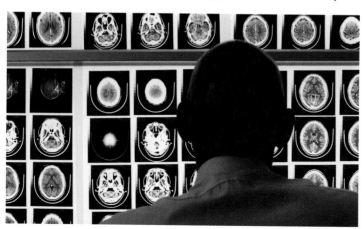

Our BEST ADVICE

The American College of Radiology (ACR) compiles and publishes "appropriateness criteria" for the value of imaging tests for specific conditions, assigning each a ranking from 1 (inappropriate) to 9 (appropriate). Unfortunately, a poll found that just one-third of radiologists use the criteria. If the test recommended by a doctor rates a 3 or less, ask whether you really need it or if some other test is more appropriate. You can see the appropriateness ratings yourself at www.acr.org. Also, if you need an x-ray or CT scan, find out if the facility is accredited by the ACR, which can help ensure that the procedure will produce a high-quality image without exposing you to excessive radiation.

91 percent of people who undergo whole-body scans have at least one positive test result. However, the vast majority of these ominous images turn out to be meaningless. The human body is full of benign nodules, clumps of scar tissue, and other harmless bumps and blobs that may turn up on a whole-body CT scan. A minuscule *2 percent* of people who test positive actually have a disease. Worse, whole-body scans may miss potential problems, so a clean test could cause a false sense of security. ■

How Much Radiation Is Too Much?

Computed tomography (CT) scans, which use high-speed computers to process multiple x-rays taken from different angles, produce exquisitely detailed cross-sectional images of organs and are now widely used in diagnosing many different conditions. But are they overused? Some scientists say yes.

After all, radiation harms cells, and CT scans expose the body to a sizable dose. For example, a CT scan of the abdomen produces at least 50 times more radiation than an x-ray. Exposure to large amounts of radiation causes a small but significant increase in the risk of cancer, particularly leukemia and cancers of the breast, lung, and thyroid.

The threat of cancer to someone undergoing a single CT scan is small, but people with conditions such as kidney stones and cancer may undergo repeated CT scans. The authors of a recent study published in the *New England Journal of Medicine* estimated that CT scans may *cause* up to 2 percent of cancer cases in the United States.

The authors of the study point out that the benefits of CT scans in medicine far outweigh the risks, but they argue that up to one-third of CT scans may be unnecessary. If your doctor says you need a CT scan, consider asking if another imaging method, such as MRI or ultrasound, would provide similar information. If you have a CT scan and you're given a copy on CD, don't lose it. It may help you avoid having a repeat scan.

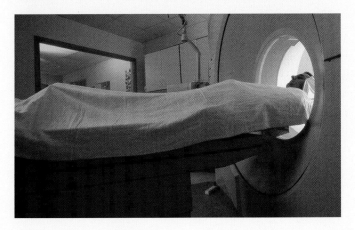

TALLYING YOUR RADIATION EXPOSURE

Some diagnostic tests expose you to more radiation than others. Here's a look at the dose a patient receives with several common tests as measured in units called millisieverts. For perspective, each year the typical person is exposed to about three millisieverts of radiation in the environment, which comes from cosmic rays, television, smoke detectors, tobacco smoke, and other sources.

TEST	RADIATION*
Dental x-ray	0.004
DXA bone scan	0.01
Limb or joint x-ray	0.06
Chest x-ray	0.1
Mammogram	0.7
Cardiac CT (for calcium score)	2
Coronary angiogram	4.6 to 15.8
Barium enema	7
CT scan, head and chest	11

*Dose in millisieverts

Sources: The Radiological Society of North America;
The Health Physics Society.

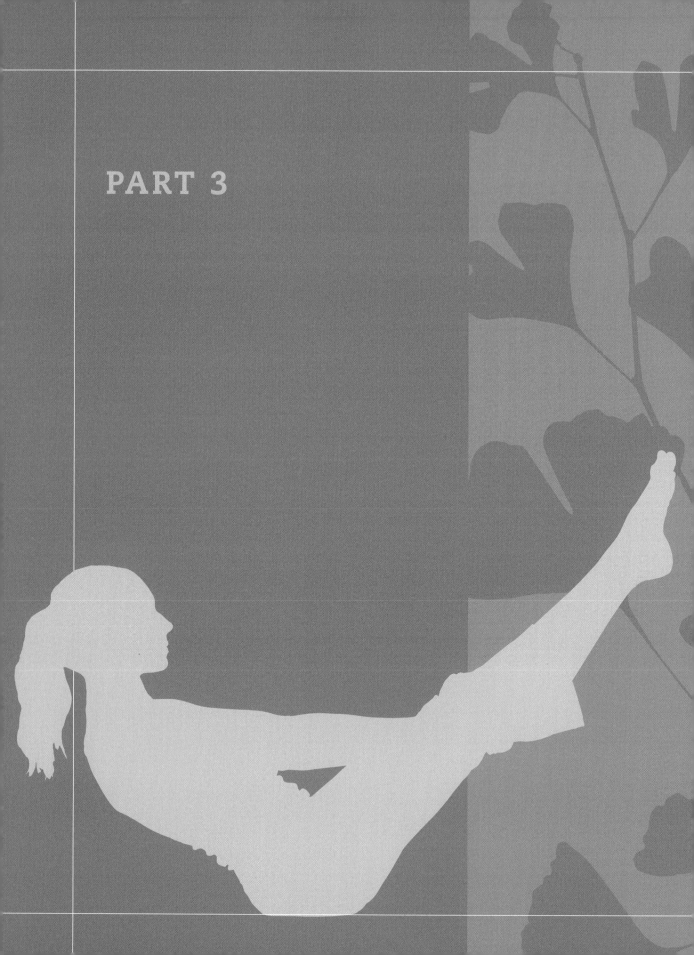

PART 3

treating
what ails you

ACNE

Acne

Chocolate and pizza don't cause acne. Neither does less-than-perfect face washing. Yet surveys show that many adults, and a whopping 41 percent of medical school students, still believe these myths. The truth? Blame your ancestors for your acne-prone skin. British researchers who studied more than 1,500 pairs of twins report that genetics accounts for 81 percent of acne cases. Until someone develops gene therapy for blemishes, a smart mix of drugstore remedies and prescription-strength medications can help in almost every case.

WORKS

✔ Acne products containing salicylic acid

Creams and cleansers containing salicylic acid—or similar chemicals such as resorcinal and lactic acid—break down the gunky mixture of skin cells and oil that clogs pores. In one small study, salicylic acid was more effective than benzoyl peroxide for reducing the number of pimples on volunteers' faces.

✔ Acne creams containing benzoyl peroxide
This drugstore remedy kills acne's main culprit: the bacterium *Propionibacterium acnes*. Recommended as a first step for teens and adults with mild, moderate, and even severe acne, it can work as well or even better than prescription antibiotic pills and creams.

In one large study, researchers split hundreds of acne sufferers among five different regimens that included benzoyl peroxide, antibiotic creams and pills, and placebo creams and pills. After 18 weeks, 60 percent of the group that used benzoyl peroxide plus a placebo pill had at least a moderate improvement. A cream combining benzoyl peroxide and the antibiotic erythromycin worked even better: 66 percent of people in this group saw clearer skin. In contrast, just 54 percent of those who took the antibiotics with a placebo had significant improvement. The bonus for your wallet: Benzoyl peroxide was one-twelfth the cost of some of the antibiotics used in the study.

Benzoyl peroxide comes in several strengths; start with the lowest to minimize side effects like redness, irritation, and peeling. Increase the strength if you're not happy with the results.

✔ Retinoid creams

Creams, gels, and washes that contain a prescription medicine such as adapalene, tazarotene, or tretinoin all work by speeding the shedding of dead skin cells. This in turn helps prevent pores from clogging. These treatments may also cool inflammation, easing redness and swelling. Expect results in 8 to 12 weeks. In one review of five well-designed studies involving 900 people with acne, tretinoin and adapalene each reduced the number of pimples on volunteers' faces by about 54 percent. In another study, tazarotene produced similar results. Other research suggests retinoids may clear up 70 percent of blemishes.

✔ Antibiotic creams

Prescription-strength antibiotic creams cleared up 35 to 66 percent of red, bumpy, inflamed blemishes in seven well-designed studies involving more than 1,600 people with acne. Volunteers got results when they used the creams for at least 12 to 15 weeks.

Azelaic acid, a cream that stops the growth of bacteria and decreases the skin's production of pore-clogging keratin, cleared up 73 percent of inflamed blemishes in one well-designed Swedish study and worked as well as tetracycline capsules in another. This remedy's advantage: It's not a true antibiotic and doesn't cause the antibiotic resistance that can make acne flare again, as antibiotic creams, pills, and capsules can.

✔ Accutane

The biggest gun in the acne arsenal, isotretinoin (Accutane) can eliminate stubborn cystic acne when nothing else works. This vitamin A derivative, usually taken for 15 to 20 weeks, cleared up 90 percent of blemishes in a well-designed study of people with severe nodular acne. But Accutane can also cause birth defects in the babies of women who become pregnant while taking it—and there's growing concern that it may raise the risk of depression and even suicidal thoughts among teens. Use only in close consultation with your doctor.

WORKS FOR SOME

● Light therapies

In a small Harvard Medical School study, people with moderate to severe acne were treated with pulses of light from an erbium glass laser. The result: They had 78 percent fewer blemishes—and their skin stayed clear until their next appointment in six months. Those who got a second treatment then had an 80 percent improvement; those who didn't began to see blemishes return.

Lasers work by killing bacteria and possibly reducing oil production, but not all methods work equally well. In a University of Michigan study, patients who received treatment with a pulsed-die laser showed no significant improvement after 12 weeks.

DON'T BOTHER

✘ Long-term antibiotic use

Once the mainstay treatment for stubborn chronic acne, antibiotic pills kill bacteria and ease inflammation caused by your immune system's reaction to the presence of infection. Studies show that these drugs can "erase" up to 67 percent of inflamed, bumpy pimples. But acne bacteria mutate cleverly and develop resistance to oral antibiotics, especially if you take them for months or years. The disappointing result: Acne blemishes will return. Experts estimate that up to half of people with acne in Europe and the United States harbor antibiotic-resistant strains. ∎

Our BEST ADVICE

More blemish-fighting power, less antibiotic resistance. That's the thinking behind the double-remedy treatment trend for acne. Some dermatologists recommend using a benzoyl peroxide cream or gel plus an antibiotic. The combination works better than either remedy alone. Others recommend adapalene, a cream that kills bacteria and unclogs pores, plus a cream containing the antibiotic clindamycin. Another proven combination is isotretinoin cream plus an antibiotic cream or gel.

Allergies

Once upon a time, you had a choice: Suffer with your allergy symptoms— The sneezing! The watery eyes! The itchy nose!—or take an antihistamine and crawl into bed before it knocked you out. Today there are more allergy pills and treatments out there than you can shake a dandelion at, and many of them really work. Among the biggest developments: Two prescription antihistamines are now sold over the counter. A growing stack of research suggests there's an effective, painless alternative to allergy shots. And other studies show that many drugstore remedies are every bit as effective as their pricier prescription-only cousins.

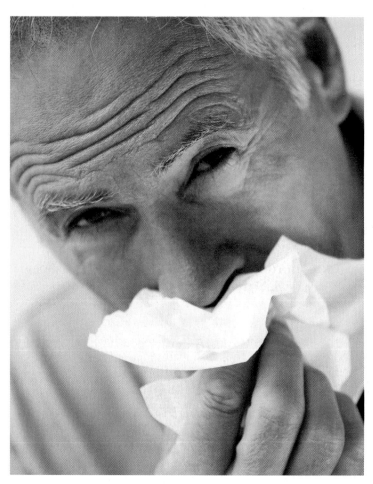

WORKS

✔ A saltwater rinse

Rinsing your nose with an over-the-counter or homemade saline solution washes out allergens and thins mucus. In one Italian study of children with pollen allergies, those who rinsed their nasal passages with saline three times a day during allergy season had less congestion, sneezing, and itching—and as a result, took fewer antihistamines than those who didn't rinse. Don't just spray a little into your nose—gently wash using a clean bulb-type ear syringe, a neti pot (from a health food store), or a waterpik device with a special nasal adapter. In a University of Michigan study of 127 adults with stuffed-up noses, 60 percent of those who rinsed thoroughly got relief, compared to 40 percent of those who just sprayed.

The University of Michigan researcher's own saline rinse recipe: Mix 1/2 teaspoon salt, 1/2 teaspoon baking soda, and

16 ounces warm tap water. To use, lean over a sink and turn your head so your left nostril faces down. Using a bulb syringe, gently flush your right nostril with 8 ounces of saline, letting the water drain out through your left nostril. Then gently blow your nose and repeat with your other nostril. Finally, clean the syringe.

✔ **Antihistamines** An antihistamine may be all you need if your symptoms are infrequent (less than four days a week or lasting for less than four weeks total) or so mild that they don't interfere with sleep or daytime activities. That's the conclusion of allergy experts from the University of Washington who reviewed 55 allergy studies. Antihistamines are second only to prescription steroids in their ability to ease the full range of allergy symptoms.

Good choices are loratadine (Claritin) and cetirizine HCl (Zyrtec), two formerly prescription drugs that are now sold over the counter and cause little or no drowsiness. These last longer than older antihistamines like diphenhydramine (Benadryl) and are less likely to cause sleepiness. That said, the older drugs, including Benadryl and brompheniramine (Dimetapp), provide stronger relief from allergy symptoms, based on the few head-to-head comparisons that have been conducted. For best results,

take an antihistamine *before* you are exposed to something you're allergic to.

Is there any reason to buy prescription-only antihistamines anymore? For most people, the answer is no. Until recently, the advantage of prescription varieties was the convenience of a pill that lasted 24 hours without sedating side effects, but now OTC pills offer the same benefits.

✔ **Antihistamine eyedrops** These drops are the most effective and safest way to relieve the symptoms of an "ocular allergy"—the itching, tearing, light sensitivity, redness, "grittiness," and eyelid swelling that can happen if you're allergic to pollen and/or mold. You can buy

antihistamine eyedrops over the counter, but you're better off with a prescription version. Best of all are prescription drops that combine antihistamines with mast-cell stabilizers. These ease symptoms quickly and need to be used only twice a day, compared to four times a day for drops containing antihistamines alone. They're also a great alternative to corticosteroid eyedrops, which are effective but can have dangerous side effects. Doctors prescribe steroid eyedrops mostly for chronic and severe eye allergy symptoms or to battle eye infections.

✔ **Decongestants** These over-the-counter pills and nasal sprays unclog

NEEDLE-FREE ALLERGY "SHOTS"

If your allergies don't respond to medications, your allergist may recommend a series of allergy shots. The process is long: Immunotherapy usually involves weekly shots for three to six months, then monthly shots for three to five years. The result: Many people with allergies to pollen, dust mites, mold, pet dander, and insect venom get relief within a year or two of starting the shots. Some become allergy-free once treatment ends, while others must continue the shots beyond five years.

Now researchers say that needle-free immunotherapy—in which tiny doses of specific allergens are placed under your tongue—work, too. In an Italian review of 70 studies of needle-free immunotherapy in children, symptoms improved for 44 percent of participants, and use of allergy medicines dropped by 24 percent. Under-the-tongue therapy was most effective for pollen allergies that lasted more than 18 months. Least effective were shorter courses of therapy and treatments for dust mites.

Interested? Ask your doctor if he can put you on a program.

ALLERGIES

congested nasal passages by shrinking swollen tissues and blood vessels. They're effective, but oral decongestants can cause insomnia and anxiety. Because they raise blood pressure, they aren't recommended for people with some forms of glaucoma or blood pressure problems. Decongestant nasal sprays won't keep you awake at night the way tablets will, but they cause "rebound" congestion if you use them for more than three days in a row.

Doctors often prescribe decongestants with antihistamines for more complete allergy relief—or recommend over-the-counter drugs that contain both. Which is better? In one Taiwanese study comparing a popular over-the-counter combination remedy with a widely prescribed combination remedy, the two were equally effective at relieving allergy symptoms. Conclusion? Start first with an over-the-counter version.

✔ Steroid nasal sprays
These sprays are prescription-only, but they're a far better choice than over-the-counter decongestant nose

sprays because they provide a wider range of benefits and can be used more frequently without the side effects of decongestants. These spritzes reduce inflammation and are the most effective remedy for all five major allergy symptoms: sneezing; runny nose; congestion; itchy nasal passages; and itchy, watery eyes, according to Australian allergy-treatment reviewers.

Steroid nasal sprays also perform better than antihistamine pills and sprays. In one Pennsylvania State University study of 44 people with respiratory allergies, those who used steroid nasal spray had less congestion than those who used antihistamine spray. As a result, they slept better and felt less groggy during the day. And when 348 people either used a steroid spray or took an antihistamine daily for four weeks, the steroid group got more relief from allergy symptoms. Be patient: These drugs start improving your symptoms within 10 hours of the first use but can take up to two weeks to be fully effective.

✔ Mast-cell stabilizers
To stop an allergy almost before it starts, consider an inhaled mast-cell

stabilizer, such as cromolyn (Intal) or nedocromil (Tilade). When taken as soon as you feel symptoms beginning, or even when you know the pollen count is rising, a mast-cell stabilizer prevents the release of inflammatory compounds, including histamines and leukotrienes, from the immune system's mast cells. In one study of 177 people with ragweed allergies, researchers found that 74 percent of those who took a mast-cell stabilizer during the three-week pollen season said the drug was effective. The catch: You have to use it up to six times a day.

✔ Leukotriene modifiers
These prescription asthma drugs can ease daytime and nighttime allergy problems because they block production of immune system chemicals called leukotrienes that help trigger congestion, itching, and watery eyes and nose. One type, montelukast (Singulair), is approved in the United States for allergies. But is it worth the extra cost and hassle of a doctor's prescription? Probably not. Two studies suggest that over-the-counter remedies work

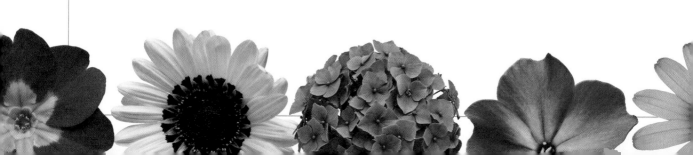

just as well for a fraction of the cost. In one University of Chicago study, the over-the-counter decongestant Sudafed was just as effective for easing congestion. And in a University of Illinois study comparing Singulair to the widely available antihistamine Claritin, the two were virtually identical.

✔ **Butterbur** Compounds in the leaves of butterbur can ease congestion by decreasing the body's production of histamines and leukotrienes responsible for allergy symptoms. In one study, butterbur extract worked as well as the prescription drug fexofenadine (Allegra) to dry up runny, congested noses in 16 volunteers. In a Swiss study of 236 people with hay fever, butterbur worked as well as the antihistamine cetirizine (Zyrtec) to ease symptoms.

Buy only butterbur extracts labeled "PA-free." These have had the plant's pyrrolizidine alkaloids, which are potentially harmful toxins, removed during processing. Also, skip this herb if you're allergic to ragweed, marigolds, daisies, or chrysanthemums.

✔ **Freeze-dried nettle** Stinging nettle leaves—freeze-dried and put into capsules—eased allergy symptoms for 55 percent of the volunteers in one recent study. Participants took 300 milligrams a day, and 48 percent said this botanical worked better than their previous allergy medicine.

DON'T BOTHER

✖ **Air filters** If all you do is plug in an air filter, you won't get much allergy relief. Canadian doctors who reviewed air filter studies concluded that filtered air didn't improve lung function and improved symptoms like coughing, sneezing, watery eyes, and runny nose only a little. If you have a pet and you use an air filter in the bedroom, at least give the filter a fighting chance by keeping the pet out of the room at all times. (Sorry, Whiskers.)

✖ **Vacuum cleaners with specialized air filters** Think you can erase allergens from your carpet with a high-quality vacuum? Think again. Vacuuming, no matter what the quality of the vacuum, usually stirs up dust, dander, and pollen, adding to your misery. When British researchers put particle-trapping devices on their noses and then tested vacuum cleaners, they found that all types sent clouds of cat dander and dust mites flying into the air. ■

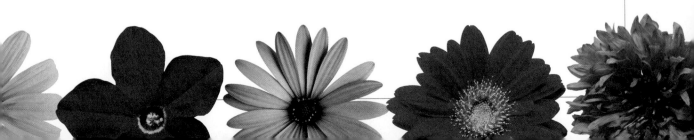

Alzheimer's Disease

An avalanche of new research has revealed that at any age, the brain is capable of regenerating itself—with the right encouragement. And while neither age-related cognitive decline (the memory lapses and fuzzy thinking that grow more common after age 65 or so) nor Alzheimer's disease is entirely preventable, you can help keep your brain sharp with these strategies.

WORKS

✔ **Exercise** When researchers in Seattle followed 1,700 adults age 65 and older for six years, those who exercised at least three times a week were about one-third less likely to develop Alzheimer's. They weren't athletes—in fact, those who were the least fit at the start of the study lowered their risk the most. They did it by walking, biking, hiking, swimming, or doing strength training or aerobics for at least 15 minutes three times a week.

Aerobic exercise may even improve memory. When 11 adults embarked on an exercise routine that included 40 minutes on an exercise bike, treadmill, stair climber, or elliptical trainer four times a week, scores on memory tests improved, and scans revealed better blood flow to brain regions associated with recall.

Lab studies suggest that exercise boosts production of brain-derived neurotrophic factor (BDNF), a sort of "Miracle-Gro" that encourages nerve cells to multiply and create more connections with each other.

✔ **A healthy weight** Extra pounds dimmed brain wattage in a recent study from Toulouse University Hospital and the National Institute of Health and Medical Research in France. Researchers checked the body mass indexes (BMIs) and cognitive skills of 2,223 women and men, ages 32 to 62, twice over five years. People with high BMIs scored lower on memory tests and experienced greater declines in mental abilities. Being overweight increases the risk of arterial plaque, which may reduce blood flow to the brain.

✔ **Fruits, vegetables, and whole grains** In a French study of 1,640 healthy adults, those who ate the most flavonoids—antioxidants found in fruits and veggies as well as coffee, tea, chocolate, and wine—had the smallest drops in brain function over 10 years. What's more, beans, greens, and whole grains are all rich in folate, a B vitamin that improved memory and information-processing speed in a study of 819 adults by researchers at Wageningen University in the Netherlands.

Finally, a diet rich in these foods, along with regular exercise, helps combat insulin resistance. Research is turning up evidence that problems with insulin usage encourage brain changes that lead to Alzheimer's disease.

✔ **Fish three times a week** High blood levels of a type of omega-3 fatty acid called docosahexaenioc acid (DHA), found in fatty fish like salmon, sardines, and mackerel, cut dementia risk by 47 percent in a Tufts University study of 899 older adults. Eating three fish meals a week led to the highest DHA levels. If you hate fin food, try fish-oil

capsules. A Swedish study found that they cut the rate of mental decline in people with mild Alzheimer's disease.

✔ **Mental stimulation** While it's not clear that it will help you remember your granddaughter's birthday, studies suggest that staying mentally active reduces Alzheimer's disease risk by as much as 33 percent for some people. When researchers at the Rush Alzheimer's Disease Center in Chicago followed 700 people age 65 and older for 4 1/2 years, those who got the most daily mental stimulation (from activities like doing crossword puzzles and reading the newspaper) were 47 percent less likely to develop Alzheimer's than those who had the least stimulation.

DON'T BOTHER

✘ **Antioxidant supplements** While diets rich in the antioxidant vitamins C (found in citrus fruits, strawberries, red bell peppers, and other fruits and veggies) and E (found in nuts and whole grains) seem to protect the brain, studies haven't found any benefit from taking these antioxidants in pill form.

Statin drugs These cholesterol-lowering medicines didn't lower the odds of developing Alzheimer's disease in a large study that followed more than 900 people for 12 years. ■

What to Expect from Alzheimer's Drugs

Used in the right combination and early in the the disease, these drugs can slow the course of Alzheimer's, though they won't work for everyone, and side effects may keep patients from using them. While some experts say the side effects outweigh the benefits, medication may ease the burden on patients and their caregivers for a few months or years and may delay the need for a nursing home.

1. DONEPEZIL (Aricept)

USED FOR: Mild cognitive impairment

SUCCESS RATE: Slowed progression to Alzheimer's disease by 58% the first year and 36% in the second year of a 3-year study of 769 people. By the 3rd year, there was no improvement.

SIDE EFFECTS: Nausea, diarrhea, cramping, lack of appetite

2. RIVASTIGMINE (Exelon)

USED FOR: Mild to moderate Alzheimer's symptoms

SUCCESS RATE: Improved attention span by 67% and reduced anxiety, apathy, and agitation by about 60% in a study of 2,119 people.

SIDE EFFECTS: Nausea, vomiting, loss of appetite, weight loss, dizziness

3. GALANTAMINE (Razadyne)

USED FOR: Mild to moderate Alzheimer's

SUCCESS RATE: In a study of 240 people who took galantamine for 36 to 48 months, one-third showed little decline and one-third declined significantly.

SIDE EFFECTS: Nausea, vomiting, weight loss

4. MEMANTINE (Namenda)

USED FOR: Moderate to severe Alzheimer's

SUCCESS RATE: Improved cognitive skills and slowed mental deterioration by 5% in one study.

SIDE EFFECTS: Dizziness, headache, constipation, confusion

Anxiety

Everyone gets anxious at times. Usually, there's a clear stimulus: flying, public speaking, a new job, being in a crowd. Often a series of slow, deep breaths will help, as will listening to soothing music if you have access to it. If you find that you're anxious or worried almost every day, though, for no obvious reason, you could have an anxiety disorder such as generalized anxiety disorder (GAD), which may also cause rapid breathing and insomnia. It's a serious health concern that merits a visit to a doctor.

WHAT WORKS

✔ Antidepressants

These medications are most commonly used for treating depression. But they are usually the first drugs to be prescribed for GAD as well, mainly because they work well and cause relatively few side effects. The top three, according to studies, are imipramine (Tofranil), extended-release venlafaxine (Effexor), and paroxetine (Paxil), although only the latter two have been officially approved in the United States to treat GAD.

How effective are they? One study found that 72 percent of people who took paroxetine for eight weeks improved. Overall, 36 percent of the paroxetine group saw their symptoms disappear.

✔ Buspirone (BuSpar)

This drug works about as well as benzodiazepine tranquilizers (described on the next page) for relieving anxiety, but it can be used longer than those drugs and is much less likely to lead to addiction issues. If you've been taking a benzodiazepine, be sure to wait at least 30 days before taking buspirone; otherwise, it may not be as effective. Downsides are that you have to take it three times a day and that it won't help with depression, which often occurs along with anxiety disorder.

✔ Cognitive behavioral therapy

In this form of psychotherapy, you learn to reframe how you view the world and to look at things that are worrying you more logically. For instance, if you constantly worry about money, you may learn to more realistically evaluate your expenses and income. Studies find recovery rates of 51 percent in people who receive cognitive therapy for six months, and the few official guidelines that exist for GAD treatment recommend this therapy in addition to medication. Generally, you need weekly sessions of one to two hours for four months.

✔ Kava

This herbal remedy works similarly to prescription anti-anxiety medications but without the mental "slowing" or memory problems that can occur with the drugs. One review of 11 studies that included more than 600 patients found that kava worked better than placebos for managing anxiety in the

WHEN PANIC ATTACKS

If you are among the majority of people who only occasionally have anxiety attacks, you certainly don't need powerful drugs to deal with the problem. Here's what major health groups recommend you do when life suddenly fills you with anxiety.

- Sit down and close your eyes.
- Shift your focus away from the stimulus of your anxiety.
- Scan your entire body for tense muscles, then relax them.
- Allow thoughts to flow through your mind, but don't focus on them.
- Breathe deeply, slowly, and regularly.

short term. Use a preparation that is standardized to 70 percent kavalactones and take it as directed; improper use of kava can harm your liver.

✔ Applied relaxation

This approach involves doing relatively simple things like deep breathing techniques, progressive muscle relaxation, guided imagery, and systematic desensitization, in which you confront your fear a little at a time. One five-month study compared GAD patients who practiced relaxation techniques with those who received anti-depressants and found that both experienced about the same improvement.

✔ Yoga

Studies find that people with GAD who practice yoga regularly have lower levels of the stress hormone cortisol and need fewer anti-anxiety drugs. Yoga helps in a few ways: The controlled breathing helps relax your mind and fuel your body, and the specific postures relax your muscles and divert your attention.

WORKS FOR SOME

● Meditation

Meditation hasn't been widely studied, but one study found that people who practiced mindfulness meditation, in which you focus on simply being in the moment, for 8 weeks got less relief from their anxiety than those who participated in cognitive behavioral therapy for 12 weeks. However, both approaches improved mood, quality of life, and overall ability to function to about the same degree.

● Virtual reality exposure therapy

In this relatively new form of therapy, people are exposed to a feared object or situation via computer in order to desensitize them to it. Studies find it's more effective than therapy in which you just imagine the feared situation and just as effective as therapies in which you actually experience it (such as sitting in an airplane if you have severe anxiety about flying).

The improvements appear short-lived, however. One study showed that after six months, people who used the exposure therapy were on a par with those who used a placebo treatment. Nevertheless, the therapy has been successfully used for people with post-traumatic stress syndrome, those with a fear of heights, and musicians scared of performing.

● Benzodiazepines

These tranquilizers, which include alprazolam (Xanax), chlordiazepoxide (Librium), and diazepam (Valium), were the first drugs used to treat anxiety and are still used quite often. They're not recommended for long-term use, however, although many doctors do prescribe them that way. Using them for more than two or three weeks can bring on depression, dependence, grogginess, and memory problems.

DON'T BOTHER

✖ Typical psychotherapy

Traditional "talk" therapy, in which you focus on your childhood and other life-shaping events, doesn't do much when it comes to anxiety disorders. A review of studies found recovery rates of just 4 percent in people using this form of therapy.

✖ St. John's Wort

While this herbal remedy is fairly effective for depression, there's no evidence it does much, if anything, for anxiety.

✖ Valerian

A cup of valerian tea or a few valerian tablets may help you relax enough to sleep, but there's very little evidence that the herb has any significant effect in relieving serious anxiety (though there's no harm in trying it). ■

Arthritis

Osteoarthritis is to older adults what ear infections are to children: common, frustrating, painful, a rite of passage. Except that people don't grow out of arthritis—they grow into it. Genes play a role in causing joint-cushioning cartilage to break down, but past injuries, too much or too little exercise, and even a crooked gait can speed up the destruction. There's no cure yet for osteoarthritis, but research is zeroing in on what brings relief.

WHAT WORKS

✔ **Acetaminophen (Tylenol)** Cheap, relatively safe when taken as directed, and with little risk of causing gastrointestinal bleeding the way other painkillers can, acetaminophen should be your first choice for treating mild to moderate arthritis pain. One review of seven trials found that people taking acetaminophen scored about four points lower on a pain scale than those taking placebos—a statistically significant difference. Meanwhile, evaluations of studies comparing acetaminophen with aspirin found that both provided similar pain relief, though ibuprofen appeared to work better than either. Acetaminophen is less likely than aspirin, ibuprofen, or naproxen to cause stomach bleeding, however. Doses up to 4,000 milligrams a day may be safe in people who don't have kidney or liver damage, but talk to your doctor first, as taking too much acetaminophen does have the potential to cause problems over time.

✔ **Acupuncture** The simple act of inserting a needle into the skin and underlying tissue of your knee can help relieve the pain of arthritis. Over and over again, whether researchers were comparing real acupuncture to fake acupuncture or even to conventional arthritis treatments, they found that the ancient Chinese treatment not only relieved pain but in some instances also improved joint function. For instance, in one study, 283 participants received either education about arthritis or 26 weeks of either fake or real acupuncture. Those who received the real thing improved 23 percent more on pain scores, 150 percent more on physical function scores, and 74 percent more on their overall ability to function compared with the other groups.

✔ **Devil's claw** This anti-inflammatory herb seems to work similarly to prescription painkillers known as COX-2 inhibitors, such as celecoxib (Celebrex). However, they don't have the potential COX-2 inhibitor side effects, including increased risk of ulcers, stomach pain, and heart attack.

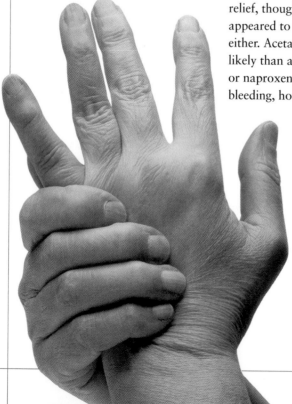

Studies in which participants took a daily dose containing 60 milligrams of harpagoside (the active ingredient in devil's claw) found the herb helped reduce the pain of arthritis in the hip, knee, and spine.

✔ **Weight loss** Losing weight is one of the best things you can do in terms of both preventing arthritis and reducing the pain, swelling, and disability it causes. That's because excess weight puts excess pressure on joints. It doesn't take much weight loss to see your condition improve: Each pound of weight you lose reduces the stress on your knees by 4 pounds. In one major study, it took only about a 10 percent weight loss (that's 18 pounds if you weigh 180) to significantly improve participants' knee and hip function. For instance, they were able to walk farther in six minutes and climb stairs faster than those who didn't lose the weight.

✔ **Corticosteroid injections** Injecting corticosteroids directly into an arthritic joint helps reduce pain and stiffness by reducing inflammation. An analysis of 10 studies found that people who received the injections were 66 percent more likely than a control group to have less pain and greater function in their arthritic knees up to 24 weeks after the treatment. Similar positive results have been documented for shoulder injections.

While these shots can relieve underlying inflammation that's responsible for the pain, they can't do anything to improve the bottom-line cause of the pain—that degenerating cartilage. And their effects are generally short-lived. They also have to be used judiciously, since long-term use can lead to thinning skin, weight gain, facial puffiness, increased blood pressure, cataracts, and osteoporosis.

✔ **Exercise** No matter how hard it is or how much it hurts initially, you need to get out there and move if you want to improve your joint function. Study after study shows that exercise is an important and successful therapy for relieving the pain and limited function that arthritis can cause.

Which exercise is best? The smart approach—endorsed by most doctors, arthritis organizations, and researchers—is a gentle mix of three types.

Range-of-motion exercise like stretching and dancing to help maintain your joints' full range of motion and flexibility

Strength exercise to keep the muscles that protect and support your joints strong

Aerobic or endurance exercise to control weight, reduce inflammation, and maintain joint function

Ideally, you should start by working with a physical therapist or trainer who understands arthritis and can develop a program tailored for you.

✔ **Capsaicin cream** Capsaicin is the substance that gives hot peppers their bite. As an ingredient in a cream to rub over painful joints, it can also relieve your arthritis pain. One study randomly assigned people with arthritis to receive either the real thing or a placebo cream. They graded their own levels of pain and stiffness the week before the treatment started, then applied the cream daily for 28 days, ranking their pain and stiffness over time. The results: Pain levels dropped by about 16 percent in the placebo group but by 77 percent in the capsaicin group, with major differences beginning in the second week. Even better, stiffness fell by 18 percent in the placebo group but by about 86 percent in the capsaicin group, beginning the first week. Interestingly, another study found that even if researchers told patients that capsaicin was less effective than other medicines, patients still preferred the cream to any other pain relief option. The main reason? Fewer side effects.

WORKS FOR SOME

● **Glucosamine and chondroitin** Despite huge initial promise—and major sales of the supplements around the world—this duo of natural remedies probably isn't as useful for arthritis as we once hoped, either separately or together. When researchers evaluated 15 studies looking at its use for arthritis, all pointed to the same conclusion: Glucosamine is not effective. Then the largest, most thorough study ever conducted on the use of glucosamine and chondroitin, published in the *New England Journal of Medicine,* found that the combination wasn't any more effective than a placebo for reducing mild to moderate knee pain.

The only exceptions were that people taking chondroitin alone responded better than those taking glucosamine alone and that the supplements seemed to have some measurable benefit for the subset of participants whose arthritis pain ranked higher than moderate. The general conclusion: For most people with arthritis, there is little benefit to the pills; for those with more severe pain, it can be considered as part of a broader treatment program.

● **Hyaluronic acid injections** In this treatment, hyaluronic acid is injected to replace a natural substance called hyaluronan that works like motor oil in the joint to let the cartilage surfaces of bones glide over each other smoothly. For some people, injections of this thick liquid can help reduce pain for a year or longer. And clinical studies show that the therapy is as effective in providing pain relief as nonsteroidal anti-inflammatory drugs (NSAIDs) like aspirin and ibuprofen. But these injections don't work for everyone, must be given relatively frequently, and are expensive. For this reason, most doctors consider the injections (also called joint fluid therapy) only as a backup plan if other remedies don't work.

● **Ginger** It's great for certain types of nausea, but there is also evidence that this anti-inflammatory herb can help with the pain, swelling, and stiffness of osteoarthritis, particularly in the knee. In one study of 261 people with knee osteoarthritis, volunteers received either a sugar pill or ginger extract. The result: 63 percent of the ginger group experienced pain relief compared to 50 percent of the placebo group. Even better: Unlike some painkillers, ginger causes few if any stomach problems. Use fresh ginger liberally in your cooking, make tea by boiling several slices of fresh ginger, or for maximum benefit, take 500 to 1,000 milligrams of powdered ginger root daily.

● **Willow bark** White willow bark—the original source of salicin, the active ingredient in aspirin—appears to provide some relief from arthritis pain, though it won't work as well as traditional painkillers.

● **SAM-e** This somewhat controversial supplement has a fair amount of scientific support as a pain reliever for arthritis. SAM-e is short for S-adenosyl-methionine, a naturally occurring chemical in the body that has many functions. In test-tube and animal

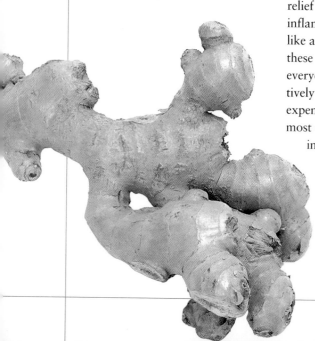

research, it protects cells that produce cartilage and stimulates them to produce joint-lubricating chemicals. Sold as a drug in some countries and as an over-the-counter supplement in others, it has proven as effective as some COX-2 inhibitors for relieving arthritis pain, but it takes longer to act. An analysis of 14 SAM-e studies showed it is also effective for improving mobility in people with osteoarthritis. However, high doses of SAM-e can cause several side effects, and it interacts with many medications. Use it only after talking with your doctor.

● **Osteotomy** This form of surgery repositions or reshapes the bones in the knee to shift weight away from the damaged arthritic area. A review of numerous studies found that while it does improve knee function and reduce pain in people with arthritis of the knee, there's no evidence yet as to whether it's more effective than conservative approaches such as exercise and pain medication.

DON'T BOTHER

✖ **Arthroscopic surgery** In this type of surgery, the surgeon makes tiny incisions in the knee, then uses small tools to either clean out debris and remove or sand down rough, torn pieces of cartilage (arthroscopic debridement) or flush out debris and calcium phosphate crystals (arthroscopic lavage). But in a major study in which 180 people were treated with either one of the two procedures or a fake arthroscopic procedure, researchers found that the surgeries not only didn't work but were potentially harmful. The researchers followed patients for two years after the surgery and found that those who had the fake surgery actually climbed stairs and walked slightly faster than those who got the real thing.

✖ **Topical pain relievers** There is little evidence that aspirin-containing creams like Aspercreme are effective for treating arthritis pain. A review of nine studies found that while the creams tend to work fairly well for one-time aches and pains (such as soreness from raking leaves), they're not very good at relieving the chronic pain of arthritis.

✖ **Vitamin E** Some natural healing practitioners theorize that vitamin E and other antioxidants reduce inflammation and ease arthritis pain. Vitamin E has been evaluated in five high-quality clinical trials. Although two concluded the vitamin worked better than a placebo for reducing pain, and one found it worked as well as an NSAID, the two largest and longest trials found no difference between the vitamin and a placebo in terms of reducing pain from osteoarthritis of the knee. Also, recent studies show that taking daily supplements of vitamin E at a dose of 400 milligrams or more can be dangerous. ■

Asthma

When you have asthma, your airways are always vulnerable. All sorts of irritants, from pollen and pet dander to tobacco smoke and even cold air, can inflame the sensitive linings of the "breathing tubes" in your lungs. The tubes can swell, clog, and spasm, leaving you gasping for breath. Asthma is on the rise, and it can be deadly if inadequately treated. Unfortunately, many people don't realize they have it—or they underestimate how serious it can be. Control yours with a plan that includes medications, regular at-home breathing checks with a peak flow meter, and smart drug-free strategies.

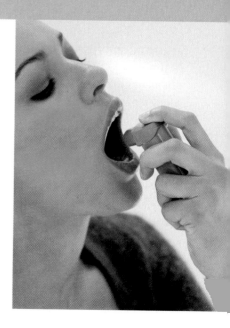

WORKS

✔ **A personalized asthma management plan—in writing** Half of all people with asthma don't recognize warning signs of an impending attack, and 75 percent aren't taking the long-acting controller medications (such as inhaled corticosteroids) that prevent attacks. Sitting down with your doctor to work out a treatment plan pays off. In one analysis of 17 well-designed studies, researchers concluded that people with an asthma action plan are 40 percent less likely to wind up in the hospital due to breathing problems. The right plan will also help you end coughing and wheezing and lead a normal life. Your plan should include the following information.

- How to take the medicines you'll use on a daily basis.

- When to use fast-acting "rescue" medications for asthma attacks.

- When and how to use a peak flow meter to help you recognize early if your asthma is worsening.

- How to avoid personal triggers like pet dander.

As part of your plan, ask your doctor for a chart showing the names of the medications you'll be taking, the doses, when and how often to take them, and the circumstances that could change the size or timing of your doses. An estimated 40 to 50 percent of people with asthma don't take their meds correctly; asthma experts at Columbia University

say using a chart can prevent this from happening to you.

✔ **Avoiding your asthma triggers** Pet dander, mold, dust mites, pollen—all of these can trigger an asthma attack if you're sensitive to them. In one large study of Europeans with asthma, researchers found that people with the worst asthma were three times more likely to be sensitive to mold than people with the mildest asthma. Finding your triggers (get tested for allergies) and controlling them are key steps in your treatment plan.

In one study of nearly 1,000 asthmatic kids, published in the *New England Journal of Medicine*, those whose families controlled dust mites by putting special covers on mattresses and pillowcases and vacuuming carefully had one more symptom-free day every two weeks than children in families that didn't use those methods.

What you should do depends on your triggers, of course. Allergic to pet dander? Ban Fido and Fifi from the bedroom and consider removing carpets, which are "reservoirs" of stored dander. Mold a problem? Lower your home's humidity to stop its growth. Another option is to try allergy shots to reduce your body's response to your triggers.

✔ A diet full of fruits, vegetables, and whole grains

Asthmatic lungs need antioxidants, the cell-protecting molecules that neutralize oxygen molecules called free radicals, which make inflammation worse. Studies suggest a connection between a diet rich in antioxidants and a lower risk of developing asthma or experiencing an asthma attack. The best way to bolster your antioxidant defenses? Aim for seven to nine servings of colorful fruits and veggies each day. To get plenty of vitamin C, go for citrus fruits, strawberries, red bell peppers, and broccoli. For vitamin E, aim for three daily servings of whole grains. Also include apples (with the skin) and tomatoes; one large British study found that people who ate five apples per week and a

tomato every other day had the greatest lung capacity.

✔ Salmon and mackerel

These fish are packed to the gills with omega-3 fatty acids, beneficial compounds that fight inflammation. Studies suggest that people who get plenty of them from their diets have healthier lungs than people who don't get as much. Like anchovies? They're also a good source of omega-3's.

✔ Breathing exercises

When 57 Australians with asthma learned one of two breath control techniques—one featured shallow breaths through the nose, the other steady, slow inhalations and exhalations through the mouth or nose—both groups had an 86 percent drop in their use of

rescue inhalers. Volunteers did their breathing exercises twice a day for 30 weeks.

✔ Coffee

It's certainly not a first-line strategy, but if you like coffee, here's a reason to keep drinking it: A strong cup or two of coffee may help prevent asthma attacks. In an Italian survey of 72,284 people, those with asthma who drank one cup of coffee per day had 5 percent fewer asthma attacks than those who drank none; drinking two cups a day cut the rate by 23 percent, while three cups cut it by 28 percent. The researchers suspect that the caffeine in coffee acts as a bronchodilator, expanding airways that become constricted when you have asthma.

DON'T BOTHER

✘ Supplements of vitamin C or E, fish oil, magnesium, or selenium

Even though some studies have found connections between getting enough of these nutrients and a lower risk of developing asthma (or of having an attack if you already have asthma), taking *supplements* doesn't seem to help.

✘ Acupuncture

When researchers at Imperial College of London reviewed 11 studies that used this ancient Chinese healing art for asthma relief,

they concluded that there was no evidence that it helped.

✘ Air filters and ion-generating air purifiers

Studies show that filters, especially high-intensity particulate air (HEPA) filters, can reduce levels of lung-irritating particles in the air, but there's little proof that people with asthma get any relief as a result. And you should avoid ion-generating devices completely. They convert oxygen into ozone, which damages lung tissue and causes coughing and shortness of breath. ∎

Back Pain

Given that back pain is the fifth most common reason people go to the doctor, you'd think we'd have figured out what to do for it decades ago. But old strategies such as ice packs and bed rest have proven ineffective. In fact, the exact opposite strategies—heat and exercise—are likely to be your tickets to relief. No matter what they do, most people feel better in a month anyway. About one-third of people with back pain, however, wind up with chronic pain lasting a year or more. Here's what may—and may not—help.

WORKS

✔ Herbal remedies

There's relatively good evidence for the use of two herbal remedies: devil's claw and white willow bark. A review of 10 studies found that doses of devil's claw (standardized to contain 50 to 100 milligrams of the active ingredient harpagoside) or white willow bark (120 to 240 milligrams) worked better to soothe back pain than the prescription pain reliever rofecoxib (Vioxx), which was withdrawn from the market because of safety issues.

✔ Massage

We're not talking about relaxing Swedish massage here but rather the type of deep tissue massage designed to break up knots known as adhesions. Studies find that when combined with exercise and education about managing and preventing back pain, it really helps reduce chronic back pain. Expect to experience some discomfort during this intense massage. Studies also support acupressure massage over Swedish massage for back pain.

✔ Heat wrap therapy

Yes, turn on the heat. A review of studies on heat for back pain found that it does help, at least a bit. In one study, it significantly reduced lower-back pain after five days compared to a placebo pill. Try a heating pad, a hot towel, a hot water bottle, or a press-on heating pad from the drugstore. Keep in mind that moist heat works better than dry heat.

✔ Capsaicin cream

Capsaicin, the stuff that gives chile peppers their heat, can also help relieve your pain. Over time, applying creams that contain it depletes the body of a substance that transmits pain signals. You'll need to use the cream for a week or more before you experience any significant relief, and it may initially cause a burning sensation, but that should wear off in time.

✔ Acupuncture

If your back pain is chronic, by all means try this ancient Chinese form of medicine. A review of 39 clinical trials found it was significantly more effective at relieving pain and improving function than no treatment or fake treatment, and it increased pain relief when added to other therapies such as ibuprofen, exercise, and behavior modification. As for acute (as in it just happened) pain, there's not enough evidence yet to say how well it works.

✔ Reading a book

A good one to try is *The Back Book* by the Royal College of General Practitioners. In a study of 162 people with back pain, those who received the book engaged in more physical activity and improved sooner than those who didn't receive it. The results were so significant that the American College of Physicians and the American Pain Society recommend that physicians treating back pain give it to their patients. You can get the book from online booksellers.

✔ **Exercise** It may seem counterintuitive to tell you to exercise when your back hurts so much that getting off the sofa seems like a challenge. But if you have chronic back pain, exercise can reduce pain and improve physical function about as well as commonly used pain relievers. The best exercises seem to be those designed to stretch, strengthen, or stabilize your core muscles—the ones that an inner tube worn around your waist would cover. That makes Pilates a good option, but aerobics also helps. Any form of exercise seems to work best if tailored for you by a trainer or physical therapist.

✔ **Back schools** The evidence isn't overwhelming, but it *is* strong enough to recommend back school, in which you learn proper ways to sit, stand, lift, and manage back pain. Studies find that back school can improve your overall function and get you back to work faster than doing nothing or getting plain old advice from your doctor. Your doctor can refer you to a physical therapy center that offers back school.

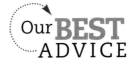
Our **BEST** ADVICE

Thanks in large part to heavy advertising by drug makers, people may believe that prescription nonsteroidal anti-inflammatory drugs (NSAIDs) work better for back pain than generic ibuprofen. But a review of more than 50 clinical trials found no difference in effectiveness. Our advice? Buy the cheapest store brand. Ibuprofen and other NSAIDs (which include naproxen, or Aleve) tend to work slightly better than acetaminophen (Tylenol) for relieving lower-back pain.

WORKS FOR SOME

● **Opioid analgesics** Also known by their out-of-favor name, "narcotics," these drugs are morphine-like substances used for pain, such as codeine, hydrocodone (Vicodin), and oxycodone (OxyContin and Percocet). They're an option for your doctor to consider when you've just injured yourself and acetaminophen and nonsteroidal anti-inflammatory drugs (NSAIDs) like ibuprofen can't control the pain. But they're definitely not for long-term use.

● **Muscle relaxants** If you've ever gone to your doctor with acute, severe back pain, chances are you've been prescribed a muscle relaxant. Many of these drugs, which include diazepam (Valium) and cyclobenzaprine (Flexeril), are approved for the treatment of other medical conditions (like anxiety and high blood pressure) but are used "off label" for muscle spasms. An analysis of 30 trials found that they're better than placebos for soothing acute back pain, but all have potentially dangerous side effects, primarily drowsiness, dizziness, and nausea.

● **Prolotherapy injections** In this treatment, various substances are injected into the painful area to trigger inflammation. This inflammation in turn stimulates cells called fibroblasts to create collagen, a protein that makes up ligaments and tendons. Adding collagen to existing ligaments and tendons makes them tighter and stronger, providing more support along the spine. Two studies that measured pain and disability levels in participants before prolotherapy and six months afterward found more than 50 percent improvement in pain and function. However, two other studies of the treatment found no differences between those receiving prolotherapy and control groups.

● **TENS** In transcutaneous electrical nerve stimulation (TENS), electrical impulses are

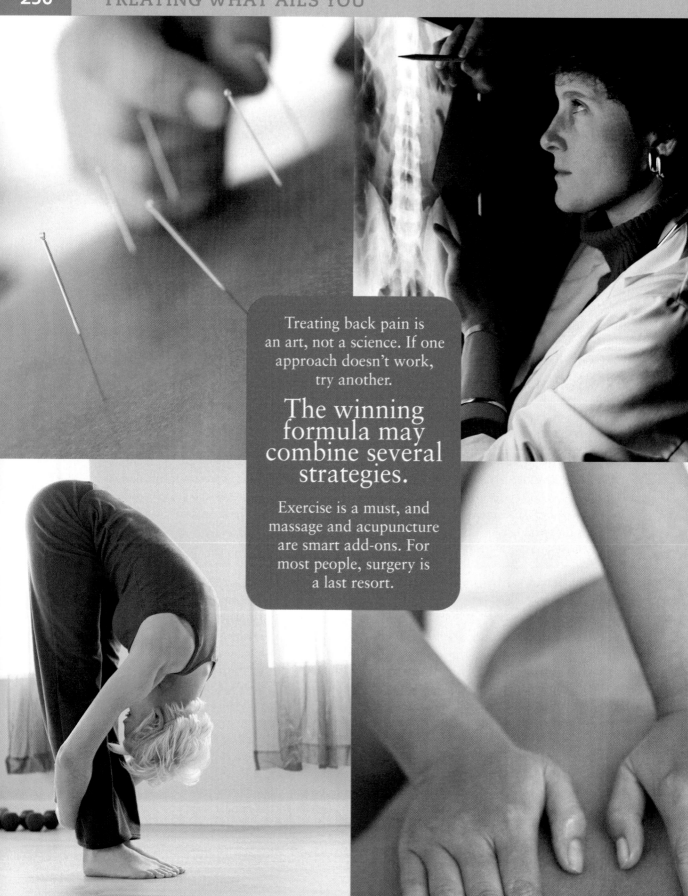

Treating back pain is an art, not a science. If one approach doesn't work, try another.

The winning formula may combine several strategies.

Exercise is a must, and massage and acupuncture are smart add-ons. For most people, surgery is a last resort.

sent through the skin to your back to relieve pain. Only two high-quality clinical trials have evaluated TENS in people with back pain. While one showed an improvement in pain, the other didn't, so it's a tossup as to whether TENS works.

● **Surgery** If your back pain is due to a condition called degenerative spondylolisthesis with spinal stenosis, in which cartilage between the vertebrae disintegrates, leading the vertebrae to slip over one another, surgery seems to be your best option. A major government-sponsored study published in the *New England Journal of Medicine* compared 372 people diagnosed with the disease who underwent decompressive laminectomy, in which bone and soft tissue are removed to relieve pressure on the nerves, with 235 who received physical therapy, steroid injections, and pain relievers. After two years, those who didn't receive surgery had modest improvement, but those who had the surgery had much greater pain relief and improved function. Plus, the surgical patients felt better quickly, many within six weeks of the procedure.

SKIP THE X-RAYS

There's no evidence that they can help diagnose uncomplicated lower-back pain. All you're doing is exposing yourself to unnecessary radiation—a lot of it. Computed tomography (CT) scans and MRIs are just as worthless unless your doctor suspects something else is going on (like cancer) or you're showing severe neurological deficits, including problems speaking, loss of feeling or balance, or abnormal reflexes. If your doctor *does* order a scan and then tells you that you have disk degeneration, don't assume that's the cause of your pain. Sixty percent of people between 40 and 60 and most people over 60 have some level of disk degeneration; most carry on just fine without even realizing they have it.

DON'T BOTHER

✖ **Bed rest** Although it was standard advice for decades, when researchers finally asked whether bed rest worked for back pain, the answer was a resounding no. Researchers evaluated 11 studies involving 1,963 patients with acute lower-back pain and found that people told to rest in bed actually recovered about 30 percent *less* function than those who stayed active.

✖ **Cold therapy** Hold the ice! There's just no evidence that cold therapy does anything to relieve back pain.

✖ **Chiropractic** A review of 39 clinical trials found no benefit from spinal manipulative therapy for acute or chronic lower-back pain when compared with conventional care (exercise, physical therapy, pain management), back school, traction, bed rest, topical gels, or even no care.

✖ **Antidepressants** An estimated one in four doctors prescribe these drugs for back pain, but an analysis of 10 major studies found that antidepressants don't help.

✖ **Back braces** Those back supports you see movers and stockroom workers wearing might as well be girdles for all the good they do in terms of preventing back pain or minimizing existing pain.

✖ **Insoles** Those cushioned inserts that you slip into your shoes are touted for reducing back pain by realigning your spine and preventing shock waves from traveling from the ground to your back. Alas, a review of all available studies (there were only six) found that none showed any benefit. ■

Bad Breath

Researchers confirm that most bad breath is the vaguely rotten-egg odor of sulfur compounds released by bacteria thriving on food residue left on your teeth and tongue. This residue can be removed with regular brushing, tongue scraping, and rinsing, giving you more hours of fresh breath every day. If none of the advice here works, see your dentist and your doctor; you may have gum disease or even a gastrointestinal or respiratory infection. And stop smoking!

WORKS

✔ **Brushing your teeth and tongue** Levels of stinky sulfur compounds fell 53 percent in people who brushed their teeth and tongues for a full minute twice a day for two weeks, report New York University dentists who studied 51 pairs of twins. Brushing removes bacteria that feed on the film of microscopic food bits that coats our teeth and tongues after a meal.

✔ **A tongue scraper** In two small but well-designed studies, tongue scrapers bested tongue brushing at removing food residue. As with other approaches, however, the effects may not last long. Fortunately, a toothbrush and tongue scraper are easy to carry in a purse or briefcase.

✔ **Antimicrobial mouthwash** The effects of mouthwash wear off fast, but you should get longer results with a germ-killing rinse. In a Dutch study, volunteers who gargled once a day with a mouthwash containing chlorhexidine, cetylpyridinium chloride, and zinc lactate cut their emission of sulfur compounds nearly in half after two weeks, while a control group that gargled with a placebo mouthwash had no change. Other studies suggest that mouthwashes containing just cetylpyridinium chloride make a dent in bad breath, too. Avoid mouthwashes that contain alcohol, which dries the mouth and could make the problem worse.

If you're willing to spend a little extra, try a mouthwash containing chlorine dioxide. In one study of 5,000 people, it not only eliminated odor-causing bacteria but also reduced proteins in the mouth that bacteria use for food.

✔ **Toothpaste with triclosan** In one manufacturer-sponsored study, toothpaste containing this germ-killing ingredient reduced sulfur compounds by 56 percent, while a "breath-freshening" toothpaste without triclosan cut them by just 10 percent.

✔ **Rinsing your mouth between meals** This will remove some of the food particles that bacteria live on.

WORKS FOR SOME

● **Sugarless gum** In a small French study, chewing gum reduced halitosis a little for about an hour but didn't really get rid of nasty sulfur compounds. Still, many dentists recommend sugarless gum or gum containing the sweetener xylitol (technically, a sugar alcohol, which bacteria can't feed on) because it boosts saliva production.

DON'T BOTHER

✖ **Breath mints** The minty smell tells the world you're trying to cover up unpleasant breath, but the sugar in most mints gives odor-causing bacteria more to feed on. ∎

Breast Cancer

You've heard the statistic: Over the course of a lifetime, one in eight women will get breast cancer. Thanks to early detection with mammograms, more and more cases are found in their most treatable stages. As a result, breast cancer death rates have been falling steadily for more than a decade. Wonder whether there's anything you can do to stop this cancer before it starts? While there have been plenty of conflicting studies, emerging research suggests that a healthy lifestyle does offer some protection.

WORKS

✔ **Getting regular mammograms** They could detect a breast mass at least two years before you or your doctor would be able to feel it. The sooner a cancer's caught, the more likely it can be successfully treated. Mammograms can also detect precancerous changes in breast tissue, allowing for treatment to begin before a tumor even exists. See page 228 for advice on when to start getting them.

✔ **Maintaining or achieving a healthy weight** Staying—or getting—slim is one of the smartest do-it-yourself strategies for sidestepping breast cancer. When Harvard School of Public Health researchers reviewed the health histories of more than 80,000 female nurses, they found that those who gained 55 pounds or more after age 18 had a 45 percent increase in breast cancer risk after menopause, compared to women whose weight stayed at healthy levels through their twenties, thirties, and forties. In another study, women who gained more than 60 pounds after age 18 tripled their risk of invasive breast cancer compared to women who'd put on 20 pounds or less. More body fat equals higher levels of estrogen, which fuels breast cancer growth.

The good news: Women who lost 22 pounds or more after menopause and were able to keep the weight off were almost 60 percent less likely to develop breast cancer than overweight women who didn't lose weight.

✔ **Breastfeeding** Delaying pregnancy until after age 25 raises cancer risk slightly, but nursing can help even the score, say University of Southern California researchers. They found that older moms who breastfed their babies had fewer cases of estrogen-sensitive invasive cancer than those who did not. Why it works: Nursing lowers levels of cancer-related hormones, including estrogen.

✔ **Cutting the fat in your diet** Nobody can say for sure that eating less fat lowers your breast cancer risk. On the other hand, after decades of research, experts have a strong suspicion that eating *more* fat increases your risk. In the largest study ever on the connection between dietary fat and breast cancer, researchers from the National Cancer Institute found that women whose diets included the most fat were 15 percent more likely to develop breast cancer than women who ate the least fat.

The high-fat eaters got 40 percent of their daily calories from fat; if you eat 2,000 calories a day, that's 800 calories' worth, the amount in seven tablespoons of butter or oil or eight ounces of cheese. Women who got about 20 percent of their calories from fat had no added

BREAST CANCER

risk. Of course, it makes sense to lower your intake of saturated fat anyway to cut the risk of heart disease and diabetes.

✔ A diet centered on fish and vegetables

Scientists studying breast cancer rates in Asia compared the diets and breast cancer rates of more than 3,000 postmenopausal women in Shanghai. Higher cancer risk was found in women who ate a more Western diet—and whose plates contained more foods like pork, poultry, organ meats, beef, and lamb, along with candy, desserts, breads, and milk. Women at lower risk ate more vegetables, soy-based products, and fish.

✔ Stopping smoking

While some studies suggest that cigarettes have little to do with breast cancer, cutting-edge research suggests that for some women, smoking increases the risk. When scientists at Emory University in Atlanta reviewed 50 studies, they found a pattern: Women who smoked and whose genes made their bodies slow to detoxify carcinogenic aromatic amines in cigarette smoke were at 2.4 times higher risk for breast cancer than those whose bodies neutralized the toxins quickly. The longer the women smoked, the higher their risk.

ENJOY SOY, SENSIBLY

For years, researchers have pondered whether diets high in soy explain why women in Asian countries have relatively low rates of breast cancer. Now, the largest-ever review of studies on soy foods and breast cancer has concluded that *most* women who eat soy products have a slightly reduced cancer risk. The exceptions are high-risk women. If you're at above-average risk due to a personal or family history of breast cancer, experts suggest you skip soy products "fortified" with extra isoflavones, avoid soy and isoflavone supplements, and have just a few servings of soy foods such as tofu and soy milk each week. If you're taking tamoxifen or another breast cancer prevention drug, have even less. Some animal and test-tube studies suggest that at high doses, soy isoflavones could stimulate the growth of estrogen-sensitive breast tumors.

The researchers say all women should avoid soy supplements. For more on soy, see page 149.

WORKS FOR SOME

● **Cancer-prevention drugs** These can help women at high risk for breast cancer, including those who've recently been treated for cancer, reduce their risk. The drugs block the effects of estrogen on breast tissue. In one landmark study, women at high risk who took tamoxifen cut their odds of developing breast cancer over the next seven years by 42 percent. And when researchers followed thousands of women who'd already been treated for estrogen receptor–positive breast cancer, just 10 percent of those who took trastuzumab (Herceptin) plus tamoxifen saw cancer spread after four years, compared to 26 percent who received tamoxifen alone. After just two years, Herceptin cut the risk of death from cancer by 33 percent.

These lifesaving meds do have side effects: Tamoxifen raises the risk of endometrial cancer and blood clots, and Herceptin increases the odds of congestive heart failure. You may also go into premature menopause. Other drugs used for breast cancer prevention include Arimidex (anastrozole) and Evista (raloxifene). ■

Bruises

When you bang into something, tiny blood vessels break under your skin, and blood forms puddles that turn all the Technicolor hues of a bruise in a predictable progression: reddish (the color of the blood), purple-blue, green, and yellow. Aging makes you more vulnerable as skin and blood vessels become more fragile and the fat layer beneath the skin shrinks. So do medications that thin the blood, including aspirin, warfarin (Coumadin), and diuretics, and birth control pills.

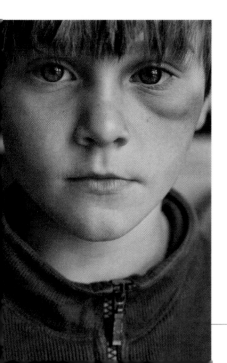

WORKS

✔ Cold compresses

Elevate the bruised area if possible and apply a cold compress to reduce leakage of blood from damaged blood vessels. Leave the compress in place for 15 to 20 minutes, then remove it so your skin isn't damaged. Wait at least two hours before reapplying; the skin continues to cool after you remove the compress.

✔ Bromelain Derived

from pineapple stems, bromelain eases bruising, possibly by breaking down proteins that trap fluids in tissues after an injury. In one study of 74 boxers with bruises on their faces and bodies, those who got bromelain had no sign of their bruises within 4 days; those who got a placebo had visible bruising for 10 days. Take 500 milligrams two or three times a day; for a big bruise, double the dose for the first 24 hours.

✔ Horse chestnut gel

Compounds in horse chestnut called saponins may reduce swelling and inflammation by sealing leaky capillaries or strengthening blood vessel walls. In Japan, an injected form of horse chestnut is widely used to reduce inflammation after surgery or injury. But you should use the herb in cream or gel form, available under brand names such as Venaforce.

WORKS FOR SOME

● **Arnica** The evidence is mixed on this popular bruise treatment, which comes in gel or cream form and as homeopathic tablets. Some studies show it helps; others don't.

● **Citrus fruit** Oranges, grapefruit, lemons: Delicious citrus is a rich source of flavonoids, antioxidant compounds that may decrease the tendency to bruise. In one French study of 96 people with fragile capillaries, half took placebos and half took supplements containing diosmin and hesperidin, flavonoids found in citrus fruit. After six weeks, the capillaries of the flavonoid group were about 60 percent stronger than those of the placebo group. Other research suggests that having a glass of orange juice plus a half grapefruit every day provides enough vitamin C to cut the risk of bruising. ■

Colds

Scientists have discovered distant planets and created cows able to produce skim milk, but finding a cure for the common cold is beyond their ability, at least so far, thanks to the hundreds of different virus strains that can cause colds. Coping with a cold is still a matter of easing symptoms. Most of the cold relief strategies here apply primarily to grownups: Researchers say that kid-strength pain relievers, plenty of fluids, and a bowl of chicken soup are your best bets for a child or even a teen. In fact, you shouldn't give cold medicine to kids (see page 192).

WORKS

✔ Decongestants

Decongestants work by shrinking swollen blood vessels in the lining of your nose. A single dose can help clear blocked nasal passages for 3 to 10 hours (but after three days, decongestants seem to lose effectiveness). The downsides: Oral decongestants can cause insomnia, nervousness, and heart palpitations; nasal spray decongestants can dry nasal membranes, causing nosebleeds, and can even lead to rebound congestion if used for more than three to four days. (Also see our note about the decongestant phenylephrine, on page 264; it doesn't work.)

✔ Aspirin or ibuprofen
Taking a nonsteroidal anti-inflammatory (NSAID) pain reliever like ibuprofen or aspirin can do more than ease the low-grade fever that sometimes accompanies a cold. Symptoms like congestion, sneezing, and sore throat are caused by inflammation that results as the immune system battles invading cold viruses. This may explain the success of a British study that found that cold sufferers who took an NSAID pain reliever plus a decongestant got more symptom relief than those who took either remedy on its own. (See our cautions on page 191 about taking multiple remedies when you have a cold.)

✔ Andrographis
Popular in Scandinavia as a cold and flu treatment, this herb is less well known than other botanicals purported to fight colds, but it may be the best of the bunch. In one well-designed Chilean study of 158 adults with colds, those who took 1,200 milligrams of andrographis extract daily for five days were 28 percent less tired, and the severity of sore throats and congestion fell by more than half.

✔ Chicken soup
The Egyptian Jewish physician and philosopher Moshe ben Maimon (Maimonides) recommended chicken soup for respiratory tract symptoms in the 12th century—and generations of mothers and grandmothers have followed suit. In one study, Nebraska Medical Center researcher Stephen Rennard, MD, found that his mother-in-law's chicken soup recipe reduced by about 75 percent the movement of neutrophils, white blood cells that fight off cold viruses but are also responsible for cold symptoms like congestion. Canned soups worked, too.

✔ Astragalus for prevention
Long recommended by Chinese healers for bolstering immunity, astragalus has proven itself in lab and test-tube studies. And in one human study that compared astragalus to echinacea and licorice extracts, astragalus triggered the strongest immune response. In another well-designed study, volunteers who took two 100-milligram tablets a day for three months had half as many colds as volunteers who took placebos.

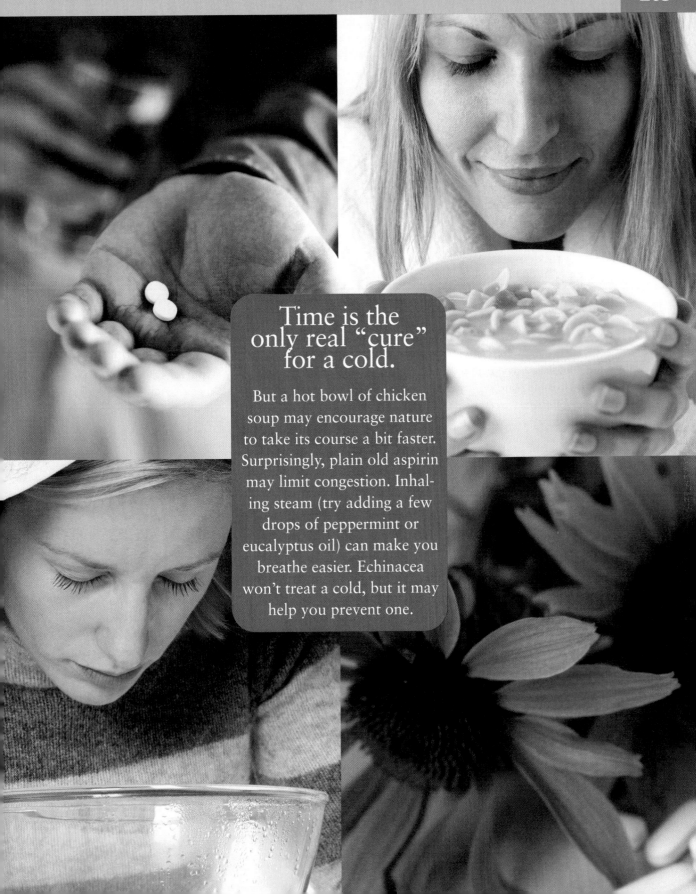

Time is the only real "cure" for a cold.

But a hot bowl of chicken soup may encourage nature to take its course a bit faster. Surprisingly, plain old aspirin may limit congestion. Inhaling steam (try adding a few drops of peppermint or eucalyptus oil) can make you breathe easier. Echinacea won't treat a cold, but it may help you prevent one.

COLDS

WORKS FOR SOME

● **Zinc nasal gels** In a Cleveland Clinic study of 78 volunteers with colds, those who used a zinc gel shortened the duration of cold symptoms from 6 days to 4.3. Not all studies on zinc nasal gels have shown a benefit, but in those that did, people started using the product within 24 to 48 hours of the start of cold symptoms and applied a new dose every 4 to 6 hours.

Don't overuse zinc nasal gels. For a small percentage of people, they can damage the sense of smell temporarily—or even permanently. If you feel a burning sensation or notice a change in your ability to detect smells, stop using the gel immediately.

● **Echinacea for prevention—but not treatment** A recent analysis of 14 studies of this wildly popular herb found that it may help prevent colds (though other reviews say it doesn't).

Already have a cold? It's too late. Echinacea failed on that front in a string of recent well-designed studies.

DON'T BOTHER

✖ **Vitamin C** Nobel Prize–winning scientist Linus Pauling, PhD, was convinced that C could ward off a cold, but science has proven him wrong for the most part. While a few studies suggest that a big dose of C at the start of a cold may shorten symptoms by about 8 percent (less than a day in the three- to seven-day course of an average cold), a definitive analysis of 29 well-designed studies involving more than 11,700 people concluded that C supplements have no power to prevent a cold. Your best bet is to get plenty of the vitamin from the produce in your diet.

✖ **Zinc lozenges** For every study showing that zinc lozenges are effective, another shows that they aren't. The two best studies to date concluded the lozenges have little benefit for cold sufferers. Zinc nasal gels, for whatever reason, seem to work better. If you opt for lozenges, follow the package directions carefully; you could become nauseated if you take too much zinc.

✖ **Cold remedies containing phenylephrine** Reformulated cold remedies that contain this decongestant have been appearing on store shelves ever since pharmacies began keeping pseudoephedrine products behind the counter. But this new kid on the block doesn't work very well. One review of eight studies found that the legally allowed dose of phenylephrine in the United States—10 milligrams—does nothing to unblock clogged nasal passages.

✖ **Antibiotics** Colds are caused by viruses, not by bacteria. We can't say it plainly enough: Antibiotics won't cure a cold.

✖ **Cold medicine for kids** An expert panel of the FDA has recommended that cold remedies be banned for kids under age 6 because they don't work and in some cases can cause serious side effects—such as liver damage if a child gets too high a dose of acetaminophen in some combination remedies. Meanwhile, the American College of Chest Physicians recommends not giving cough-and-cold remedies to kids under the age of 15.

A better plan: Keep kids well hydrated and give them child-strength pain relievers (never aspirin if there's a fever) to make 'em comfortable if they're really miserable. ■

Cold Sores

If you're prone to cold sores, you know that these painful, itchy blisters can appear at the most inconvenient moments. The trigger? It could be sunburn or added stress or even your menstrual cycle, fatigue, a cold, or dental surgery. Once you've been exposed to the herpes simplex virus that causes cold sores, the virus is with you for life. Most of the time, it lies dormant in nerve cells. Start treatment at the first sign of tingling and itching to increase your odds of short-circuiting a full-blown blister.

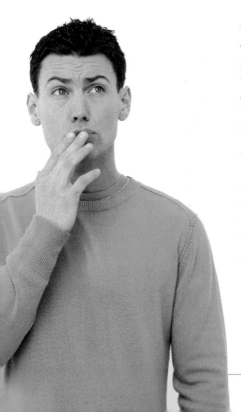

WORKS

✔ **Oral antiviral drugs** If you're prone to frequent and/or severe outbreaks, ask your doctor about prescription virus-fighting pills. Taken at the first sign of a cold sore, then repeated as directed, the drugs valacyclovir (Valtrex), acyclovir (Zovirax), and famciclovir (Famvir) can halt an outbreak before blisters form. Taken a little later, they can speed healing time. In one study, valacyclovir healed blisters in 3 days compared to 4.3 days for placebo pills. In another study, famciclovir reduced the size of blisters that appeared by 50 percent.

These drugs can also be taken to prevent an outbreak, either long term if you're prone to cold sores or short term when you know you'll be exposed to triggers such as bright sunlight. In a study published in the *Journal of the American Medical Association,* 147 recreational skiers took acyclovir or a placebo before ski trips. Just 7 percent of the drug group got cold sores compared to 26 percent of the placebo group.

✔ **Prescription antiviral creams** Oral antiviral drugs work much better than these creams, but for people who don't want to use the pills or can't take them, acyclovir and penciclovir creams are another option, though they need to be used often—up to six times a day—to be effective. They work by suppressing the cell-to-cell spread of the herpesvirus. In one Canadian study of 3,057 people with cold sores, those who applied penciclovir cream six times a day the first day and every two hours during the day for the next four days saw blisters heal 31 percent faster than those who used a placebo cream.

✔ **Sunscreen for prevention** The sun's ultraviolet (UV) rays reactivate dormant herpesvirus particles, leading to an increased risk of blisters after a day in the sun. Using a lip balm with an SPF of 15 or higher can help stop an outbreak before it starts. The proof: In one National Institutes of Health study of 38 people prone to cold sores, those who wore sunblocking lip balm had no breakouts after exposure to UV light, while 71 percent of those who used a placebo cream got blisters.

COLD SORES

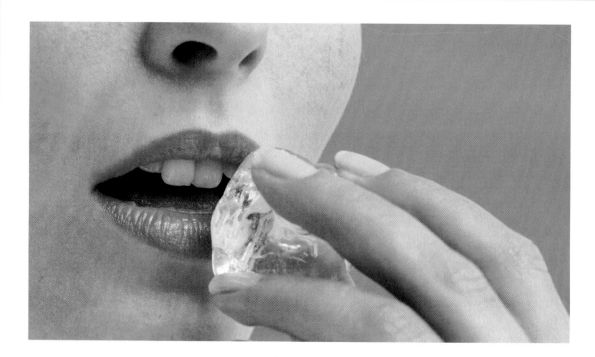

WORKS FOR SOME

● **Over-the-counter cream with docosanol (Abreva)** Applied to cold sores five times a day, this drugstore remedy healed cold sores nearly a day sooner than did a placebo cream in one study of 437 people with cold sores. The cream seems to work by preventing the virus from fusing with cell walls, which stops it from entering cells and replicating.

● **Ice** Applying ice (preferably wrapped in a towel so skin doesn't freeze) at the first tingle or itch can stop some outbreaks. Try this remedy when you have 1 1/2 to 2 hours to spare; that's how long it took for ice to work in one study of 14 people. (Leave the ice on for a few minutes, remove it for a few minutes, then repeat over and over again.) Ice users were cold sore–free within two days.

● **Creams containing** *Melissa officinalis* Extracts of this herb, better known as lemon balm, speeded healing and eased stinging and itching slightly faster than a placebo cream in one German study of 61 people. In test-tube studies, melissa extracts prevent the virus from attaching to cells. A well-studied brand you may find in a health food stores is Cold Sore Relief, made by Enzymatic Therapy.

DON'T BOTHER

✖ **Lysine tablets** Supplements of this amino acid are popular for cold sores, but there's little evidence that they protect against outbreaks. Studies that do show positive results in preventing recurrences tend to involve relatively high doses, from 1,000 to 3,000 milligrams a day. If you want to try high doses of lysine for prevention, check with your doctor first.

✖ **Creams and ointments containing salicylic acid** This acid—the same compound that's the active ingredient in aspirin—damages skin and can actually slow healing after an outbreak. ■

Colon Cancer

Since studies emerged showing that fiber doesn't prevent colon cancer, you might think all bets are off when it comes to reducing your risk of this disease. You'd be wrong. There are still plenty of things you can do to prevent colon or rectal cancer, beginning with regular screenings. In fact, colorectal cancer is one of the few cancers that can be completely cured—even before it is officially deemed a cancer.

WORKS

✔ **Colonoscopy** Catching colon cancer early is far and away the best strategy for "preventing" it. Guidelines call for a colonoscopy once every 10 years starting at age 50. For the procedure, you're sedated while the doctor threads an instrument with a small camera attached to the end through your rectum and colon, looking for precancerous growths called polyps. If the doctor sees any, he can cut them out, effectively "curing" a cancer before it begins. (For more on colon cancer screening tests, see page 223.)

✔ **Aspirin and other nonsteroidal anti-inflammatory drugs (NSAIDs)** There is compelling evidence that regular long-term use of aspirin and other NSAIDs like celecoxib (Celebrex) can prevent colon cancer. One of the most convincing studies involved more than 80,000 women who were followed for 20 years. Those who took at least 325 milligrams of regular aspirin twice a week for at least 10 years were 33 percent less likely to develop colon cancer than those who used aspirin less frequently. The same held true for nonaspirin NSAIDs. However, the study also found that high aspirin use increased the risk of gastrointestinal bleeding, with the highest risk in people taking more than six aspirin a week.

Don't start taking extra aspirin or any other pain reliever without talking to your doctor, though; taking these drugs on a regular basis can pose significant risks.

Statin drugs Taking a cholesterol-lowering medication such as atorvastatin (Lipitor), simvastatin (Zocor), or pravastatin (Pravachol) for at least five years could slash your risk of colon cancer nearly in half, according to a study involving about 4,000 people. Statins could reduce cancer risk by decreasing inflammation and/or by inhibiting an enzyme that's involved with cholesterol production and possibly with the development of colorectal cancer. Of course, statins have potential side effects and aren't right for everyone. You and your doctor should weigh the risks and costs against the benefits.

DON'T BOTHER

✘ **Fiber** For years we were told that a high-fiber diet reduces the risk of colon cancer. Then researchers sat down and pooled the data from 13 major studies and found that it's not true. That doesn't mean you should throw out your whole-grain cereal; such diets *are* related to lower risks of heart disease and diabetes.

✘ **Exercise** Don't get us wrong—exercise is still critical to good health. But according to a study of nearly 32,000 women, it won't lower your risk of colon cancer. ■

Constipation

Don't obsess if you don't "go" as often as you think you should—what's normal for one person is unusual for someone else. If you're really constipated, you'll know it. You'll struggle to pass hard, dry stools, and you may have a stuffed, uncomfortable feeling. Here's what can help get things moving again.

WORKS

✔ **High-fiber foods plus water** The best approach to preventing—and over the longer term, solving—constipation is to eat more fruits, vegetables, beans, and whole grains and wash everything down with lots of water. Don't try one without the other; studies find that either alone does little to help relieve constipation. And be patient: It may take several weeks to see an improvement. (For more immediate relief, try prunes or prune juice, hot coffee, or a cup of warm milk with a teaspoon of ground flaxseed mixed in; all are said to help.) Aim to get at least 25 grams of fiber a day. A bowl of bran cereal will deliver as much as 10 grams, and 1/2 cup of red kidney beans will net you more than 8 grams. A cup of raspberries? An easy 8 grams.

WORKS FOR SOME

● **Fiber supplements and osmotic laxatives** Some people who try fiber supplements for constipation get relief—but not everyone. About half of the people who try them eventually stop using them for two main reasons: because of bloating and because they aren't working. A task force for the American College of Gastroenterology found that only fiber supplements containing psyllium (such as Metamucil) are effective for chronic constipation.

For briefer episodes, some studies find that osmotic laxatives can help. These products (including milk of magnesia) contain ingredients such as magnesium hydroxide or citrate, sodium phosphate, or polyethylene glycol, which induce the intestines to secrete water that can be absorbed by stool, softening it. Use them for only short periods (a week or two) and expect them to take a few days to work.

● **Biofeedback** If you're chronically constipated, biofeedback could help. It teaches you to relax your pelvic floor muscles and the muscle that controls the anus when you're trying to go. Studies suggest it works in up to 70 percent of patients with a form of chronic constipation called dyssynergic defecation, in which you can't control the

Our **BEST** ADVICE

Use stimulant laxatives, such as Ex-Lax, senna, Senokot, Dulcolax, and castor oil, only after talking with your doctor. These are strong medicines that force the bowel muscles to contract. If you use them too much, your colon may come to rely on them. It's better to try gentler remedies first.

coordination of your muscles to push stool out. It doesn't work as well for people who have slow-transit constipation, which typically occurs in young women who have one or fewer bowel movements a week. ■

Coughs

There are scratchy, dry coughs; wet, phlegmy ones that make people on the bus move away from you; and the lung-busting variety that's so forceful it hurts. Believe it or not, your best bet may be to skip the drugstore (two major panels of cough experts—one American, one British—have recently concluded that there's little evidence that *any* cough preparation works) and brew up an old-fashioned steaming cup of tea with honey and lemon.

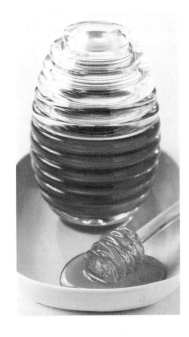

WORKS

✔ **Honey** This age-old folk remedy finally has a little science behind it. In one Pennsylvania State University study of 105 coughing kids who received buckwheat honey, a honey-flavored preparation containing dextromethorphan (the ingredient in many cough syrups), or no treatment at all, parents reported that kids who got honey saw the greatest reduction in coughing severity and frequency. Don't give honey to children under the age of 1, though; it's not safe for them.

✔ **Cough or allergy remedies containing a "first-generation" antihistamine plus a decongestant** This combo earned an "A" from a committee of cough experts convened by the American College of Chest Physicians (ACCP), who called its benefits "substantial." The proof:

In a University of Massachusetts study, the combination of brompheniramine (an antihistamine) and sustained-release pseudoephedrine (a decongestant) reduced coughing by 20 to 30 percent in three days in people whose coughs were due to the common cold. Harvard University experts recommend that for coughs due to a cold or an allergy, try an allergy medicine containing the antihistamine brompheniramine, diphenhydramine, or chlorpheniramine combined with a decongestant. But be careful: These first-generation antihistamines (so-called because they were some of the first on the market) can cause drowsiness. And British cough experts say that combining them with a decongestant can lead to dry mouth, dizziness, headache, and insomnia—all of which may be worse than putting up with a cough.

✔ **Cough drops** Maybe it's because they're so simple and commonsense, but hardly anyone has studied the effectiveness of good ol' cough drops to temporarily soothe dry, scratchy coughs. That said, if you put one in your mouth and your coughing quiets, you'll know they work. Try a brand with lemon, honey, or slippery elm.

WORKS FOR SOME

● **Inhaled ipratropium (Atrovent)** For a serious cough that won't stop—from a cold or bronchitis—experts recommend the prescription drug ipratropium in an inhaler.

COUGHS

DON'T BOTHER

✖ Cough remedies containing dextromethorphan The ACCP committee gave this cough suppressant a "D" and ruled it has no benefits. An analysis of four studies involving 710 people with coughs due to the common cold did show that this drugstore remedy can reduce the frequency and severity of coughs—but only by about 14 percent. And it can make you nervous or restless. Not a great bet.

✖ Cough remedies for children Skip them if your child's under age 15. "No medication available in the United States has been shown to effectively treat cough in children," noted University of Pittsburgh Medical Center doctors who reviewed 38 studies of cough and cold remedies. In one definitive Pennsylvania State University study of 100 kids ages 2 to 18 with upper respiratory infections, dextromethorphan and diphenhydramine were no better than a placebo at stopping nighttime coughing.

✖ Nonsedating antihistamines like loratadine The cough panel ruled against products (such as Claritin and Tavist) containing this newer, nondrowsy antihistamine.

✖ Mucus-thinning guaifenisen The research on this expectorant cough medicine is mixed: One study of 239 people with colds found that those who took it had fewer and milder coughs, but another found no benefit. Studies in people with bronchitis were also mixed, leading the chest doctors to give this remedy low marks. And by the way, never take a product that contains both guaifenisen (an expectorant designed to bring up phlegm) and dextromethorphan (designed to suppress coughs). These work at cross purposes, so the combination makes no sense. ∎

Our BEST ADVICE

A stubborn cough could be a holdover from a serious head cold (in which case, it could last about four weeks), but a longer-lasting cough warrants a trip to the doctor. The cause could be acid reflux, chronic obstructive pulmonary disease (COPD), an iron deficiency, or even medications like ACE inhibitors, often used to treat high blood pressure.

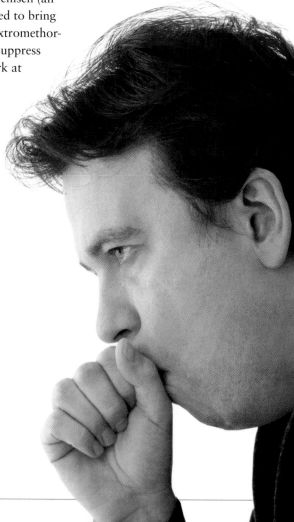

Depression

Depression is far more serious than just a few days of feeling down. It significantly increases the risk of heart disease and heart attack. It also tends to go hand in hand with chronic health conditions like asthma, diabetes, pain, arthritis, and obesity. Yet it's one of the most treatable mental health conditions. The key is patience as you and your doctor work to find the right treatment—or combination of treatments—for you. Don't try to work through depression on your own; doing so can be dangerous, and it's just not necessary.

WORKS

✔ Antidepressants

Not every antidepressant works for every person, but with more than 38 different antidepressants available worldwide, chances are good that one will work for you if you need one. Two of the main drug classes—tricyclics like amitriptyline (Elavil) and imipramine (Tofranil) and selective serotonin-reuptake inhibitors (SSRIs) like fluoxetine (Prozac) and paroxetine (Paxil)—work equally well. But the SSRIs tend to have fewer side effects such as weight gain and dry mouth, and studies find that patients are more likely to stick with them. New data suggests that two SSRIs together often work significantly better than one alone.

One of the newest antidepressants is venlafaxine (Effexor). Unlike an SSRI, which works only to increase the amount of the mood-related chemical serotonin in the brain, Effexor increases the amounts of serotonin *and* norepinephrine. When researchers pooled data from eight well-designed studies that compared Effexor to SSRIs or a placebo, they found that scores on three depression scales declined more in people taking Effexor than in those taking SSRIs or placebos.

✔ Hypnotherapy and cognitive behavioral therapy (CBT) Worrying too much and ruminating too long on your troubles often underlies depression, and both of these therapies can help change such habits. When researchers assigned 84 people diagnosed with depression to receive 16 weeks of hypnotherapy or cognitive behavioral therapy (a form of psychotherapy aimed at changing thoughts and behaviors that may be contributing to depression), participants in both groups improved significantly compared to a control group. The people who got hypnotherapy did slightly better than the CBT group.

✔ SAM-e The only major review of studies on this supplement found that SAM-e improved symptoms of depression 27 to 38 percent better than placebos. The review also found that SAM-e was as effective as tricyclic antidepressants.

FINDING THE RIGHT ANTIDEPRESSANT

You may have to try several drugs or drug combinations to find one that relieves your depression without unacceptable side effects. That said, some doctors are too quick to switch patients from one antidepressant to another without first increasing the dosage or giving it more time to work. Generally, if you don't show any improvement within two to four weeks of taking the highest recommended dose (which could be six weeks or more after you start taking the drug), it's time to switch. Note that most side effects abate within one to two weeks of starting the medication.

DEPRESSION

✔ **St. John's wort** This herb has been shown in studies to be as much as 71 percent more effective than placebos for treating mild to moderate depression. Trials comparing St. John's wort to antidepressants found they both worked about the same, although patients were less likely to drop out of the trials if they took the herb, because it has fewer side effects.

✔ **Electroconvulsive therapy (ECT)** It may bring up memories of the movie *One Flew Over the Cuckoo's Nest,* but ECT, in which short bursts of electricity are sent into the brain to "reboot" brain cells, is not only quite safe, it's also very effective in treating patients for whom antidepressants don't work.

✔ **Psychotherapy** This works best when combined with medication. It's also effective at preventing a relapse. Look for a therapist who practices cognitive behavioral therapy (described on page 271) or interpersonal therapy, in which you learn to cope better with stress, improve your interactions with others, and deal with the effects of depression. Studies find these two forms work best.

✔ **Exercise** The same endorphins that contribute to "runner's high" can provide

FISHING FOR RELIEF?

The same fish-oil pills that can help your heart may have the power to ease depression. In countries where fish consumption is high, depression rates tend to be low. Conversely, in places where fish isn't as popular, depression rates are often much higher. The omega-3 fatty acids found in fish like salmon play a crucial role in the healthy development and maintenance of the brain. Supplementing with omega-3 fatty acids, primarily in the form of fish oil, may relieve mild to moderate depression. One review of 10 studies found that high doses of fish oil improved depression significantly better than placebos, though the researchers noted that more large-scale, well-controlled trials are needed due to problems with the existing studies. You may need to take as much as 4 grams daily; check with your doctor before starting.

natural relief for depression—and help prevent a relapse, if you can manage to get yourself off the couch. In one study that pitted brisk walking or jogging against sertraline (Zoloft) or a combination of the drug plus the exercise, after 16 weeks, all three groups had about the same improvement, but at six months, the people who kept up the exercise had the lowest rates of remission. Just 50 minutes of exercise a week reduced the risk of relapse by 50 percent.

It doesn't seem to matter what form of exercise you do; aerobics, strength training, and flexibility exercises like yoga all seem to provide similar benefits.

✔ **Qigong** One exercise worth trying, particularly if

you're 60 or older, is qigong (pronounced *chee-guhn*), an ancient Chinese martial art that combines steady, slow movement with breathing patterns. In a Hong Kong study, people diagnosed with depression who participated in 16 weeks of qigong surpassed the control group in every measure after 8 weeks.

DON'T BOTHER

✘ **Vagus nerve stimulation** Researchers have concluded—and doctors agree—that this therapy, in which a stimulator implanted under the skin sends electrical impulses to the left vagus nerve in the neck, just doesn't work. ■

Diabetes

Diabetes isn't going away any time soon. Caused by a combination of genetics and lifestyle factors, it's preventable up to a point, though you might not know it given the increasing number of people with the disease. But treating it once you're diagnosed is even more challenging, especially as the disease progresses and medications stop working as well. Good blood sugar control is critical to avoiding problems like nerve damage and catastrophes like blindness and amputation. But taking care of your heart is equally key since most people with diabetes eventually die of heart disease—so it's essential to make sure your blood pressure and cholesterol are under control.

WORKS

✔ **Oral medications** At first, your doctor may have you try to bring down your blood sugar by improving your diet and adding regular exercise, but unfortunately, the percentage of people who can stay off medication is low. There are many different drugs available, and your doctor may use them alone or in combination. It's agreed that metformin (Glucophage) is the best one to use first. In a review of 29 clinical studies, it reduced the risk of complications like retinopathy and neuropathy as well as death, and it worked better than anything else for controlling blood sugar, cholesterol, blood pressure, and weight.

Because diabetes is a progressive disease, most drugs, including insulin, become less effective the longer you take them. Your doctor may increase your dosage or change your regimen altogether if you aren't seeing good results.

✔ **Insulin** If your insulin-producing cells (located in the pancreas) begin wearing out, you'll eventually need injections of this hormone. In terms of taking animal vs. human insulin, either is fine, although animal insulin is usually cheaper. An analysis of 45 studies found no significant differences between blood sugar control or episodes of low blood sugar in people taking either purified porcine (pig) insulin or semi-synthetic human insulin, the two forms most often studied, and no differences in negative side effects.

✔ **Exercise** It won't "cure" your diabetes, but it can make your cells more sensitive to insulin, which naturally lowers blood sugar. Fourteen clinical trials comparing people with type 2 diabetes who exercised with those who didn't found that the exercisers dropped their A1c levels (a long-term measure of blood sugar control) by 0.6 point—a significant amount. People who exercised also became much more sensitive to insulin, reducing the strain on the pancreas, and their triglyceride levels dropped.

If you're wondering whether you should do aerobic exercise or lift weights, the answer is yes to both. A1c scores dropped an average of 0.51 point after two weeks in people who walked on treadmills or rode bikes and an average of 0.38 point in those who worked out on weight machines. Those who did both got an *additional* 0.46 point drop.

Since exercise gobbles up blood sugar, if you're using insulin, you may even be able to substitute an exercise session for an injection. Talk to your doctor.

✔ **Weight loss** Drop about 10 percent of your body weight, and your fasting blood sugar level could drop by 26 percent, along with big reductions in cholesterol, blood pressure, and triglycerides. That adds up to a lower risk of heart disease and

DIABETES

other diabetes complications. If you're extremely over-weight, consider bariatric surgery, in which a surgeon cinches your stomach into a small pouch so it holds less food. The surgery effectively cured the disease in 73 percent of people with recent-onset diabetes. It's not to be entered into lightly, however, since it carries significant risks.

Cinnamon Laboratory studies find that this aromatic spice has insulin-like effects on cells, helping them take up more glucose from the blood-stream. While just a handful of clinical trials have evaluated its use in people with diabetes, most found that supplementing with cinnamon does lower blood sugar levels. One study found that people taking 1 gram a day of cinnamon (about 1/4 teaspoon) had glucose levels averaging 156.5 mg/dl after 40 days, compared to 223.2 mg/dl in those taking a placebo. Stick to 1 gram; two other studies showed similar effects even at higher doses.

WHAT DIET STRATEGY IS BEST?

Here's a sad fact: We don't really know. That's the conclusion of reviewers who analyzed 18 studies involving 1,467 partici-pants who followed any of a number of different diets, including low-fat/high-carbohydrate, high-fat/low-carbohydrate, and low-calorie regimens. All that the reviewers could say after evaluating these studies was that exercise works for maintaining blood sugar control and that there is an "urgent need" for studies looking at diet. That said, hardly any doctor or nutritionist would argue against a diet rich in fruits and vegetables, beans, and whole grains and low in saturated fat.

✔ **Laser surgery for eye complications**
Having diabetes puts the eyes at risk; a condition called dia-betic retinopathy can even cause blindness. A procedure known as pan-retinal laser pho-tocoagulation, in which a laser is used to make hundreds of tiny cuts or burns in the eye to reduce the growth of abnormal blood vessels, can stem the loss of vision. And if you develop macular edema, or swelling of the retina from leaking blood vessels, focal retinal laser sur-gery, which aims to close the leaking vessels, is the procedure recommended to preserve your vision.

✔ **Antidepressants plus capsaicin cream for nerve pain** There are no medications specifically marketed to treat diabetic neuropathy, which can cause excruciating pain. But based on analysis of 25 studies, reviewers recommended starting with an antidepressant and a cream containing capsaicin, the ingre-dient in hot peppers that interferes with the nerves' ability to transmit pain signals. Tricyclic antidepressants such as desipramine (Norpramine), imipramine (Tofranil), and amitriptyline (Elavil) worked much better than newer antide-pressants for relieving pain.

WORKS FOR SOME

● **Chromium** Small doses of this mineral may help some people with diabetes maintain blood sugar levels. A recent analysis of 36 studies found that supplementing with about 200 micrograms of chromium picolinate a day reduced A1c levels by about 0.6 point, about as much as some oral medications. The researchers admit, however, that some of the studies were of poor quality. Some research suggests that chromium helps nor-malize blood sugar only in people who are deficient in the mineral.

● **Fish-oil supple-ments** They won't help control your blood sugar, but these pills can help lower the risk of a heart attack—which is

An Arsenal of Diabetes Drugs

Deciding what drug or combination of drugs is right for you is a complicated process for your doctor, as different drugs work through different pathways and have unique side effects. Below is a snapshot of the drugs available and how well they work according to one review.

Metformin

Blood pressure: Average reduction of 5 mmHg systolic and diastolic
LDL cholestrol: Average decrease of 10 mg/dl
HDL cholestrol: No effect
Triglycerides: Average decrease of 10 mg/dl
Hypoglycemic episodes: Possible
A1c: Average reduction of 1 point
Weight: No effect
Side effects: More gastrointestinal problems (nausea, gas, vomiting, and abdominal pain) than with any other agent

Second-generation sulfonylureas
Glipizide (Glucotrol), glyburide (Micronase, Diabeta), micronized glyburide (Glynase)
Blood pressure: Average reduction of 5 mmHg systolic and diastolic
LDL cholestrol: Typically reduced levels
HDL cholestrol: No effect
Triglycerides: Not studied
Hypoglycemic episodes: 4 to 9% more frequent than in people receiving metformin or thiazolidinediones. Slightly higher risk with glyburide than with other sulfonylureas
A1c: Average reduction of 1 point
Weight: Increase of 2.2 to 11 pounds
Side effects: Diarrhea, nausea, abdominal pain, constipation, itching, vomiting, rash, dizziness, headache, hypoglycemia

Alpha-glucosidase inhibitors
Acarbose (Precose), miglitol (Glyset)
Blood pressure: Not studied
LDL cholestrol: No effect
HDL cholestrol: No effect
Triglycerides: Average decrease of 10 to 30 mg/dl (acarbose)
Hypoglycemic episodes: Possible
A1c: Average reduction of 1 point
Weight: No effect (acarbose)
Side effects: Gas, diarrhea, hypoglycemia

Meglitinides
Nateglinide (Starlix), repaglinide (Prandin)
Blood pressure: Not studied
LDL cholestrol: No effect
HDL cholestrol: No effect
Triglycerides: Not studied (nateglinide), Average decrease of 10 to 30 mg/dl (repaglinide)
Hypoglycemic episodes: Possible (nateglinide), 4 to 9% more frequent than in people receiving metformin or thiazolidinediones (repaglinide)
A1c: Average reduction of 0.5 point (nateglinide), 1 point (repaglinide)
Weight: Not studied
Side effects: Hypoglycemia, weight gain, nausea, headache

Thiazolidinediones
Rosiglitazone (Avandia), pioglitazone (Actos)
Blood pressure: Average reduction of 5 mmHg systolic and diastolic
LDL cholestrol: Average increase of 10 to 12 mg/dl (drug class). Average increase of 10 to 15 mg/dl (rosiglitazone)
HDL cholestrol: Average increase of 1 to 5 mg/dl (pioglitazone)
Triglycerides: Average decrease of 15 to 52 mg/dl (pioglitazone). Average increase of 6 to 13 mg/dl (rosiglitazone)
Hypoglycemic episodes: Possible
A1c: Average reduction of 1 point
Weight: Increase of 2.2 to 11 pounds compared to metformin, 6.6 pounds compared with acarbose and repaglinide
Side effects: Increased risk of heart attack and hospitalization for gallstones and foot and leg swelling (pioglitazone). Slightly greater risk of congestive heart failure and mild anemia than with other medication. May increase risk of loss of bone mineral density more than other drugs

Source: Systematic Review: Comparative Effectiveness and Safety of Oral Medications for Type 2 Diabetes Mellitus, *Annals of Internal Medicine*, September 2007.

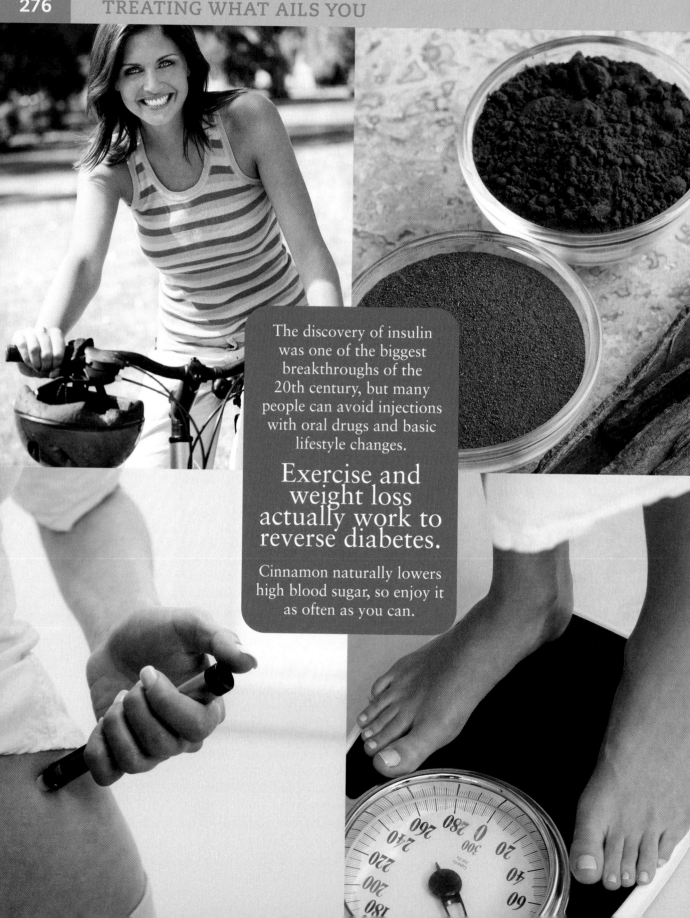

The discovery of insulin was one of the biggest breakthroughs of the 20th century, but many people can avoid injections with oral drugs and basic lifestyle changes.

Exercise and weight loss actually work to reverse diabetes.

Cinnamon naturally lowers high blood sugar, so enjoy it as often as you can.

critically important since most people who have diabetes die of heart disease. One way fish oil helps is by lowering levels of blood fats called triglycerides. An analysis of 18 clinical studies found that people taking fish-oil doses ranging from 3 to 18 grams a day reduced their triglycerides by an average of 50 mg/dl. Note that some studies suggest that fish-oil capsules may actually slightly raise LDL, or "bad" cholesterol, but as David Katz, MD, a preventive medicine specialist at Yale University School of Medicine, explains, "The overall influence on the lipid profile is decidedly positive."

FOR PREDIABETES: EXERCISE AND CALORIE CUTTING

If you have insulin resistance, or prediabetes, you're at increased risk of developing full-blown diabetes. Following a low-fat, low-calorie diet and exercising for 2 1/2 hours a week can reduce your risk by about 58 percent. In a seminal study on preventing diabetes in high-risk people, just 14 percent of those assigned to a diet and exercise program developed diabetes over three years compared to nearly 30 percent of those taking a placebo and 22 percent of those taking the diabetes drug metformin (Glucophage). The diet/exercise combination was even more effective in people 60 and older, cutting their risk by 71 percent.

The problem with prescribing diet and exercise to prevent diabetes is that most people won't do it. That's why your doctor is much more likely to write you a prescription for metformin. The same study found that taking metformin could reduce the risk of developing the disease by 31 percent over three years, but it was far less effective in people 60 and older.

DON'T BOTHER

✖ **Chinese herbs** Specifically, this means Chinese and Thai herbs like holy basil leaves, Xianzhen Pain, Qidan Tongmai, traditional Chinese formula (TCT), Huoxue Jiantang Pingshi, and Inolter. Numerous studies of these herbs show they reduce blood sugar so much that people end up with hypoglycemia.

✖ **Pioglitazone (Actos)** This oral drug is used by millions of people with diabetes, but a major analysis found it does little to improve health, and it has significant side effects. The review showed that more people taking the drug were hospitalized for leg and foot swelling and heart failure than those who didn't take it and that people gained an average of about eight pounds while taking it.

✖ **Rosiglitazone (Avandia)** Major studies have found that this drug increases the risk of heart attack by 43 percent and the risk of death from any cardiovascular cause by 64 percent. It also reduces bone density. Plus, rosiglitazone doesn't work any better than any other oral medications at reducing blood sugar levels. If you're taking this drug, talk to your doctor about other options. ■

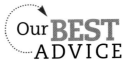

Our BEST ADVICE

Depression and diabetes go together like airline travel and frustration. People with diabetes are more likely to be diagnosed with major depression, and people with major depression are more likely to develop diabetes. One analysis of 27 studies found that the worse a person's depression, the worse their blood sugar levels, disease severity, and diabetes-related complications. If you suspect you're depressed, talk about it with your doctor.

DIARRHEA

Diarrhea

When "the runs" have you running to the bathroom, your best bet may be to simply let diarrhea, um, run its course. Your main challenge is to prevent the dehydration that often results. If you use an over-the-counter diarrhea remedy, keep in mind that it will shorten your bout by only a day or less. For more details, see the Diarrhea Medications entry on page 194. While you're recovering, stick with a bland diet; rice, bread, dry crackers, and bananas work well.

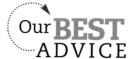

Our BEST ADVICE

To keep yourself hydrated during a bout of diarrhea, drink plenty of clear liquids, including water, tea, and broth. Avoid milk and other dairy foods. You might also try a rehydration solution such as Rehydralyte or, for kids, Pedialyte.

WORKS

✔ **Loperamide (Imodium)** Loperamide slows the movement of food through the digestive tract, giving the small intestine more time to absorb fluid and nutrients. Studies find that it relieves diarrhea within 18 to 28 hours on average compared to 40 to 45 hours with placebos.

✔ **Pepto-Bismol** The "pink stuff," officially known as bismuth subsalicylate, may not work quite as well as loperamide, but it does work. One study found it led to 109 loose stools after 4 to 24 hours of use, compared to 165 loose stools with a placebo. Another study, of tourists struck with traveler's diarrhea, found that diarrhea in people who took Pepto-Bismol improved within 24 to 25 hours, compared to 31 to 34 hours for those who got a placebo. Taking a tablespoon of Pepto several times a day may also help prevent traveler's diarrhea.

✔ **Antibiotics for traveler's diarrhea** When you visit developing countries, chances are fair that you'll end up with diarrhea from eating food or drinking water contaminated with bacteria from the local water supply. Of course, you can reduce the risk by taking the usual precautions (such as avoiding tap water, raw fruits and vegetables that you haven't peeled yourself, ice, etc.). But for extra insurance, consider asking your doctor for a prescription. Some antibiotics administered in a once-a-day dose are 90 percent effective at preventing traveler's diarrhea. They can also help once you have it.

If you get watery diarrhea without fever, take rifaximin (Xifaxan) three times a day for three days. If you have a fever and are passing bloody stools, take azithromycin (Zithromycin) as directed instead. Consider asking your doctor for a prescription for nine 200-milligram tablets of rifaximin and another for four 250-milligram tablets of azithromycin—and fill the prescriptions before packing your suitcase.

WORKS FOR SOME

● **A liquid diet** Some people swear by a clear liquid diet when they have diarrhea. But in the one study we found, in which 71 people with diarrhea followed a liquid-only diet or ate anything they wanted for 24 hours, there was no difference in how long participants' diarrhea lasted. ∎

Ear Infections

Achy ears are a rite of passage for many kids—and their distraught parents. But before you dole out the antibiotics, consider this: Pain relievers may be all most kids need, and sometimes antibiotics are ineffective against middle ear infections anyway. Often the culprit is a mixture of bacteria and viruses—which don't respond to antibiotics. Here's what *can* help.

WORKS

✔ A wait-and-see approach In a landmark study of 283 kids with ear infections, 62 percent of those whose parents waited 48 hours before filling a prescription for antibiotics never needed the drugs; the children felt better in two days or less without them. Parents who followed this wait-and-see strategy, endorsed by the American Academy of Pediatrics, opted for antibiotics only if their children had stubborn fever or ear pain or, in the case of babies and toddlers, were extremely fussy. The benefits of waiting: Kids avoid antibiotic side effects like diarrhea, vomiting, allergic reactions, and a higher risk that antibiotic-resistant bacteria will take up residence, making it more difficult to treat a serious infection like pneumonia or meningitis if one crops up in the future.

✔ Pain relievers Treat the pain and fever with ibuprofen or acetaminophen and anesthetic eardrops (available in the United States only by prescription). That's what parents who avoided antibiotics did in the wait-and-see study. Choose a pain-relief formula appropriate for your child's age and follow dosing and timing directions precisely.

✔ Antibiotics first— for young babies and severe infections The American Academy of Pediatrics recommends giving amoxicillin or other antibiotics to babies six months or younger who have ear infections. Older kids with high fevers or rampant ear infections (your doctor will decide what qualifies) may need them as well, the academy says, but parents can try two days of wait-and-see therapy for these kids, too.

✔ Herbal eardrops An Israeli study of 171 kids ages 5 to 18 with ear infections found that those who received an eardrop solution containing extracts or oils of calendula, garlic, lavender, mullein, and St. John's wort experienced a 93 percent decrease in pain after 30 minutes; those who got anesthetic eardrops had an 80 percent drop in pain.

WORKS FOR SOME

● Xylitol-sweetened gum for prevention Made with a sweetener derived from wood, this gum cut the risk of ear infections nearly in half in a Finnish study of 306 preschoolers. Xylitol discourages the growth of bacteria in the mouth, so there's less that can travel up a child's Eustachian tubes. The Finnish kids chewed often—two pieces of gum five times a day.

DON'T BOTHER

✘ Antibiotics for all ear infections The American Academy of Pediatrics estimates that 80 percent of kids with middle-ear infections will get better without antibiotics. In the wait-and-see study, kids who got antibiotics right away recovered about nine hours sooner than those who didn't, meaning they didn't need pain relievers. But 23 percent had diarrhea thanks to the drugs. ■

Eczema

The itchy, flaky, red skin of eczema isn't just kid stuff. While most of the 15 to 20 percent of babies and children who have it grow out of it (and thank goodness, since British researchers say families with a child who has eczema feel as much stress as those caring for a kid with diabetes), eczema remains a problem for at least 3 percent of grownups. It appears to have a genetic link and also seems to stem from an oversensitive immune system that produces a response just short of a true allergic reaction to triggers, which may include certain foods.

WORKS

✔ **Moisturizers** If you have eczema, you know how dry, itchy, and sensitive your skin is—and that dryness makes itching and rashes even worse. That's why major dermatology groups recommend applying a thick layer of moisturizer once or twice a day to seal in the water. Keeping your skin hydrated may mean you'll need less steroid cream to control rashes. In a Spanish study of 173 kids with eczema, those who were slathered daily with moisturizer needed 42 percent less high-potency steroid cream.

Thick moisturizer from a tub is better than lotion, say some dermatologists, who recommend products like Aquaphor Ointment, Eucerin Creme, Vanicream, Cetaphil Cream, and Moisturel Cream. But studies have found that moisturizers containing ingredients such as petroleum jelly, glycerol, and oat extracts also

work well. For maximum hydration, apply after soaking in a tepid (not hot) bath, then patting your skin dry, suggest dermatologists at the National Jewish Medical and Research Center in Denver. If baths make your skin itch more, opt for short showers.

✔ **Topical steroids** Steroid creams, ointments, gels, and lotions can't cure eczema, but they're the best choice for controlling flare-ups. It's true that overusing them can lead to thinning of the skin, but it's rarer than people think. In fact, some researchers say that fear of steroid creams can have worse side effects than the creams themselves. In one British study of 200 people with eczema, 73 percent admitted to being worried about using a cream, and 24 percent admitted to skimping on or skipping the treatment as a result. But studies show that smart use brings relief, usually without problems. When British researchers followed 174 kids and teens with mild to moderate eczema for 18 weeks, they found that treating for three days with a strong cream (0.1 percent betamethasone valerate) worked as well as seven days of treatment with a weak cream (1 percent hydrocortisone) for treating flare-ups. Both groups had the same number of scratch-free

PREGNANT? CONSIDER PROBIOTICS

Researchers haven't proved it definitively, but consuming these "beneficial bacteria," found in yogurt with active cultures and also sold as supplements, could help your baby avoid eczema, especially if it runs in your family. These bacteria benefit the immune system and seem to affect inflammation in ways that keep the body from overreacting to allergens. Talk to your obstetrician about taking probiotic supplements during your pregnancy and then ask your pediatrician about supplementing infant formula or breast milk with a probiotic powder.

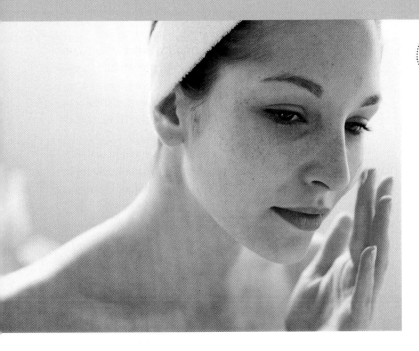

Slather generously. Using too little moisturizer and/or steroid cream can backfire. In one German study of 30 adults with eczema, those who applied as much of both as their doctors recommended saw their itching, dryness, and skin crusting improve about 20 percent more than those who skimped. If you're using a moisturizer and a steroid cream, always apply the steroid cream first. Also, avoid scratching as best you can; it only makes the itching worse.

days and the same number of relapses—and neither showed signs of thinning skin.

✔ **Immunomodulator creams** First introduced as an alternative to steroid creams, tacrolimus (Protopic) and pimecrolimus (Elidel) reduce eczema symptoms by 50 percent or more, say British researchers who reviewed 31 studies involving more than 8,000 people. A 0.1 percent tacrolimus cream was about 42 percent more effective than pimecrolimus, and pime-

crolimus was judged less effective than some steroid creams. But there are bigger concerns—and a controversy.

The FDA now requires "black box" warnings on both of these drugs, saying they may raise the risk of skin cancer and lymphoma. Other experts say there's no link, and major medical organizations, including the American Academy of Dermatology and the National Eczema Association, say the evidence for such a link is weak. These creams are not intended for kids under the age of 2.

✔ **Phototherapy** Stubborn, severe eczema that isn't healed by creams or steroid pills may respond to exposure to ultraviolet (UV) light. In one study of 73 people with moderate to severe eczema, those who got twice-weekly "narrow-band UVB" treatment for 12 weeks saw a 28 percent reduction in itching, oozing, and crusting. See a dermatologist about UV therapy.

DON'T BOTHER

✖ **Borage oil** Despite the marketing claims, at least two studies of people with eczema have found these capsules provide no benefit.

✖ **Antihistamines** Antihistamines won't relieve itchy skin, say dermatologists at the State University of New York at Stony Brook, who reviewed

16 studies on this popular remedy. That said, older, sedating antihistamines like diphenhydramine (Benadryl) may help you sleep if itching is keeping you awake. ∎

FATIGUE

Fatigue

Stuck in an energy crisis? First, rule out lack of sleep. If you have insomnia, see page 301. Next, you and your doctor should rule out depression—a common cause of fatigue—along with diabetes and sleep apnea. You'll find information on all three in this book, too. Other medical causes of fatigue include hypothyroidism, heart disease (especially in women), and hepatitis C. Everyday fatigue should respond to the measures outlined here.

WORKS

✔ **Exercise** It sounds counterintuitive, but it's true: Expending energy creates more of it. Dozens of studies show that sedentary people who start an exercise program report 30 percent more energy than people who sit on the couch. Just 15 minutes could give you a burst of energy, but a regular routine (30 minutes most days of the week) can lead to lasting improvement.

✔ **Caffeine in small, strategic doses** An effective way to thwart an afternoon slump is to sip a mere two ounces of coffee each hour from midmorning until midafternoon, Harvard Medical School researchers say. Drink too much caffeine, though, and you may find yourself unable to sleep at night. It takes three to seven hours for just half of the caffeine in a cup of coffee to leave your body, say Stanford University experts.

✔ **Sunlight** Australian volunteers who got five hours of exposure to bright light from sunshine or sitting near a lamp designed to simulate sunlight performed better on tests of mental alertness and reported feeling more awake than people who were exposed to dim lights. Can't stay outside all afternoon? In a Japanese study, 16 women performed better on alertness tests after sitting near a sunny window for 30 minutes compared with sitting in a dimly lit room.

✔ **A short nap**
A 20-minute nap boosted performance on computer tests in one small study. Even better was the nap plus a small cup of coffee or tea. In another recent study, researchers concluded that a mere 10-minute nap produced immediate improvements in

MEDICAL CAUSES OF FATIGUE

If your fatigue is new or dramatic, prolonged or unexplained, you may have a serious medical problem. If everyday pick-me-ups don't help, ask your doctor about these conditions.

Underactive thyroid: This is a relatively common cause of fatigue, especially in women. A simple blood test can diagnose it.

Heart disease: New research suggests fatigue is a distinct characteristic of women's cardiovascular disease. Ask your doctor to check your cholesterol, blood pressure, and blood sugar—diabetes and prediabetes also raise heart disease risk.

Lupus: This autoimmune disease affects mostly women and is usually diagnosed between ages 15 and 45. Pain due to inflammation is a common symptom.

Hepatitis C: If you ever used IV drugs, snorted cocaine through a straw, got a tattoo from a shady tattoo parlor, had a blood transfusion before 1992, or got abnormal results on a liver function test, ask your doctor about a hepatitis C test. This virus attacks the liver and often causes no symptoms for 20 to 30 years, at which point liver damage makes you feel tired.

fatigue levels and cognitive performance that lasted for up to 155 minutes.

✔ **Acupressure** When University of Michigan researchers taught college students acupressure points believed to be either stimulating or relaxing (the students weren't told which were which), they found after five days that volunteers felt more energetic when they pressed the stimulating points once a day. Press firmly for three minutes at the base of the skull, one finger-width from the side of the spine; on the pad between the joints of the thumb and index finger; and on the sole of the foot, one-third of the way from the toes.

WORKS FOR SOME

● **Iron supplements** If you think you're iron deficient, see your doctor for a blood test. While fatigue can be a sign of iron deficiency, never take iron supplements on your own—for some people, they can be dangerous.

● **Vitamin B$_{12}$ supplements** Most people get plenty of B$_{12}$ from food, though you can be deficient (and feel tired as a result) if you have a gastrointestinal disorder that blocks absorption. Ask your doctor if deficiency could be causing your fatigue. ■

Flatulence

It doesn't matter how prim you consider yourself, you still pass gas. Gassiness comes from swallowing air, from the bloodstream, from chemical reactions in the intestine, and from the fermentation of food in your digestive tract. To reduce gas—and its obvious release—here's what works.

WORKS

✔ **Standing up** If you're feeling gassy, stand tall and let gravity do its work. Standing up helps gas pass more easily, reducing the likelihood that gas will make an embarrassing noise. Exercise offers the same benefits. Our recommendation? A walk outside.

✔ **Beano** This over-the-counter product (it comes in tablets or drops) contains a naturally occurring intestinal enzyme that can reduce gas production from a meal of beans or other gas-producing complex carbohydrates. Take it just before you eat.

WORKS FOR SOME

● **Simethicone** This chemical, found in products like Maalox, works by reducing the "foaming" of gas bubbles, supposedly allowing gas to pass more easily (i.e., discreetly) and reducing bloating. While studies found it works better than placebos at reducing gas and bloating, many of them were poorly designed or used a lactose placebo, which could have made the symptoms of the placebo group worse. A 1996 analysis of studies concluded there was no "convincing evidence" that simethicone reduces flatulence.

● **Activated charcoal products** These supposedly work by absorbing intestinal gas. Several studies in which healthy volunteers were fed gas-producing foods found that it did reduce hydrogen levels in their breath (a sign of gaseousness) and the number of "flatus events." However, other studies found no benefit. And no studies have been conducted with people who already had gas.

● **Rice** Adding rice to a gas-producing meal may reduce gas according to one study. ■

FLU

Flu

Anything you can do to fight the flu is worth the effort. This viral infection not only triggers high fevers and body aches, it can also leave you feeling deeply tired for weeks—and even pose a deadly threat to people who are elderly or have a weakened immune system or chronic disease. It can also leave you more prone to developing pneumonia. Here's the latest on how to protect yourself and speed your recovery if you catch the flu despite your best efforts.

WORKS

✔ **Antiviral drugs** At the first sign of the flu, call your doctor and ask for a course of oseltamivir (Tamiflu) or zanamivir (Relenza), flu fighters that can ease symptoms and shorten your recovery period. These drugs work by preventing viral particles from being released from infected cells, thereby limiting the spread of the virus inside your body. The catch: The drugs are effective only if you start treatment within 24 to 48 hours of your first symptoms.

They do work. In a study of more than 4,000 people ages 13 to 97 with the flu, those who received oseltamivir recovered in about five days compared to six for those who received a placebo shot. The oseltamivir group also felt 29 percent less fatigue, had 26 percent fewer body aches, and had 57 percent fewer fevers after 48 hours. The drug cut recovery time nearly in half for people with heart disease and chronic obstructive pulmonary disease—good news because flu can be fatal for people with chronic health problems.

A safety note: If a child or adult in your household is taking oseltamivir, pay attention to their behavior. Japanese researchers report that some kids and teens taking the drug have developed delirium and tried to injure themselves.

✔ **Sambucol** In one well-designed Norwegian study, this liquid elderberry extract helped flu sufferers recover in three to four days versus seven to eight days for those who got a placebo. Experts suspect that antioxidant compounds called anthocyanins in elderberry (they're responsible for the berry's gorgeous, dark purple hue) bolster immunity and prevent the influenza virus from attaching itself to cells in the body. A typical dose is one tablespoon four times a day for three to five days.

✔ **Flu vaccines for prevention** Flu shots aren't perfect, but they're worth getting. At best, a flu vaccine provides 70 to 90 percent protection against the strains of influenza virus that are common in a particular year. At worst, the vaccine may be just 40 to 50 percent effective. The reason: Constantly mutating flu viruses may change between the time each year's vaccine formula is established and the start of flu season. Still, being vaccinated is worth it, especially for older

FLU SHOTS FOR THE WHOLE FAMILY?

Kids' flu symptoms are often overlooked. In one Vanderbilt University study of 4,539 preschoolers, parents, doctors, and even healthcare practitioners in emergency rooms missed flu symptoms in four out of five children. The danger? Kids can transmit the virus for up to three weeks. This groundbreaking study prompted the FDA to recommend flu shots for all kids ages 6 months to 5 years. But experts suggest considering shots for the entire family—children and parents—to alleviate misery and avoid spreading the virus to older relatives and those with weakened immunity.

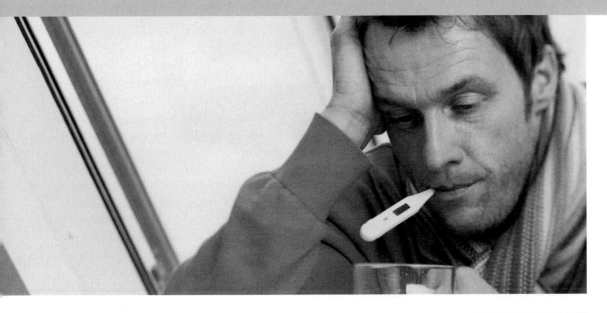

people. A 10-year study of thousands of older people found that flu vaccines cut the risk of being hospitalized with flu-like illnesses by 27 percent and reduced the risk of dying from the flu by 48 percent.

✔ **Antiviral drugs for prevention** People who took either oseltamivir or zanamivir after someone in their household caught the flu reduced their risk of getting it themselves by 75 to 81 percent, report researchers at Seattle's Fred Hutchinson Cancer Center. Ask your doctor for a prescription.

Hand washing for prevention The influenza virus can survive for hours on hard surfaces like metal, glass, and plastic—and even on cloth, paper, and tissues. For protection, wash your hands regularly with soap and water. It's more effective than using an antimicrobial hand gel.

DON'T BOTHER

✖ **The antiviral drugs amantadine and rimantadine** The US Centers for Disease Control and Prevention (CDC) recommends against their use because they're effective against just one of three major classes of flu viruses. Even more troubling: The virus develops resistance to these drugs swiftly; in one year, the CDC found that the percentage of flu infections resistant to these drugs rose from 1.9 to 14.5 percent.

Antibiotics Since the flu is caused by viruses, not by bacteria, antibiotics do nothing to fight off an infection or ease symptoms. So skip 'em! ■

IS IT THE FLU … OR JUST A COLD?

SYMPTOM	COLD	FLU
Fever	Rare	Yes; usually high and sudden
Headache	Rare	Severe
Aches and pains	Slight	Dramatic
Fatigue, weakness	Some	Significant
Stuffy nose	Yes	Sometimes
Sneezing	Yes	Occasionally
Sore throat	Yes	Sometimes
Chest discomfort	None to mild	Yes
Cough	Hacking	Sometimes severe

HEADACHE

Headache

"Headache" sounds so innocuous. But when you feel like a hammer is pounding your skull from inside your head or as if your brain is caught in a vise, pain relief is all you can think of. If your headache is the garden-variety tension type, a standard painkiller should do the trick, especially if you wash it down with some caffeine. If your headaches are frequent or especially bad, there's help for you, too (for migraines, see page 308).

WORKS

✔ **Ibuprofen and other painkillers** Wondering which pain reliever is best for your pounding head? The truth is, ibuprofen, naproxen, aspirin, and acetaminophen all bring relief, though ibuprofen may have a slight edge: It bested acetaminophen in one study published in the *Journal of Clinical Pharmacology* and tied with aspirin in another study reported in the journal *Headache*. And when Dutch researchers reviewed 41 pain-relief studies, they concluded that ibuprofen was slightly better than naproxen because it was less likely to cause side effects.

For fastest relief, take ibuprofen in liquid gel capsules, which brought relief in 24 minutes for volunteers in one study. Acetaminophen took 29 minutes—a small difference, but every second counts when your head hurts.

✔ **Caffeine** A 200-milligram dose of caffeine—about the amount in a large mug of coffee—lifted tension-headache pain 30 minutes faster than ibuprofen in a study of 345 people conducted at the Diamond Headache Clinic in Chicago. Nearly 60 percent of people who got ibuprofen or caffeine got complete relief, but combining the two strategies was even better: It erased pain for 71 percent of study volunteers and kept them pain-free for more than four hours. Caffeine may ease head pain by shrinking swollen blood vessels, the researchers say.

Another way to use caffeine to battle a big headache: Take a product that combines acetaminophen, aspirin, and caffeine. Studies show that this combo is effective against tension headaches and works better than acetaminophen alone.

Our BEST ADVICE

If you take medicine for head pain more than 15 times each month, it's time to lay off the pain reliever. "Medication overuse headaches" happen when the first dose of the day wears off and blood vessels begin to swell again. Pain returns, so you take something to relieve it, and a vicious cycle begins. The best remedy: Quit your pain reliever. It'll hurt, but once the rebound effect wears off, your doctor will be able to treat the underlying cause of your headaches.

✔ **Botox for killer head pain** Botox is more than a wrinkle eraser. This toxin, injected into the muscles around the eyes and forehead and sometimes the jaw, can help relieve headaches when nothing else can. In one study, people with tension headaches, chronic daily headaches, or migraines who'd already tried up to three other pain remedies received one to four Botox treatments at three-month intervals. They rated their improvement on a 5-point scale, with 1 being no change and 5 being excellent. The result: 84 percent said things had improved. Among those who had four Botox treatments, 92 percent rated the improvement at 4 or higher.

Botox partially paralyzes muscles for about three months. For patients whose headaches involve the entire head, additional injections are given in the upper back area of the neck and shoulders.

✔ **Sumatriptan (Imitrex) for cluster headaches** This migraine medicine, taken as a nasal spray or injection, can halt the excruciating pain of cluster headaches fast. Injections stopped pain within 15 minutes for 96 percent of volunteers in one study. In another study,

47 percent of headache sufferers who used a sumatriptan nasal spray were pain-free in 30 minutes.

✔ **Verapamil for recurrent cluster headaches** Cluster headaches are also known as "alarm clock" headaches because they're cruelly predictable: 80 to 90 percent of people with cluster headaches experience a string of vicious daily headaches for a week to a year, followed by a remission period. Another 20 percent have these headaches every

single day with scarcely a break. Either way, see your doctor for help. Several medications can interrupt the cycle. One of the most popular, verapamil, is effective but carries risks. Researchers from London's National Hospital for Neurology and Neurosurgery found that some people taking it developed irregular heartbeats or slower-than-normal heart rates. The scientists say that people who choose this medication should have their heart rates monitored by their doctors.

WORKS FOR SOME

● **Cold packs** A cold pack applied to the forehead or back of the head for 15 minutes could ease a throbbing noggin. In one University of Illinois study of 45 people with migraines plus tension headaches, cold packs completely erased pain for 9 percent and were mildly to moderately effective for 55 percent.

● **Relaxation techniques** Meditation, progressive muscle relaxation, or simply lying in a darkened room as you take slow, steady breaths could all melt the muscle tension that contributes to headaches. In one study of 94 headache sufferers, learning and using relaxation techniques such as these eased pain for 39 percent of volunteers. If you

have chronic tension headaches, consider biofeedback, a system that uses computers or other devices to help you stay focused on relaxation. In the same relaxation study, 56 percent of volunteers who used biofeedback got relief.

● **Acupuncture** It may or may not make your headache go away, but if you have

chronic daily headaches, it could help you cope better. When 74 people with chronic headaches tried either 10 acupuncture treatments over six weeks plus standard medications or medications alone, the acupuncture group reported that they were 3.7 times less likely to "suffer" with their headaches, though they didn't experience any less pain.

DON'T BOTHER

✖ **Antibiotics and decongestants for sinus infections** Think a sinus infection is the cause of your head pain? Think again. In a study of 2,991 people who thought they had sinus problems, researchers from the Headache Care Center of

Springfield, Missouri, found that 97 percent were most likely having migraines.

✖ **Melatonin** Study results are conflicting, so experts have deemed this remedy not ready for primetime. ∎

Heartburn

That burning sensation in your chest and throat could be heartburn or, if it occurs frequently, gastroesophageal reflux disease (GERD). Behind both: A faulty valve at the lower end of the esophagus that lets stomach acids back up into your food pipe. To ease the discomfort, start with the lifestyle changes and over-the-counter medicines recommended here. Move up to more serious treatments for GERD, also listed here, if your doctor says your esophagus has been damaged and you need stronger relief.

Our BEST ADVICE

Skip the sleeping pills. According to a large health survey, people who took benzodiazepines such as diazepam (Valium), alprazolam (Xanax), and triazolam (Halcion) in order to fall asleep were 50 percent more likely to have heartburn at night than those who didn't take the sleep aids. Other research has shown that these drugs loosen the lower esophageal sphincter, the ring of muscle that's supposed to keep stomach acids where they belong.

WORKS

✔ **Antacids** Antacids such as Maalox, Mylanta, Gelusil, Rolaids, and Tums absorb and neutralize stomach acid. Experts suggest trying these first, along with lifestyle changes, to ease the discomfort of mild to moderate heartburn. For best relief, choose an antacid, such as Gaviscon-2 or Genaton, that contains an alginate, an ingredient that forms a protective coating over the food in your stomach (or look for "alginic acid" on antacid labels). When Baylor College of Medicine experts reviewed 10 clinical trials, they concluded that antacids with added alginates improved mild heartburn by 60 percent, while antacids alone eased discomfort by just 11 percent.

Take antacids after you eat; they go to work fast and could be less beneficial if taken on an empty stomach. If heartburn won't let up, see your doctor. Overuse of magnesium-based antacids can lead to diarrhea, while overuse of aluminum-based types can cause constipation. Before you take large doses of any heartburn remedy, see our warnings on page 203.

✔ **H$_2$ blockers** If you're still having pain after a few weeks, add an over-the-counter H$_2$ blocker, such as cimetidine (Tagamet), famotidine (Pepcid), or ranitidine (Zantac), which reduces acid production. They ease symptoms for 70 percent of people in just a few weeks. Take H$_2$ blockers at least 30 minutes before you eat.

✔ **Proton-pump inhibitors (PPIs)** These drugs, available over the counter and by prescription, are serious medicine. They block acid production, buying time for damaged esophageal tissue to mend itself. They also stop the pain. Take one only if your doctor suggests it and use it for the shortest time possible; these drugs can completely stop the production of stomach acids you need for digesting food. PPIs include esomeprazole (Nexium), lansoprazole (Prevacid), and omeprazole (Prilosec).

The new thinking about PPIs: More and more digestive disease specialists recommend starting treatment with these powerful drugs if you have severe GERD. After eight weeks, your doctor may cut your dose in half and may check to see if your esophageal damage is improving.

Your doctor may prescribe both an H$_2$ blocker and a PPI; the drugs work in different ways (and are taken on different dosing schedules).

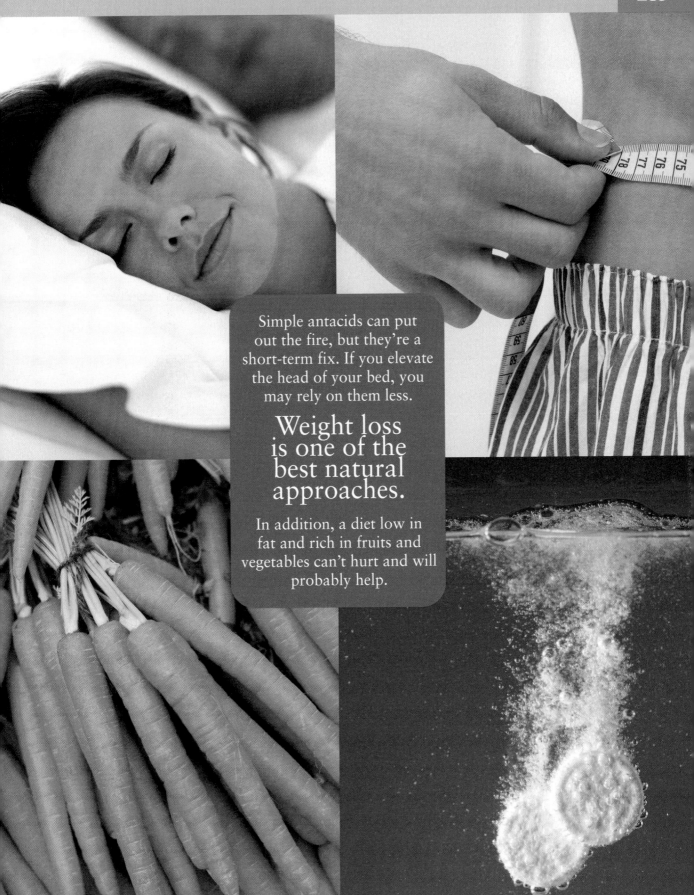

Simple antacids can put out the fire, but they're a short-term fix. If you elevate the head of your bed, you may rely on them less.

Weight loss is one of the best natural approaches.

In addition, a diet low in fat and rich in fruits and vegetables can't hurt and will probably help.

HEARTBURN

✔ **Acupuncture** When drugs don't work, doctors tend to simply double the dose. But a study from the University of Arizona suggests a different approach: Stick with your current dose and add a course of acupuncture. When 30 people with persistent heartburn received either a double dose of PPIs or twice-weekly acupuncture plus their regular dose for four weeks, the acupuncture group had a significant decrease in daytime and nighttime GERD. The group that simply got more drugs didn't see much improvement.

✔ **Weight loss** Weight gain leads to a decrease in pressure at the gastroesophageal junction—and an increase in reflux. Dropping 27 pounds cut reflux episodes by 40 percent in one study.

✔ **Sleeping with your head elevated** Propping yourself up about 11 inches on a wedge pillow or by raising the head of your bed could cut reflux episodes dramatically and shorten those you do have.

✔ **Reclining on your left side** In one study published in the *Journal of Clinical Gastroenterology*, people who slept on their right sides had twice as much reflux as left-side sleepers. Because of the position of the stomach, acid is more likely to reflux when you lie on your right side.

DIET AND HEARTBURN

There's plenty of conflicting advice out there about what to eat and what to avoid if you have heartburn. Here's what the most recent research suggests.

Eat more fiber and produce and less fat. When researchers at the Houston Veterans Affairs Medical Center did esophageal scans of 164 people, they found that those who ate more fruits, veggies, whole grains, and beans were 20 percent less likely to have signs of esophageal erosion caused by the acid backwash of reflux. At higher risk: People who took in more fat, protein, and calories.

Sip fewer soft drinks. Researchers who polled more than 15,000 people about their lifestyle habits and history of GERD found that those who had more than one carbonated, caffeinated drink per day were 24 percent more likely to have sleep-disturbing nighttime reflux than those who drank fewer.

Follow your tummy's lead on other foods. When researchers from Stanford University reviewed more than 100 studies of lifestyle remedies for acid reflux, they exploded a lot of myths about old-time diet no-nos for heartburn sufferers. Avoiding chocolate, mint, spices, greasy foods, and late-night noshing, they found, doesn't help most people. What it means for you: Don't put any food on the off-limits list until you've found that eliminating it works for you.

WORKS FOR SOME

● **Cutting out coffee** When 15 intrepid GERD sufferers sipped coffee or plain warm water after meals for 24 hours—and had their acid backwash measured via a tube inserted in their throats—researchers concluded that coffee made little difference in GERD symptoms. Yet other studies have found that large quantities of java can bring on reflux even in people who aren't prone to GERD. It could be that some people are more sensitive to coffee's heartburn side effects.

DON'T BOTHER

✘ **Sipping a glass of milk** It feels cool and soothing going down, but milk doesn't have any special heartburn-relieving properties. In fact, experts say, the fats and protein in milk can stimulate the stomach to produce more acid. ∎

Heart Disease

To prevent coronary artery disease, you'll need to keep your cholesterol (see page 297) and your blood pressure (see page 293) low, for starters. The disease builds for decades before you notice signs, most commonly mild chest pain called angina that occurs when you're exercising and goes away with rest. Preventing blood clots with medication, opening clogged arteries, and sidestepping a heart attack are the goals of heart disease treatment.

WORKS

✔ **Blood thinners** If you have "stable" cardiovascular disease, that is, some artery blockage and angina but no immediate risk of a heart attack, taking medication like aspirin and blood thinners to prevent blood clots is likely your best bet. A major study that many cardiologists called "blockbuster" followed more than 2,000 patients at 50 sites throughout North America for 4 1/2 years. Researchers found that the rate of heart attacks and deaths in patients taking medication were nearly identical to those in patients taking medication *and* undergoing angioplasty for blocked arteries. While the angioplasty initially improved patients' angina more than the medication, the improvement wasn't that significant, and it disappeared over time. The study shocked cardiologists, primarily because the majority of patients receiving angioplasty have stable heart disease.

✔ **Coronary artery bypass surgery and angioplasty** Bypass surgery is typically performed when one or more coronary arteries are blocked, putting you in imminent danger of a heart attack, or after you've had a heart attack. It involves taking a piece of artery from another part of your body and using it to create a detour around the blocked artery. For years, bypass was the gold standard for treating heart disease. Then came angioplasty, a much less invasive procedure in which a balloon is inserted through a catheter to open the artery, and a tiny metal tube called a stent is placed to keep it open. With the advent of angioplasty, doctors dropped bypass surgery in droves.

Maybe they shouldn't have. At least two major reviews of dozens of studies found that bypass is often superior to angioplasty, particularly in patients with several blockages or more severe blockages. In one review of 23 clinical studies in which the patients were randomly assigned to have either bypass or angioplasty, patients in both groups were just as likely to be alive in 10 years, but angioplasty patients were much more likely to continue to have angina from blockages. Plus, 5 years after angioplasty, patients needed 33 percent more procedures to unblock reclogged arteries than bypass patients. One caveat: Patients undergoing bypass had a slightly higher risk of stroke, but the overall benefit, researchers said, still pointed to bypass as the better choice. An obvious downside to the more invasive procedure: a longer hospital stay.

Based on your particular case of heart disease, your doctor will recommend which procedure is right for you.

✔ **Drug-eluting stents medicated with sirolimus** Stents work like tiny scaffolds to prop open arteries after the gunk that clogs them has been cleaned out. But even with stents, those arteries can clog again. Newer stents that release clot-busting drugs are meant to prevent this problem. An analysis of 38 clinical trials including 18,000 patients who

HEART DISEASE

were followed for up to four years found that those who received stents embedded with the drug sirolimus had the lowest risk of heart attack compared with those who received stents embedded with the drug paclitaxel or bare-metal stents. Patients who received paclitaxel stents also required more additional procedures to unblock arteries than those who got either sirolimus or bare-metal stents; sirolimus patients had the lowest risk of needing additional procedures.

Recently experts were concerned that using drug-eluting stents could slightly raise the risk of potentially fatal blood clots and heart attacks, especially when used in patients who were much sicker than patients the stents were meant for (those with newly diagnosed stable coronary disease). But a major study found that such concerns are unwarranted.

WORKS FOR SOME

● **Off-pump bypass surgery** For nearly 30 years, most bypass surgeries were performed with the aid of a heart/lung bypass machine, which takes over for the heart during the surgery. The use of the pump is believed to be a reason behind surgical complications and even deaths during the procedure, as well as temporary memory problems and "fuzzy thinking" afterward and a higher risk of stroke. Now surgeons have the option of performing bypass without the pump. One of the largest studies ever to compare the procedures found that patients who underwent off-pump bypass surgery were 19 percent less likely to die in the 30 days after the procedure, 30 percent less likely to have post-procedure strokes, and 57 percent less likely to have breathing problems. They were also less likely to have cognitive problems.

Based on this and other studies, researchers suggest that if you have a high risk of stroke or are elderly or female, you may be slightly better off with the off-pump procedure.

DON'T BOTHER

✖ **Combining aspirin with other blood thinners** If you're at risk for blood clots from heart disease or other cardiovascular conditions, your doctor may prescribe aspirin along with blood thinners like heparin. But a major review of 10 studies found that taking both benefited only patients with mechanical heart valves. Otherwise, researchers found no difference in the risk of atrial fibrillation (abnormal heartbeat), heart disease, or death between people taking both drugs or just the blood thinner. However, patients receiving the combined therapy were 43 percent more likely to have major bleeding than patients receiving blood thinners alone. ■

WITH ANGIOPLASTY, TIMING IS EVERYTHING

While bypass surgery may be better than angioplasty for people with more than one blocked artery, angioplasty still has a place in treating heart disease, particularly right after a heart attack. However, timing is key. When researchers examined the effects of angioplasty compared to clot-busting medicine on 2,166 heart attack patients who had one completely blocked artery, they found that angioplasty performed more than 24 hours after the heart attack didn't make any difference in patients who weren't having additional symptoms. In fact, people who got angioplasty 3 to 28 days after their heart attacks showed an *increased* risk that the artery would become blocked again, requiring another procedure.

High Blood Pressure

If you're taking daily doses of a nonsteroidal anti-inflammatory drug (NSAID) like ibuprofen or aspirin for pain, talk to your doctor about other options. A review of studies in which participants used NSAIDs for at least four weeks found an average blood pressure increase of 3.54 mmHg systolic and 1.16 mmHg diastolic. Prolonged use of ibuprofen increased the risk of hypertension by 185 percent.

High blood pressure sounds relatively harmless, but it's not called the silent killer for nothing. It can rupture a blood vessel in the brain, causing a stroke, and damage coronary arteries in ways that make a heart attack more likely. Or the heart may become so exhausted from pumping in such "high-pressure" conditions that it begins to fail. High blood pressure is partly genetic, but it's highly treatable. If you know your pressure's high, do something to bring it down. Your life may depend on it.

WORKS

✔ **Starting treatment early** The time to nip high blood pressure in the bud is when you're diagnosed with prehypertension, or high-normal blood pressure—a systolic (the first number) reading of 130 to 139 mmHg (millimeters of mercury) and/or a diastolic (the second number) reading of 85 to 89 mmHg. If you have it, you also have twice the risk of heart attack and stroke compared to someone with lower blood pressure—meaning it's time to act.

You can certainly try to bring down your pressure by changing your diet and getting more exercise, but your doctor may also want you to take medication. According to a major study, starting treatment with a drug called an angiotensin-receptor blocker like candesartan (Atacand) could reduce the risk of developing full-blown hypertension by 66 percent over two years, though diuretics and beta-blockers are usually the first choices (more on these below).

✔ **Diuretics** These "water pills," one of the oldest medical treatments for high blood pressure, work by pulling water out of the bloodstream to be eliminated in the urine. Less water equals lower blood volume equals lower blood pressure. Diuretics fell out of favor in recent years as newer (and much pricier) drugs became available. But in 2002 a major study comparing the commonly used diuretic chlorthalidone (Thalitone) to the calcium channel-blocker-amlodipine (Norvasc) and the ACE (angiotensin-converting enzyme) inhibitor lisinopril (Zestril) found that the diuretic worked best in terms of reducing blood pressure and preventing long-term complications.

The diuretic prevented heart failure 25 percent better than amlodipine and was better than lisinopril at lowering blood pressure and preventing stroke, heart failure, and angina. Another study found that the diuretic was better than the alpha-blocker doxazosin (Cardura) for reducing blood pressure and preventing all cardiovascular complications, particularly heart failure.

HIGH BLOOD PRESSURE

✔ **ACE inhibitors and angiotensin-receptor blockers (ARBs)** If a diuretic alone doesn't work to control your blood pressure, your doctor may add or switch you to an ACE inhibitor or ARB, both of which curtail the ability of angiotensin hormones to contract the muscles that surround blood vessels and narrow the vessels. An analysis of 61 studies of the two drugs found that they're equally effective at controlling high blood pressure, although ACE inhibitors are more likely to cause a harmless but persistent dry cough.

THE LOWER-YOUR-BLOOD-PRESSURE DIET

The DASH diet has been shown to reduce blood pressure by an average of 5.5 mmHg systolic and 3.0 mmHg diastolic.

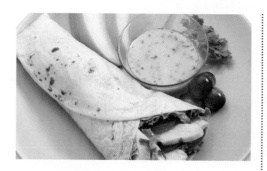

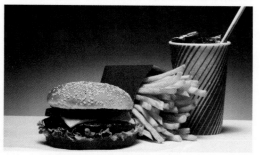

DASH is HIGH in ...

VEGETABLES
Four or five servings a day (a serving is 1 cup of greens or 1/2 cup of cooked vegetables)

FRUITS
Four or five servings a day (a serving is one piece of fruit or 1/2 cup of cut fruit)

NUTS, BEANS, AND SEEDS
Four or five servings a week (a serving is 1/2 cup of cooked beans, 2 tablespoons of peanut butter, or 1.5 ounces of nuts)

LOW-FAT DAIRY FOODS
Two or three servings a day (a serving is 1 cup of milk or yogurt or 1.5 ounces of cheese)

GRAINS
Six to eight servings a day (a serving is one slice of bread or 1/2 cup of cereal, cooked rice, or pasta)

DASH is LOW in ...

SATURATED FATS
(found in foods like hamburger and other fatty meats, ice cream, butter, and full-fat cheese)

SODIUM
(abundant in most fast food and countless processed, canned, and packaged foods)

CHOLESTEROL
(found in foods like egg yolks, fatty meats, and cheese)

✔ A diet rich in fruits, vegetables, and low-fat dairy

When researchers tested the effects of a diet high in fruits and vegetables on people with high blood pressure, they found it worked pretty well in terms of reducing blood pressure. But add low-fat dairy foods to that eating plan (known as the DASH, or Dietary Approaches to Stop Hypertension, diet), and you've turned what was a four-cylinder treatment into a six-cylinder treatment. The diet with low-fat dairy reduced systolic and diastolic blood pressure twice as much as the fruit and veggie diet did when compared to a typical Western diet low in fruits, vegetables, and dairy products.

Simply adding dairy foods won't work; they have to be low fat. One theory is that the fat content of full-fat dairy products may prevent your body from absorbing calcium, which plays a role in blood pressure control.

✔ Exercise

Doing aerobic exercise—we're talking about brisk walking, jogging or running, biking, aerobics classes, swimming—for 30 minutes on most days of the week can bring your blood pressure down by 4 mmHg systolic and 3 mmHg diastolic, on average. That may not sound like much, but a reduction of as little as 5 mmHg systolic can reduce

DO YOU SNORE?

If you answered yes (or your partner did), and you have high blood pressure, ask your doctor if you might also have obstructive sleep apnea. People with this condition stop breathing numerous times during the night, waking up just enough to take a breath before falling back to sleep. They also have a 45 percent higher risk of high blood pressure than people without sleep apnea. Treatment is pretty simple: A mask attached to a machine that uses negative pressure to force air into your nose and keep your airways open all night.

your risk of dying from a stroke by up to 14 percent, from heart disease by 9 percent, and from any cause by 7 percent.

✔ Losing 20 pounds

If you're overweight, dropping 20 pounds no matter what your starting weight can reduce your systolic blood pressure by 5 to 20 mmHg. Even a 10-pound loss is sufficient to reduce your blood pressure enough to *prevent* hypertension.

✔ Cutting back on booze

While moderate alcohol consumption is beneficial in terms of protecting you from heart disease, drinking too much works against you in several ways. If you regularly have more than one drink a day (for women) or two drinks a day (for men), you're facing a possible systolic blood pressure increase of 2 to 4 mmHg.

✔ A home blood pressure monitor

Definitely head to the drugstore for one of these. An analysis of

18 studies of people with hypertension found that those who monitored their blood pressure at home had systolic readings that were 4.2 mmHg lower than those of people who had their pressures checked only at the doctor's office, and their diastolic readings were an average of 2.4 mmHg lower. It may sound like a small difference, but it could be enough to reduce the amount of blood pressure medication you take. It's also large enough to reduce the risk or severity of a heart attack or stroke.

Our BEST ADVICE

Before you have your blood pressure taken, sit quietly for five minutes with your feet on the floor (not dangling from the exam table). It could lead to a systolic reading about 14 points lower, enough to keep you from a diagnosis of hypertension.

HIGH BLOOD PRESSURE

WORKS FOR SOME

● **Eating less sodium**
Sodium (a component of salt) and high blood pressure go together like bacon and eggs—for some people. For others, cutting back on sodium has little or no effect on blood pressure. If you have diabetes or are obese, however, you're likely to be especially sensitive to sodium, and you, more than anyone else, need to keep your sodium intake low. Aim to get no more than 2.4 grams of sodium a day—the amount in about a single teaspoon of salt. Reduce your intake even more—to 1.6 grams a day—and you could lower your blood pressure as much as if you took a blood pressure medication.

There is simply no way you can get your sodium intake that low unless you stay away from processed foods. These days, even breakfast cereals are high in sodium. And fast food? Even a relatively "healthy" grilled chicken club sandwich has almost 1,700 milligrams of sodium, nearly your entire daily allotment. The bottom line: You need to cook more meals from scratch at home and read labels scrupulously.

● **Taming chronic stress** What we know for sure is that chronic stress—feeling pressured or anxious all the time—increases the risk of high blood pressure. It's harder to prove that reducing stress lowers pressure, but it certainly can't hurt. Meditation, deep breathing, and even formal stress-reduction programs are good places to start.

● **Beta-blockers** These drugs work by blocking the effects of adrenaline on cells that play a role in the strength of your heartbeat and the movement of smooth muscles, like those in the heart and surrounding blood vessels. But research suggests that you may be better off using something else. A Swedish analysis of 16 studies comparing beta-blockers with other medications like diuretics and calcium channel-blockers found that the risk of stroke was 16 percent higher in people treated with beta-blockers and that their risk of dying from any cause was 3 percent higher. People taking the beta-blocker atenolol (Tenormin) had the highest risk of stroke (26 percent). Beta-blockers also failed to reduce the risk of heart attack.

DON'T BOTHER

✖ **Supplements** The evidence is still shaky on the benefits of supplements such as vitamin C, omega-3 fatty acids (including fish oil), coenzyme Q10, and magnesium for treating high blood pressure. While some studies find benefits, others find none. Among the supplements that show promise is arginine (see page 213 for more details). But you're probably better off focusing your efforts on getting more exercise and eating more fruits and vegetables.

✖ **Garlic** Although it may be good for your heart in other ways, it doesn't look like fresh garlic or garlic supplements have any significant effect on blood pressure. ■

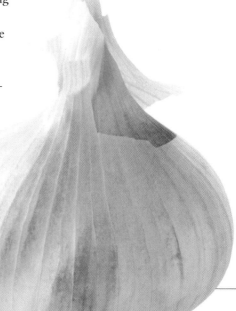

High Cholesterol

Cholesterol is essential to the body, which uses it to make cell membranes, hormones, vitamin D, and more. But its reputation as a cause of heart attacks is somewhat deserved. (Actually, many people who have heart attacks don't have high cholesterol—but lowering your levels still lowers your risk.) High cholesterol even contributes to Alzheimer's disease, strokes, and colorectal cancer. Getting your "bad" LDL cholesterol down and your "good" HDL cholesterol up is key. You also need to watch out for triglycerides, blood fats that accumulate when you eat too many calories; they provide the raw material for making artery-clogging LDL.

WORKS

✔ **Statin drugs** In the early 1990s, the treatment of high cholesterol was revolutionized by the introduction of these drugs. Today, statins are some of the most prescribed medicines in the world, and the drop in deaths from heart disease in many countries is attributed in part to their use. They can reduce LDL levels by as much as 63 percent. A recent analysis of 27 studies published in the *Archives of Internal Medicine* found that statins can reduce the risk of heart attack by nearly 30 percent in people without heart disease and lower stroke risk by 14 percent.

✔ **Oatmeal and other foods rich in soluble fiber** Starting every morning with a generous bowl of steaming oatmeal may not keep the doctor away, but it could help keep your cholesterol down. Soluble fiber, the type found in oats, dried beans and peas, most nuts, and barley, acts as a strainer in your gut, "catching" fatty acids created through food digestion and holding onto them so they leave your body along with the undigested fiber. An analysis of 67 clinical trials found that eating 2 to 10 grams of soluble fiber a day reduced total cholesterol by about 1.7 mg/dl (milligrams per deciliter) and LDL by 2.2 mg/dl. A government organization concluded that increasing your daily soluble fiber intake by 5 to 10 grams will lead to a 5 percent drop in LDL.

A half cup of cooked barley, oatmeal, or oat bran contains about 1 gram of soluble fiber. A half cup of lima beans gives you a whopping 3.5 grams. Even a large orange, grapefruit, or pear delivers 2 grams.

If you just can't seem to eat enough soluble fiber, consider taking a psyllium supplement such as Metamucil, Citrucel, or Fiberall. A typical dose is 10 grams a day.

✔ **Plant stanols and sterols** These days, you can get close to the same cholesterol-lowering bang from a glass of orange juice or a couple of tablespoons of salad dressing or margarine as you can from a statin—provided you buy versions of these foods that are enriched with stanols or sterols, natural plant compounds similar in structure to cholesterol. These cholesterol "look-alikes" occupy cholesterol receptors in your

How the Statins Stack Up

This chart compares the changes you can expect in your cholesterol and triglyceride levels from various statin drugs. The bottom line: All statins work; the key is getting the right dose. In many cases, there's simply no need to take an expensive brand-name drug; cheaper generics will work just fine.

STATIN	CHOLESTEROL			
	TOTAL↓	LDL↓	HDL↑	TRIGLYCERIDE↓
Altocor 10–60 mg Lovastatin extended release	18–29%	24–41%	9–13%	10–25%
Crestor 5–40 mg Rosuvastatin	33–46%	45–63%	8–14%	10–35%
Lescol 20–80 mg Fluvastatin	17–27%	22–36%	3–9%	12–23%
Lescol XL 80 mg Fluvastatin extended release	25%	33–35%	7–11%	19–25%
Lipitor 10–80 mg Atorvastatin	25–45%	35–60%	5–9%	19–37%
Mevacor 10–80 mg Lovastatin	16–34%	21–42%	2–9%	6–27%
Pravachol 10–80 mg Pravastatin	16–27%	22–37%	2–12%	11–24%
Zocor 5–80 mg Simvastatin	19–36%	26–47%	8–16%	12–33%

body and block the absorption of actual cholesterol from the foods you eat. An analysis of four high-quality clinical trials found that getting about 2.3 grams of sterols/stanols per day from a margarine-type spread reduced total cholesterol levels by 7 to 11 percent and LDL cholesterol levels by 10 to 15 percent. Stick with 2 grams a day; there's no evidence that higher amounts provide additional benefit.

✔ **Niacin for high triglycerides and low HDL** Also called nicotinic acid, this B vitamin works best for increasing HDL and reducing triglycerides. In fact, it's one of the few medications that increase HDL. Studies find triglyceride drops of 26.1 percent and HDL increases of 15 to 35 percent. The major side effect is flushing, but newer extended-release formulations turn that problem into a minor irritation.

✔ **Fibric acid derivatives for high triglycerides** These drugs, such as gemfibrozil (Lopid) and fenofibrate (Antara, Tricor), are best used for reducing triglycerides. In one five-year study, gemfibrozil produced an average 35 percent drop in triglycerides, with a more modest 8 percent drop in LDL cholesterol and an average 9 percent increase in HDL.

✔ **Chinese red yeast rice** This natural dietary seasoning, sold in capsule form as a supplement, contains several of the same chemicals found in the cholesterol-lowering drug lovastatin (Mevacor), which is why it's often called nature's statin. And indeed, a meta-analysis of 93 clinical trials found that red yeast rice was about as effective as lovastatin and four other commonly used statins for lowering total and LDL cholesterol and triglycerides and increasing HDL. Doses vary depending on the formulation. Don't take this supplement if you're taking a statin.

✔ **Soy** The cholesterol-lowering benefits of soy are small, even when you eat a lot of it. In one analysis of eight studies, people who ate a daily average of 50 grams of soy protein—the equivalent of a whopping 1 1/2 pounds of tofu—reduced their total cholesterol by almost 6 percent. But people who ate a more reasonable 25 grams daily lowered their total cholesterol by only 1.1 percent. It's likely that people who eat soy foods lower their cholesterol because they eat less saturated fat, not because of any special properties of soy.

✔ **Garlic** The evidence on garlic in terms of lowering cholesterol is mixed, primarily because of differences in the types of garlic used in clinical trials and the small number of participants in most trials (small trials often aren't sufficiently "powered" to show significant effects). But among studies showing a benefit, garlic pills reduced LDL cholesterol by 11.4 percent and triglycerides by 9.9 percent. Garlic may also slightly lower the risk of blood clots, which can trigger heart attacks. If you prefer real garlic to pills, use at least 1 1/2 cloves a day and let them stand for 10 minutes after chopping to allow key compounds to form.

✔ **Policosanol** This supplement is derived from Cuban sugarcane or wheat germ, but only studies using the Cuban version (not available in the United States) show a cholesterol-lowering effect. Plus, published studies have been very small, with fewer than 50 participants. That said, studies comparing 10 milligrams of Cuban policosanol with low doses of statins (10 to 20 milligrams a day) found that both reduced cholesterol levels by about the same amount. An analysis of 29 trials that compared policosanol to placebos found 5 to 40 milligrams of the supplement taken for an average of 30 weeks reduced LDL cholesterol by 23.7 percent and total cholesterol by 16.2 percent, with a 10.6 percent increase in HDL.

Our BEST ADVICE

See a registered dietitian for help if you want to lower your cholesterol by changing your diet. A review of 12 studies comparing the benefits of dietary advice from a dietitian vs. advice from a doctor or from self-help resources like books and the Internet found that participants who got their advice from dietitians or even on their own had cholesterol reductions 9.75 mg/dl lower than those of people who got advice only from their doctors.

WORKS FOR SOME

● **Bile acid sequestrants** These prescription drugs, often used in conjunction with a statin, include cholestyramine (Questran, Prevalite, and Locholest), colestipol (Colestid), and colesevelam (WelChol). They work fairly well for reducing LDL cholesterol (one major study found a 20.3 percent drop compared to a 12.6 percent drop in a placebo group). However, they can *increase* triglycerides, which is why they're recommended only for certain people (those whose triglycerides aren't already high).

HIGH CHOLESTEROL

DON'T BOTHER

✖ **Vytorin** This drug marries simvastatin (Zocor) and a different type of cholesterol-lowering drug called ezetimibe (Zetia). Unlike statins, Zetia works by blocking cholesterol absorption in the intestine. Although studies found the combination could reduce LDL cholesterol levels up to 20 percent more than a statin alone, a major study comparing its effects on plaque buildup in the major artery in the neck found no difference between patients taking Vytorin and those taking Zocor alone. While both medications prevented further plaque buildup, neither significantly reduced it. It's not yet clear whether Vytorin or Zetia reduces the risk of heart attacks or stroke.

In the meantime, since generic statins cost about one-third as much as Vytorin *and* have been shown to reduce the risk of heart attack and stroke, and since Vytorin doesn't seem to provide any more benefit

WHAT ABOUT FISH OIL?

Although fish oil does seem to provide valuable heart benefits, such as stabilizing heart rhythm and reducing inflammation in the arteries, it doesn't do much in terms of lowering cholesterol. Numerous studies find that while fish oil can reduce triglycerides by about 30 percent, reductions in LDL cholesterol and increases in HDL cholesterol are modest, and there's no proven reduction in plaque buildup. Getting the triglyceride benefit usually requires taking about 4 grams of fish oil a day; check with your doctor before taking this or any other amount.

than a statin alone in terms of the major reason for heart attacks (plaque buildup), there's no compelling reason to take it.

✖ **Guggul** This Indian herbal extract is a mainstay in Ayurvedic medicine and is often touted as a natural option for reducing high cholesterol. But clinical studies just don't show a consistent benefit. In one of the few well-designed studies on guggul, published in the *Journal of the American Medical Association*, the supplement actually *increased* LDL levels. Meanwhile, an analysis of all published studies on guggul

for high cholesterol found no significant differences in total cholesterol, HDL, or triglycerides between placebo and guggul groups.

✖ **Clofibrate (Atromid-S)** This fibric acid derivative is still on the market in many countries, but its effects on cholesterol are very modest, and in one seminal study, total deaths among people who took the drug increased slightly due to liver and intestinal cancers.

✖ **Cutting out cholesterol-rich foods** It's not the cholesterol in eggs and seafood that increases your blood cholesterol levels; it's mainly the saturated fat in foods like red meat, cheese, and ice cream, which is converted to cholesterol in your body. You can safely eat an egg or two a day without worrying that it might increase your cholesterol levels or risk of heart disease. ∎

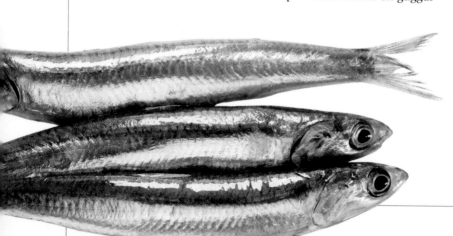

Insomnia

Staring at the ceiling at night? You're not alone. An estimated one in three adults have trouble falling asleep or staying asleep at least one night per week. Before you reach for a sleeping pill, it's smart to understand what healthy sleep really is and how it changes with every birthday. The truth is, lighter and more interrupted sleep is natural as we grow older: After midlife, sleep time drops about 27 minutes per decade. You may also need more time, up to a half hour, to find your way into dreamland. But if bedtime's a battle instead of bliss, these measures can help.

WORKS

✔ **Exercise** Walk, swim, pop in an aerobics video, or go to the gym—your choice. Just find a way to fit more exercise into your day. Some studies suggest that exercise is just as effective as sedatives.

When 2,624 women and men took a 40-hour healthy lifestyle course that encouraged them to exercise more, insomnia dropped by 64 percent and reports of restless sleep fell by 59 percent, say researchers from Brigham Young University. And in a small Stanford University study, troubled sleepers who added about a half hour of exercise (like walking or low-impact aerobics) four times a week happily reported that they fell asleep 15 minutes sooner and got about an hour more sleep each night than those who didn't exercise.

✔ **Bright light therapy** When older people with insomnia were exposed to bright light for 45 minutes a day for two months, they fell asleep faster, slept longer, and felt more energetic during the day than people who had just 20 minutes a day of light therapy. Study volunteers used special light-therapy lamps that deliver 10,000 lux of brightness. You can buy one without a prescription, but talk to your doctor first to make sure it's right for you; some experts say they're not a good idea for people with eye conditions like glaucoma or cataracts. Going outdoors at midday could have similar results by subtly resetting your body clock, say sleep experts from Ottawa Hospital in Canada.

✔ **Cognitive behavioral therapy (CBT)** If you've had insomnia for a long time, chances are you've developed sleep-related habits that all but ensure that your problem will continue. This form of talk therapy aims to break the cycle, retraining you to be ready for sleep at bedtime and to stop stressing on nights when sleep is slow to come or you do wake up.

A Harvard University study of 63 people with insomnia found that CBT worked better than prescription sleeping pills at helping people fall asleep and stay asleep. After eight weeks, the therapy cut the amount of time it took to fall asleep in half and improved "sleep efficiency" (a measure of uninterrupted sleep per night) by 17 percent, while drugs reduced nodding-off time by only about 15 percent and boosted sleep efficiency by only 3 percent. After a year, most of the therapy group members were still enjoying these sleep advantages—and 38 percent of people in the drug-treatment group asked for the training.

If you're interested in trying this, find a therapist specifically trained in CBT.

✔ **Good "sleep hygiene"** No, this doesn't mean going to bed clean (though if taking a bath or shower before bed relaxes you, by all means do it). It means

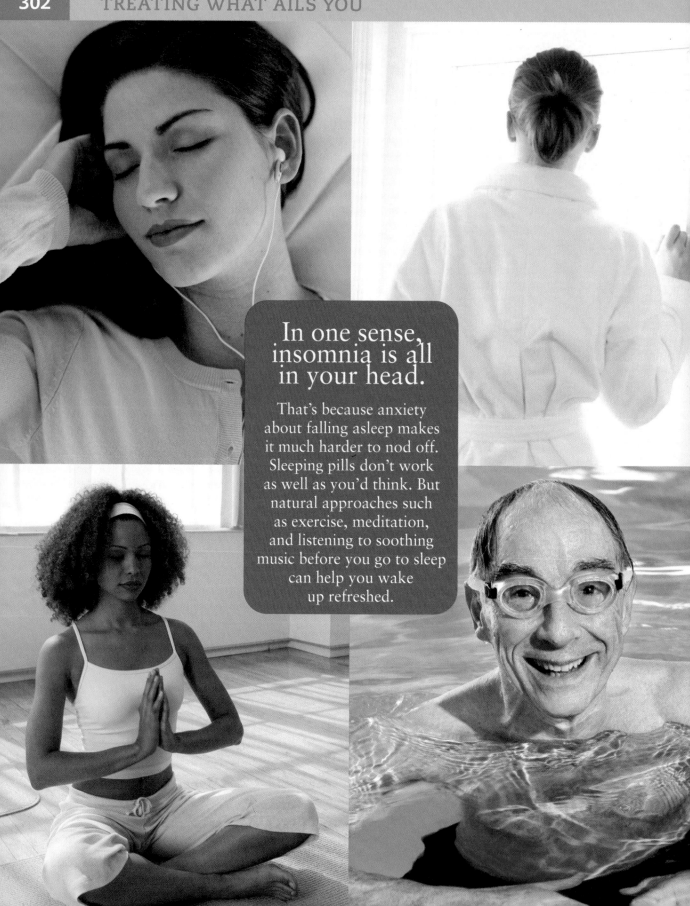

In one sense, insomnia is all in your head.

That's because anxiety about falling asleep makes it much harder to nod off. Sleeping pills don't work as well as you'd think. But natural approaches such as exercise, meditation, and listening to soothing music before you go to sleep can help you wake up refreshed.

tweaking your sleep habits to encourage better shuteye. That includes establishing a relaxing bedtime routine, banishing stressors and stimuli like that box of unpaid bills and the TV from your boudoir, going to bed and waking up at the same times each day, and leaving the bedroom if you can't fall asleep within 15 to 20 minutes, returning only when you feel really sleepy. In just a few weeks, your mind and body will associate your bed with refreshing, deep sleep. Canadian researchers who reviewed nondrug insomnia fixes say good sleep hygiene can help you fall asleep in 30 minutes or less and sleep for an extra 30 to 40 minutes per night.

✔ Listening to your favorite relaxing music
Put your bedroom CD player on a timer and drift off as quiet, soothing music plays. This strategy helped 60 problem sleepers fall asleep faster, sleep more soundly, and feel less tired during the day in a study from Taiwan.

✔ Relaxation techniques
Deep breathing, progressive relaxation, yoga—almost any type of relaxation therapy, performed at any time of day, may help you fall asleep faster and sleep more soundly. Studies show relaxation techniques can help you fall asleep 14 minutes sooner and sleep an extra 20 minutes.

✔ Silencing a snoring bed partner
Bedding down with a chronic snorer is decidedly bad for your sleep. In the Married Couples Sleep Study, researchers at Chicago's Rush University Medical Center checked on the sleep quality and habits of 10 couples and discovered just how disruptive a snoring mate can be. The spouse of one snorer was awakened eight times *every hour* by her husband's rasping night noises. If something similar is happening to you, try moving to another room or wearing earplugs and above all, asking your mate to seek medical help for snoring.

WORKS FOR SOME

● Newer insomnia drugs
The new widely advertised sleeping pills—including zolpidem (Ambien), zaleplon (Sonata), and eszopiclone (Lunesta)—are less likely than older pills to cause side effects, probably because the body metabolizes them faster. But how effective are they? A study conducted by the National Institutes of Health (NIH) found that people who took prescription sleep aids received very little objective benefit. On average, they fell asleep only about 13 minutes faster than those who took placebo pills, and they slept only 11 to 32 minutes longer. Most of the

subjects in both groups *believed* that they had slept much better, however. Some researchers speculated that sleeping medications disrupt the ability to form memories, so the pill takers didn't remember the time they spent awake or tossing and turning.

Keep in mind that no sleeping pill is meant to be taken long term; a report from the NIH warns that few prescription drugs for insomnia have been tested in long-term studies of a year or more—yet many people take them for years on end.

● Melatonin
In your body, melatonin produced by your pineal gland helps regulate your sleep-wake cycle. As a supplement, melatonin has been approved by the FDA to ease sleep disorders in blind people with circadian rhythm disorders. Experts say it may help modestly for insomnia due to jet lag or shift work.

Since the long-term effects of melatonin have not been studied, experts warn against everyday use. Be cautious about even short-term use; too much can cause sleep disruption, daytime fatigue, headache, dizziness, and irritability.

INSOMNIA

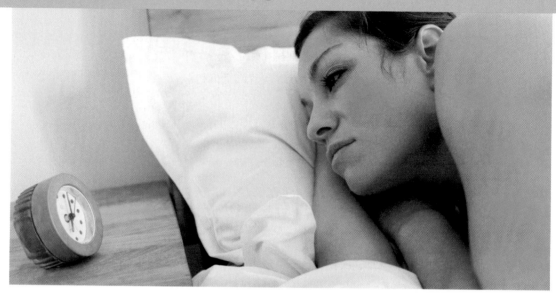

DON'T BOTHER

✖ Antihistamines

Nearly one in four people with insomnia try over-the-counter antihistamines in order to get a good night's sleep. And older antihistamines, such as diphenhydramine (the stuff in Benadryl), do make you drowsy, so they can help you fall asleep in a pinch. But these drugs can make you feel sleepy all day, and they aren't intended for long-term use, say NIH sleep experts. For older people, they may even cause hazy thinking and delirium and can lead to constipation, urinary retention, and blurred vision.

✖ Valerian

This age-old botanical is safe but probably not effective, say University of Washington researchers who reviewed 29 well-designed studies. The most rigorous studies found the least benefit, they report.

✖ Benzodiazepines

These sedatives—such as alprazolam (Xanax), chlordiazepoxide (Librium), diazepam (Valium), and lorazepam (Ativan)—ease anxiety, relax muscles, and helped people fall asleep 11 minutes faster and stay asleep 48 minutes longer in studies, Canadian researchers report. But they are habit forming, and their use has been linked with daytime fatigue, confusion, and a higher risk of motor vehicle accidents, falls, and fractures. If nondrug approaches aren't working for your insomnia, these drugs are safe to take at a low dose for a maximum of two to four weeks, say researchers from McMaster University in Hamilton, Canada. But "there appears to be virtually no evidence to support the chronic use of benzodiazepines for insomnia," they conclude.

Our BEST ADVICE

Can't sleep? Try cutting out caffeine. In a study of thousands of Australians, those who got 240 milligrams of caffeine a day—about the amount in two eight-ounce cups of coffee—had a 40 percent higher risk of insomnia than those who skipped it. It takes three to seven hours for your body to metabolize just half the caffeine in a cup of tea or coffee. If you can't live without it, drink it only in the morning.

✖ Warm milk

If drinking a soothing cup of warm milk is part of your bedtime ritual, there's no reason to stop—but the milk itself probably isn't putting you to sleep. A study at the Massachusetts Institute of Technology disproved a popular theory that milk raises levels of the slumber-promoting amino acid tryptophan. ∎

Menopause Symptoms

Technically, menopause is just one day in your life: the day 12 months after your last menstrual period started. But it's the months and years leading up to it (called perimenopause), when your estrogen levels jump up and down like a caffeinated 2-year-old, and the 5 to 10 years after it, when those levels become nearly nonexistent, that cause problems like hot flashes and vaginal dryness. Most symptoms go away eventually, and for many women, a "grin and bear it" attitude is enough to get them through. But if your suffering is bad, here are strategies that can help (and some that can't).

WORKS

✔ Hormone replacement therapy (HRT)

The truth: Nothing works as well for menopause symptoms. Reviews of studies find that HRT reduces both the frequency and intensity of hot flashes up to 90 percent compared to about 50 percent for a placebo. HRT also helps improve bone density. The caveat: A major study found higher rates of breast cancer, heart disease, and stroke in women who took an estrogen-plus-progestin drug (progestin is included with estrogen therapy to lower the risk of uterine cancer) and higher rates of stroke in women who took an estrogen-only drug.

That sounds scary, all right. But it doesn't mean that if you're dripping unbearably with sweat, you can't use HRT *in the short term* for symptoms like hot flashes. Today doctors generally advise women to use HRT for no more than a year or two, though some studies suggest you can use it for up to five years without risk. Studies find that using the lowest possible dose of estrogen, with or without progestin, not only significantly reduces the risks of any negative side effects but still provides relief from hot flashes, night sweats, vaginal dryness, and other symptoms.

If you're under 60, you may have even less to worry about with regard to HRT. Additional analysis of the data in younger women found that heart disease risks were not significantly higher in women under 60 or those who took HRT soon after menopause began. In healthy young (ages 50 to 59) postmenopausal women, HRT may even benefit the heart.

If your primary complaint is vaginal dryness and pain, urinary incontinence, or frequent urinary tract infections, HRT in pill form isn't your only option. Ask your doctor about vaginal estrogen in the form of tablets, creams, or rings. If you have "brain fog," also fondly known as menopause brain, HRT may help. Recent studies found that women who wore low-dose estrogen patches had significantly higher cognitive function (such as memory and learning ability) than women wearing placebo patches.

✔ Antidepressants

Antidepressants for hot flashes? Yes. Even in low doses, the drugs fluoxetine (Prozac), paroxetine (Paxil), and venlafaxine (Effexor) can help regulate body temperature and curb hot flashes, though they may not work as well as HRT. In one study of 87 women with a history of breast cancer, those who took Prozac averaged 19 percent fewer hot flashes than those who took placebos. In a large study of Effexor, also involving women with a history of breast cancer, 63 percent of those who received 75 milligrams a day had far fewer hot flashes compared to just 20 percent of women who received a placebo. In another study, of postmenopausal women with no history of breast cancer, hot flash scores dropped 51 percent in those who received extended-release Effexor for 12 weeks compared to a 15 percent drop in women who got a placebo. These drugs also work well for the cognitive problems associated with menopause.

✔ **Gabapentin (Neurontin)** This drug was originally developed to treat epilepsy but is used for a variety of other medical conditions, including hot flashes. An

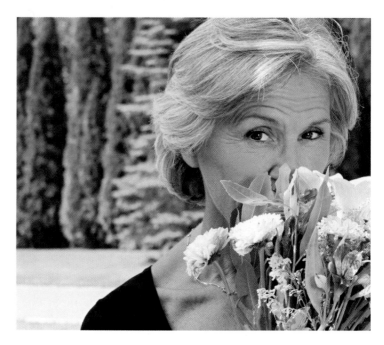

analysis of two clinical trials, including one of women with breast cancer who took tamoxifen (a drug that puts premenopausal women into menopause and can cause

severe hot flashes) found it reduced the average number of hot flashes by 2.05 a day compared with placebos.

WORKS FOR SOME

● **Clonidine (Catapres)** This blood pressure drug has a modest effect on menopause symptoms. An analysis of four major studies found that women who took it experienced an average of one fewer hot flash per day compared to those taking placebos. Studies suggest that clonidine works best in women with breast cancer who are being treated with drugs like tamoxifen and not as well in women who reach menopause naturally.

● **Black cohosh** This is one of the most-studied herbal options for hot flashes, yet there's still no clear answer on whether black cohosh works. Short-term trials (generally three to six months) showed it was slightly more effective than a placebo in women with mild to moderate hot flashes. A long-term trial, however, found no benefit after one year. If it does work for you, it may take six weeks to see results.

● **Soy** Many women and gynecologists swear by soy for

hot flashes, so we've listed it under "Works for Some." It does *seem* that soy would cool hot flashes since it contains hormone-like compounds called isoflavones that are structurally similar to estrogen. Unfortunately, most women could eat tofu until the cows come home and probably not get a lot of relief. An analysis of six trials of soy isoflavones with dosages ranging from 50 to 150 milligrams a day found that women taking them had only one fewer hot flash a day after taking the supplement for four weeks to six months than those taking placebos. And doctors and researchers who looked at 17 well-designed studies on the benefits of soy extract and red clover, an isoflavone-rich herb that's also used to fight hot flashes, found no consistent relief among women who took soy extract.

(There was even less evidence that red clover helped.)

If you want to try eating more soy, go ahead, but keep in mind that some studies suggest a high-soy diet may increase the risk of breast cancer (see page 260 for more info). Experts do not recommend isoflavone supplements.

DON'T BOTHER

✖ **Dong quai** This Chinese herb is often touted as the ideal supplement to prevent hot flashes, but studies don't support its use. One study found it had no effect on women's own production of estrogen, nor did it prevent or reduce hot flashes compared to placebos.

✖ **Vitamin E** Just one placebo-controlled study has looked at vitamin E as a treatment for hot flashes, and it found no significant difference between the number or severity of flashes in 105 women taking either daily vitamin E or placebos.

✖ **Red clover** An analysis of six trials of two types of red clover isoflavones, including the brands Promensil and

Rimostil, found that compared with placebos, they reduced the number of hot flashes in menopausal women by less than one-half a day on average.

✖ **Evening primrose** This herb contains high amounts of omega-3 fatty acids and is often recommended for menopause symptoms. The one placebo-controlled trial that evaluated how well it works combined 2,000 milligrams of evening primrose with 10 milligrams of vitamin E a day. The study found that women who received placebos actually had *fewer* hot flashes than those who received the combination treatment, although so many women dropped out of the trial because they weren't

The old standard advice for coping with hot flashes still applies: Avoid hot baths or showers and spicy foods, wear natural fabrics that breathe, and dress in layers so you can take off some clothing when you need to. At night, sleep with a fan blowing on you. For vaginal dryness, a water-based vaginal lubricant (such as K-Y Jelly) or vaginal moisturizer (such as Replens) can help.

getting symptom relief that even those results are suspect.

✖ **Wild yam cream** Despite ads you might see on the Internet, these creams don't contain progesterone, although one of the ingredients can be used to synthesize the hormone in a lab (not in your body). Studies show they have little or no effect on menopause symptoms.

✖ **Exercise** It's good for you in so many ways, including protecting your heart and shoring up your bones, which become frailer as you age, but it won't lessen your hot flashes, according to recent research. ∎

MIGRAINES

Migraines

Migraines, now thought to be caused by changes in neurological activity in the brain, can be excruciating, nauseating, and strange—some are preceded by an "aura" of flashing lights, blind spots, or tingling sensations. Many people don't even know that their head pain is a migraine. You may be having migraines if you have any of these symptoms: throbbing pain on one or both sides of your head, nausea, sensitivity to light and sound, and an ache so painful that it keeps you from regular activities.

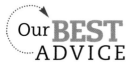

Our BEST ADVICE

Don't overdo your use of painkillers, or you could end up worse off. Using over-the-counter pain pills more than twice a week or taking migraine-easing triptans more than 17 times a month can eventually cause "rebound" migraines, warn German researchers.

WORKS

✔ **Migraine-formula pain relievers** If your migraines are fairly mild—that is, your attacks don't usually keep you from everyday activities, and you experience vomiting during an attack less than 20 percent of the time—these inexpensive over-the-counter pills may help, say pain experts at Chicago's Diamond Headache Clinic. Aspirin, ibuprofen, acetaminophen, and naproxen all work, but we recommend an OTC migraine product that contains a blend of acetaminophen, aspirin, and caffeine. These pills relieved migraine pain 20 minutes faster than ibuprofen in one study. In another, they were better than the prescription migraine stopper sumatriptan (Imitrex) for relieving the pain of moderately intense migraines, especially if taken at the first signs of an attack.

Prescription drugs that "abort" a migraine If drugstore painkillers don't do the trick, ask your doctor about the gold standard drug for stopping bad head pain: a triptan. Also known as selective serotonin-receptor agonists (brand names include Imitrex, Zomig, and Frova), these drugs can halt a migraine if taken at the first sign of an attack and can even ease pain when an attack's under way. Triptans start easing pain within one hour 24 to 45 percent of the time and provide complete relief within two hours for 23 to 42 percent of people who take them.

✔ **A very low fat diet** When 54 people prone to migraines followed an extremely low fat diet (they got just 10 to 15 percent of their calories from fat each

day) for 12 weeks, 94 percent reported having at least 40 percent fewer headaches. When they did get migraines, pain was 66 percent less severe, and the headaches were about 70 percent shorter. As a result, they used 72 percent less medicine than before the study, report Loma Linda University researchers.

✔ **Migraine-prevention drugs** If you get two or more migraines each month, you're a candidate for one of these. Experts at East Carolina University say the right remedy could cut your risk of future headaches in half—but be patient; it can take four weeks to begin seeing improvement and up to six months to see if a therapy is really working for you.

The migraine-prevention drugs with the best track record are the beta-blockers

What Triggers Your Migraines?

Steering clear of your migraine triggers can help you avert attacks. Until recently, migraines were often blamed on foods such as red wine, aged cheese, and chocolate, but now experts are less sure that specific foods set off the headaches. When researchers at the Headache Center of Atlanta asked 916 adults what triggered their migraines, here's what they said.

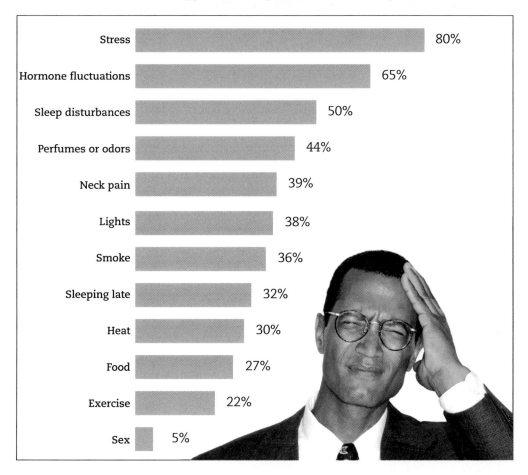

Trigger	Percentage
Stress	80%
Hormone fluctuations	65%
Sleep disturbances	50%
Perfumes or odors	44%
Neck pain	39%
Lights	38%
Smoke	36%
Sleeping late	32%
Heat	30%
Food	27%
Exercise	22%
Sex	5%

propranolol (Inderal) and timolol (Blocadren). Studies suggest that 90 percent of people who take them get relief. Other first-line choices that earned an "A" for effectiveness from the East Carolina experts include the antidepressant amitriptyline (Elavil) and the anticonvulsants divalproex sodium (Depakote), and topiramate (Topamax).

Calcium channel-blockers can sometimes work when beta-blockers don't.

✔ **Butterbur** One expert calls butterbur-based remedies "the best safety-tested herbal to date for the treatment of headache." In one study of 245 people published in the journal *Neurology*, 68 percent of those who took a butterbur product called Petadolex saw the number of migraines they experienced drop by at least 50 percent—a better result than for some first-line migraine-prevention drugs.

MIGRAINES

WORKS FOR SOME

● **Acupuncture** A British review of 13 studies concluded it's too soon to tell whether acupuncture can prevent or ease head pain. But in a study of 401 headache sufferers, most of whom got migraines, researchers at Memorial Sloan-Kettering Cancer Center in New York found that those who received 12 acupuncture treatments over three months used 15 percent less pain medication than those who didn't get acupuncture.

● **Vitamin B$_2$ (riboflavin)** When 55 people in a Belgian study took this vitamin every day for three months, 60 percent had half their usual number of migraines, German researchers report. The volunteers took 400 milligrams per day, 300 times more than the recommended daily amount of 1.5 milligrams. Longer studies are needed to be sure these amounts are safe.

● **Feverfew** This popular herb offers only "mild and transient" benefits, say British researchers who reviewed five well-designed studies of the effects of feverfew on migraines. But in a recent study of a feverfew extract containing consistent levels of the active ingredient, parthenolide, repeat migraines were reduced from nearly five per month to about three.

● **Melatonin** When 34 Brazilian migraine sufferers took melatonin before going to bed every night for three months, two-thirds said the number of migraines they experienced dropped by 50 percent, and eight were migraine-free. One caveat: People in this study knew they were taking melatonin, so at least some of the improvement could be due to the placebo effect.

● **Magnesium** Low brain levels of this mineral have been found in at least eight studies involving people who get frequent migraines. Yet when researchers have given magnesium to migraine-prone volunteers, the results have been mixed—perhaps because supplements won't help people whose magnesium levels are normal. It may work best in women who get menstrual migraines and for people who get auras before attacks, but two out of three studies of magnesium for migraines have shown no benefits.

DON'T BOTHER

✖ **Homeopathy** In a well-designed British study of 63 people, researchers found no significant difference in migraine occurrence after three months of either individually tailored homeopathic remedies or a placebo. ■

Nausea

Whether it's from motion sickness, pregnancy, cancer treatment, or anesthesia, nausea can be even worse than pain. At any rate, it's no fun, nor is its natural conclusion, vomiting. And treating it isn't always easy, though we've listed some useful strategies here. One remedy not included, which is often effective for chemotherapy-related nausea, is marijuana, but it has mind-altering side effects and is illegal in most places.

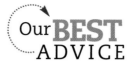

Our BEST ADVICE

If you're feeling nauseated and want to avoid vomiting, find somewhere quiet to sit still, and sip a clear sweet liquid such as apple juice or soda. Avoid orange juice, which is too acidic. It may also help to suck a Popsicle.

WORKS

✔ **Acupuncture/acupressure** These approaches seem to work for everything from chemotherapy-related vomiting to motion sickness. A review of 11 clinical trials on acupuncture, acupressure, and electrical stimulation (in which a tiny electrical current is transmitted between the acupuncture needles) found that acupressure reduced the incidence of vomiting by 18 percent, and needle and electrical acupuncture reduced it by 26 percent. The acupressure also reduced the severity of the nausea.

Acupressure is the basis for wristbands like the Sea-Band, designed so that a plastic button presses against the P6 acupressure point on the inside of the wrist. Studies find that it can reduce postsurgical nausea as well as prevent motion sickness.

✔ **Vitamin B_6** If your nausea is related to pregnancy, consider taking 10 to 25 milligrams of this vitamin three times a day. A review of 28 studies on treatments for morning sickness found that it improved nausea (although not vomiting) with few side effects.

✔ **Ginger** Ginger extracts seem to work well for pregnancy-related and postoperative nausea, though not as well for motion sickness. An analysis of five clinical trials comparing the effects of 1 gram or more of ginger with those of placebos found that ginger reduced the risk of postoperative nausea and vomiting by 31 percent. Other reviews have found it works better than placebos and as well as vitamin B_6 and dimenhydrinate (Dramamine) for preventing nausea and vomiting in pregnancy.

✔ **Over-the-counter motion sickness medications** Dimenhydrinate and cyclizine (Marezine) work equally well for reducing nausea and vomiting from motion sickness. A study comparing the two, however, found that people taking dimenhydrinate were drowsier and more likely to have other gastrointestinal symptoms than those taking cyclizine. The key is to take the drugs well before you board the ship or embark on a winding car ride.

WORKS FOR SOME

● **Prescription anti-nausea drugs** A review of more than 700 clinical studies found that while nausea and vomiting affect 8 out of 10 people after surgery, just 1 of 3 would benefit from anti-nausea drugs. Most have side effects such as headache. ∎

Nicotine Addiction

You can eat the best diet in the world and work out six days a week, but if you're still smoking, you're still destroying your health. One in three men and one in five women in developed countries smoke—not because they're ignorant of the risks but because it's so darn hard to quit. If you've tried, don't give up; studies find that it often takes multiple tries. The more therapies you use from the "Works" list below, the better your chances.

WORKS

✔ **Counseling programs and behavioral therapies** The best of these help you in three ways: They train you to solve practical problems related to quitting (for instance, if you always light up when you pour your first cup of coffee in the morning, it may help you to switch to tea); they include social support as part of treatment (such as pairing you with a nonsmoking "buddy" you can call when you feel the need to smoke); and they help you set up social support outside of therapy. Ask your doctor for a referral.

✔ **Exercise** Exercising three times a week may work even better than a behavioral therapy program (of course, doing both is ideal). One study found that nearly 20 percent of the exercisers were still smoke-free after a year compared to 11 percent of the therapy group. And there was a bonus: They gained less weight.

✔ **Nicotine-replacement therapies** These include gums, patches, lozenges, inhalers, and nasal spray. It doesn't matter if you get your nicotine fix from a prescription product or an over-the-counter one; both are equally effective. Studies find that the patch increases quit rates by about 7 percent compared to placebos, the gum and inhaler by about 8 percent, and the nasal spray by 12 to 16 percent.

✔ **Bupropion (Zyban)** This antidepressant increases the quit rate by about 10 to 13 percent compared to taking a placebo and doubles the success of the nicotine patch compared to using the patch alone. An added benefit is that it seems to reduce the weight gain so common after quitting.

WORKS FOR SOME

● **Aversive smoking interventions** This includes taking unpleasant measures like smoking very fast and puffing rapidly on a cigarette until you feel sick. Don't try this on your own; it should be used only under medical supervision. Studies find it works best in those for whom other options have failed.

DON'T BOTHER

✖ **Trying to quit on your own** If you're trying to be tough and quit smoking on your own—without any help from your physician, nicotine-replacement products, counseling, or medication—you're likely to fail even if you use self-help manuals or booklets.

✖ **Acupuncture** An analysis of 24 studies found no difference in quit rates between smokers who received real acupuncture and those who got fake acupuncture.

✖ **Hypnotherapy** The evidence just isn't there to support this approach. ■

Osteoporosis

If you've ever tripped on a step and fractured a bone, you could chalk it up to clumsiness—but osteoporosis might also be to blame. People don't always realize that these bone breaks, or even loss of height (which can result from compression fractures in the spine), may be the first sign of the disease. This condition, in which your bones lose density and become as thin as the denim in a pair of 15-year-old jeans, is both preventable and reversible with treatment.

WORKS

✔ **Bone-building drugs** Numerous drugs are available today for treating osteoporosis or its predecessor, osteopenia. A major analysis of the following three drug types found no clear "winner" in terms of preventing fractures. (Hormone replacement therapy, which reduces the risk of fractures after menopause, is no longer recommended as a front-line therapy because of possible health risks.)

Parathyroid hormone (calcitonin): This hormone stimulates bone-building cells. Studies find it works best at preventing hip and other non-spinal fractures. Once given only by injection, it's now available as a nasal spray for women who are more than five years past menopause.

Selective estrogen-receptor modulators (SERMs): Raloxifene (Evista) works like estrogen in the body, helping reduce bone loss. It not only works well for preventing fractures in women with osteoporosis but is also one of the few drugs also approved to prevent osteoporosis in post-menopausal women.

Bisphosphonates: These drugs include alendronate (Fosamax), risedronate (Actonel), ibandronate (Boniva), and others. They bind to bone to prevent it from breaking down. The only bisphosphonate approved to *prevent* osteoporosis is Boniva. Side effects can include gastrointestinal problems and even damage to the esophagus. Some patients have reported severe muscle or bone pain while using these drugs, so be sure to talk with your doctor about the risks.

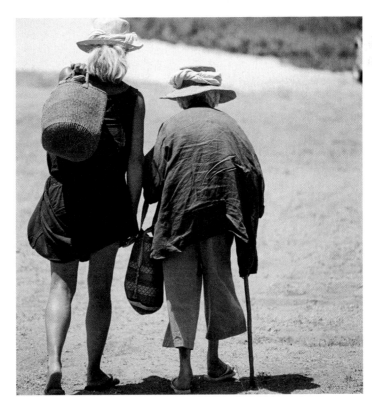

OSTEOPOROSIS

✔ **Weight-bearing exercise** The biggest bone benefits come from weight-bearing exercise done in childhood and early adulthood, but you'll still reap some benefits if you start now. Walking or jogging, doing aerobics, and lifting weights or using dumbbells all count. If you're dieting, exercise can also help offset bone loss that may result when you try to lose weight by cutting calories.

✔ **Vitamin K** Here's another reason to eat your spinach—and your kale and collard greens: They're rich in vitamin K, which some studies show can cut the risk of bone fractures. Research suggests that supplementing with 45 milligrams a day can reduce the rate of spinal fractures by 65 percent, but it's safer to get your vitamin K from food. A cup of cooked spinach contains about 1 milligram.

✔ **Fruits and vegetables** In addition to vitamin K and calcium, these provide other nutrients important in maintaining bone health and preventing fractures, including vitamins A and C, potassium, magnesium, and fluoride. If you eat at least five servings of fruit and vegetables a day (more is better), you're getting enough of most of these nutrients.

WORKS FOR SOME

● **Calcium** Calcium is no longer considered the "slam dunk" for preventing osteoporosis it was once thought to be. Some studies have failed to show any bone benefits from taking supplements. But Australian researchers who reviewed data from 29 studies involving nearly 64,000 people (mostly postmenopausal women) found that taking calcium supplements alone or with vitamin D for three to five years reduced the risk of a fracture by about 12 percent on average. People who gained the most bone protection were those whose diets were low in calcium to begin with. Talk to your doctor about whether calcium supplements are right for you.

DON'T BOTHER

✖ **Phytoestrogens** These hormone-like compounds found in soy don't seem to have any effect on bone density in premenopausal women, and the evidence is mixed in postmenopausal women. What's more, studies find that there's no way to get enough from your diet alone to affect bone density; you'd have to take supplemental soy protein or phytoestrogens, which experts recommend against.

✖ **Testosterone** There's simply no evidence that supplemental doses of this hormone strengthen bone or prevent osteoporosis. ■

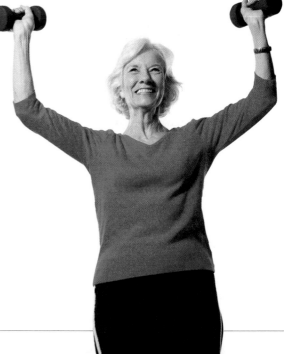

Premenstrual Syndrome

If you have premenstrual syndrome (PMS), you know that once a month, the you that is "you" disappears, and some real-life avatar takes her place, one that is crabby and depressed, with headaches, bloating, and anxiety. While the real you may return once your period begins, then you're coping with cramps and maybe heavy bleeding. Chances are you've tried over-the-counter remedies, hot compresses, and banishing your family to the basement. But what really works to combat the physical and emotional pains of PMS and menstruation? Read on.

WORKS

✔ **Vitamin B₆** It seems hard to believe, but a vitamin really can smooth this bumpy monthly transition. An analysis of nine clinical trials found that compared to those taking a placebo, women who took up to 100 milligrams of vitamin B₆ a day were more than twice as likely to have fewer premenstrual symptoms, such as bloating, breast pain, headache, and lack of energy, and 69 percent less likely to suffer from menstrual-related depression.

✔ **Calcium** The same stuff you take for your bones can also reduce those monthly symptoms that make your family cringe. In fact, PMS symptoms such as depression, problems concentrating, muscle pain and cramps, fatigue, and anxiety actually mimic those of calcium deficiency. Studies find that calcium levels drop significantly as estrogen rises in midcycle and that women with PMS tend to have much lower levels of calcium (and higher levels of estrogen) than women without it.

Studies find that supplementing daily with 1,200 to 1,600 milligrams of calcium (in two doses) can improve PMS symptoms. In the largest study, women were randomly selected to receive either 1,200 milligrams a day of calcium carbonate or a placebo for three menstrual cycles. Those who got the calcium scored 48 percent lower on a test that measured symptom severity, compared to a 30 percent drop in those who got placebos.

✔ **Antidepressants** For women who experience serious mood changes at "that time of the month," antidepressants like fluoxetine (Sarafem), sertraline (Zoloft), citalopram (Celexa), and paroxetine (Paxil) can help. These drugs, called selective serotonin-reuptake inhibitors (SSRIs), help the feel-good chemical serotonin hang around longer in your brain. Instead of taking large doses every day as one would to treat depression, women with PMS generally take small doses during the two weeks before their periods, although some take it all month long. One analysis of 15 studies found that the drugs were all better than placebos for treating serious premenstrual symptoms.

✔ **Birth control pills** These maintain steady levels of reproductive hormones. When you take them, you avoid the high premenstrual estrogen levels that trigger

PREMENSTRUAL SYNDROME

PMS. One birth control pill, Yaz, is approved specifically to treat premenstrual dysphoric disorder (PMDD), a more serious form of PMS, and is often used for PMS. One major study of the drug found that women taking it were 49 percent less likely to experience premenstrual depression, while women taking a placebo were 36 percent less likely to become depressed. Other studies find that taking any birth control pill on a continuous basis—without the seven days of placebo pills that trigger periods—ends periods in 80 to 100 percent of women. Without periods, of course, there is no PMS.

✔ **Spironolactone (Aldactone)** This prescription diuretic, taken during the 10 or so days prior to menstruation and the first 2 or 3 days, blocks a hormone that causes fluid retention. It can ease some PMS symptoms, including bloating and mood changes. Other diuretics don't seem to work as well.

WORKS FOR SOME

● **Magnesium** If your major issue with PMS is bloating or cramps, give magnesium a try. One study of 38 women found that those taking 200 milligrams of magnesium for two menstrual cycles reported much less bloating and weight gain than those who took a placebo. Don't expect immediate results; women in this and other magnesium studies needed at least two, and sometimes three, months of daily supplements before things improved. Other studies have found some improvement in mood, migraines, and menstrual cramps with supplemental magnesium doses of about 360 milligrams a day.

● **Chasteberry** This herbal remedy, thought to increase levels of the hormone progestin, has been used for centuries to treat a variety of women's reproductive issues, from heavy bleeding to infertility to menstrual cramps. There are no truly good studies on the effectiveness of chasteberry for PMS, though some studies do suggest a benefit. In the one trial that compared the herb to a placebo, 52 percent of the women who got 20 milligrams of chasteberry daily reported that their symptoms improved by 50 percent or more, compared to 24 percent of the women who got a placebo.

DON'T BOTHER

✖ **Vitamin E** There is some evidence that supplements of this vitamin, at doses of 400 IU per day, can improve breast pain and other PMS symptoms. However, vitamin E has come under scrutiny recently because of its potential to increase internal bleeding; it may even slightly increase the risk of premature death. If you want to take it, check with your doctor first.

✖ **Black cohosh** This herbal remedy has primarily been tested in menopausal women. Although it's sold to treat PMS in Germany, studies on its benefits for this condition are skimpy. In fact, no well-designed studies show any benefits for PMS. ∎

Prostate Cancer

Prostate cancer can't be prevented with a single pill or food. You simply can't fight advancing age or genetics, two major risk factors. But there's evidence that healthy lifestyle changes can reduce your risk. Start today: Scientists suspect that some habits, such as eating plenty of cruciferous veggies like broccoli and cabbage, have their most powerful anticancer effects in younger men.

WORKS

✔ **Achieving a healthy weight** In an American Cancer Society study that tracked the weight and health of 70,000 men for 21 years, researchers found that men with high body mass indexes (BMIs) were more likely to develop aggressive prostate cancer. (Ironically, overweight men were *less* likely to develop less aggressive prostate tumors.) And when researchers at Massachusetts General Hospital checked the weights of 788 patients diagnosed with advanced prostate cancer, they found that men of normal weight were less likely than overweight men to die in the five years after their diagnoses.

✔ **Selenium-rich foods** At least seven studies have found a link between selenium and a lower risk of prostate cancer. In one, researchers tracked more than 1,000 men who received either 200 micrograms of selenium or a placebo every day. After 7 1/2 years, there were 52 percent fewer cases of prostate cancer in the selenium group.

Cancer experts say it's too soon to recommend selenium supplements because studies haven't yet revealed the best and safest dose. But you can easily get the recommended daily amount (55 micrograms) by eating three or four Brazil nuts, a serving of flounder or sole, six ounces of poultry or meat, or a cup of pasta and two slices of bread. Your multivitamin probably contains another 20 micrograms.

✔ **Cruciferous vegetables** Lab studies show that sulforaphane, a compound found in cruciferous vegetables

Our BEST ADVICE

Talk with your doctor before taking calcium supplements or loading up on dairy foods. Several disturbing—if inconclusive—studies have shown that men who consume high amounts of calcium have an increased risk of prostate cancer. While the National Cancer Institute says a diet rich in dairy products and calcium increases risk just a little, nutrition experts at the Harvard School of Public Health say evidence for a link between dairy intake and fatal prostate cancer is strong. Milk may spur production of a hormone called IGF-1 that could fuel the growth of cancer cells. Harvard nutritionists suggest sticking with one or two servings of dairy a day.

such as broccoli, broccoli sprouts, bok choy, and brussels sprouts, has strong anticancer properties. In a Harvard Medical School study of 47,365 men, those under age 65 who ate five or more servings a week had a 20 percent lower risk of prostate cancer than those who had less than one serving. These veggies seem to work best early in the development of prostate cancer, a process that can take decades.

✔ **Pomegranate juice** In studies, a daily glass of this tart juice slowed the rise in

PROSTATE CANCER

levels of prostate-specific antigen (PSA) in men with prostate cancer. New research suggests that antioxidants in the juice break down into beneficial compounds that may concentrate in prostate tissue.

✔ Soy foods and dried beans

There's mounting evidence that soybeans and other legumes may lower prostate cancer risk. In fact, consumption of soy foods may be one reason that Asian men have death rates from prostate cancer that are four to five times lower than those of Western men. You can probably chalk up the benefits to phytoestrogens, which behave like weak hormones in the body. In one review of lab studies of the isoflavone genistein, 74 percent of studies showed that in animals, it reduced growth of prostate tumor cells. Aim to get your isoflavones from tofu, edamame, soy milk, soy nuts, and dried beans—not from supplements.

✔ A low-fat diet plus exercise

A low-fat, high-fiber diet and regular exercise can slow the growth of prostate cancer cells by up to 30 percent, say researchers at UCLA. Meanwhile, a diet high in saturated fat is linked with increased prostate cancer risk.

What to eat instead of fatty red meat? Try fish. The good-for-you fats in fatty fish like salmon may or may not help prevent prostate cancer directly, but fish is still good for your heart, and it's very low in saturated fat.

✔ More whole grains, less sugar

Your goal: Lower, steadier blood sugar levels. There's plenty of evidence that this eating strategy cuts the risk of diabetes and heart disease as well as growing proof that it may keep your cancer risk low. The link: Higher blood sugar means higher insulin levels—and insulin can help spur growth of cancer cells.

PROSTATE PROTECTION IN A PILL?

Wondering whether the drug you take for an enlarged prostate can protect you from prostate cancer? Johns Hopkins University researchers followed 18,882 men who took finasteride (Proscar) or a placebo for up to seven years and found that men in the finasteride group lowered their odds of developing prostate cancer by 24 percent. The downside: More of the cancers found in this group were aggressive, fast-growing types. And guys who took finasteride had some problems with low libido and erectile dysfunction. Experts say it's too soon to give it to all men to cut cancer risk.

DON'T BOTHER

✘ Overdosing on tomato products

Recent studies have deflated the popular theory that lycopene, an antioxidant in tomatoes, has special prostate-protecting powers. It's still important, of course, to eat a wide variety of fruits and veggies, experts say.

✘ Green tea

While researchers continue to study promising anticancer compounds in green tea, the FDA has turned down a request to label this beverage a cancer fighter. An FDA official who issued the ruling said it's highly unlikely that it protects against prostate cancer.

✘ Supplemental beta-carotene, vitamin E, lycopene, or any other high-dose antioxidant

Getting antioxidants from food may help lower prostate cancer risk, but it's unclear whether getting a concentrated dose in pill form helps—and it could hurt. There's some evidence that taking too much beta-carotene could raise risk. And there is proof that vitamin E could make a heart attack more likely. ■

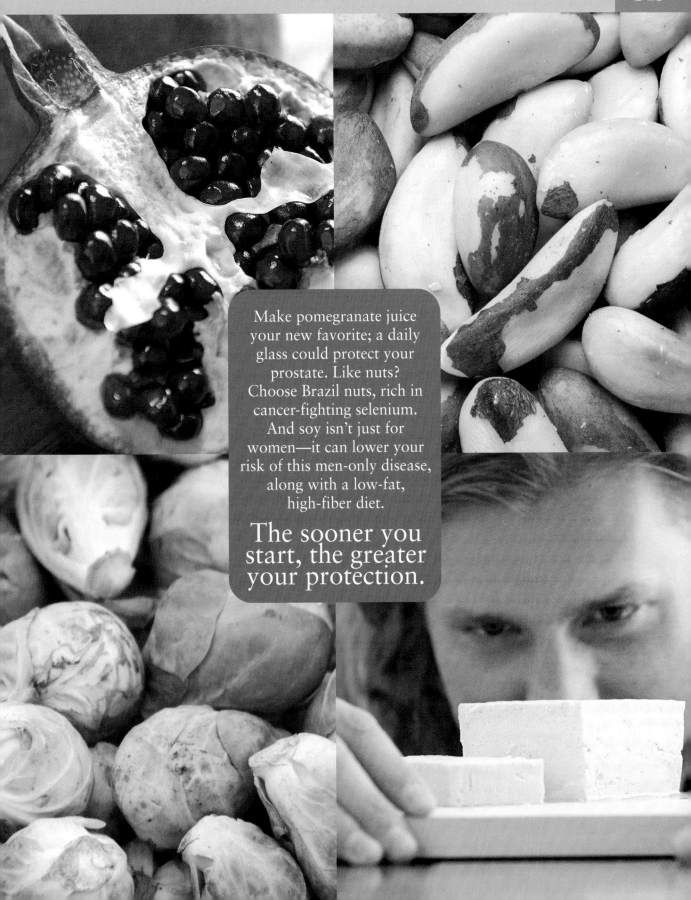

Make pomegranate juice your new favorite; a daily glass could protect your prostate. Like nuts? Choose Brazil nuts, rich in cancer-fighting selenium. And soy isn't just for women—it can lower your risk of this men-only disease, along with a low-fat, high-fiber diet.

The sooner you start, the greater your protection.

Prostate Enlargement

Are you getting up to "go" more often—and spending more time starting or finishing the job? Does your bladder sometimes still feel full? Half of all men over age 50 eventually experience problems caused by an enlarged prostate, the gland that encircles the urethra, through which urine exits the bladder. Prostate enlargement, or benign prostatic hyperplasia (BPH), isn't a sign of prostate cancer, but symptoms can be similar, so see your doctor.

WORKS

✔ **Prostate-shrinking drugs** Finasteride (Proscar) and dutasteride (Duagen) work by reducing levels of dihydrotestosterone (DHT)—a potent form of testosterone that spurs the growth of prostate cells—by 80 to 90 percent. The result: Over three to six months, your prostate deflates by about 20 percent.

The drugs work best if you have urinary problems due to a moderately enlarged prostate gland; they're not very effective for men who have symptoms of BPH despite a normal-size gland. Be patient; you may see some improvement in two or three months, but it could take a year for complete improvement. Side effects may include reduced libido and even impotence.

✔ **Alpha-blocker drugs** Your doctor may start with one of these medicines, such as tamsulosin (Flomax), which provide fast relief by relaxing the muscles around the neck of the bladder, opening the gates for better urination.

Side effects include dizziness and sudden low blood pressure when you stand up (these tend to clear up quickly once your body gets used to the drug) and fatigue. You may also have problems with ejaculation, but studies show that taking some of these drugs every other day is just as effective for improving urination and reduces ejaculation problems. Be careful about taking an erectile dysfunction drug with these meds; the combination can cause dangerously low blood pressure.

✔ **Surgery** If your symptoms don't improve with medications, or if you have ongoing complications like urinary tract infections, surgery may be your best option. Older procedures, from the most invasive (removal of the inner portion of the gland, called open prostatectomy) to transurethral resection of the prostate (TURP), ease symptoms by 88 to 98 percent. Long-term side effects may include retrograde ejaculation (in which semen flows into the bladder), impotence, and incontinence, though these are uncommon. Newer, less invasive techniques that involve inserting a stent or use heat to shrink prostate tissue are almost as successful and have fewer side effects.

WORKS FOR SOME

● **Saw palmetto** Small studies and lots of anecdotal evidence say this popular herb works as well as the drug finasteride. But a large well-designed study of 225 men, published in the *New England Journal of Medicine*, found it was no better than a placebo for shrinking the prostate or easing urinary problems. ∎

Restless Legs Syndrome

The rest of your body wants to sleep, but your legs are wide awake, torturing you with creepy-crawly sensations and causing you to kick and flail 'til the covers are nowhere to be found. If this sounds familiar, you may have restless legs syndrome (RLS). It may have a genetic basis, though iron deficiency, low folate levels, pregnancy, and other medical conditions can also bring it on. There's no treatment that works for everyone, so we've focused on those that bring relief for some.

Our BEST ADVICE

When RLS symptoms hit at night, try getting out of bed and walking around the house for 10 minutes to quiet the sensations in your legs. You might also try sitting on the edge of the bed and drawing circles with your toes.

WORKS FOR SOME

● **Getting more iron** Several very small studies suggest that correcting iron deficiency reduces symptoms and improves sleep. If you have RLS, ask your doctor to check your iron levels. You may need to take iron supplements under your doctor's supervision, or eat more iron-rich foods.

● **Changing your antidepressant** There's some evidence that RLS can start or become worse if you take a tricyclic antidepressant, a selective serotonin-reuptake inhibitor (SSRI), or lithium.

● **Avoiding caffeine, alcohol, and nicotine** There have been no well-designed studies of nondrug treatments for RLS, but experts at the University of Kentucky say that avoiding alcohol, caffeine, and nicotine may improve symptoms.

● **Getting enough folate** An analysis published in the journal *Alternative Medicine Review* suggests that for some people, low folate levels contribute to RLS and bringing levels of this B vitamin back to normal could help. You need about 400 micrograms of folate a day from foods like leafy greens, enriched rice, fortified cereals, lentils, and chickpeas. You can get there by having a half cup of lentils or pinto beans, a cup of cooked broccoli, and a cup of orange juice.

● **Ropinirole (Requip) and pramipexole (Mirapex)** In a review of seven clinical trials of the dopamine agonist Mirapex, researchers found that 60 percent of people with RLS reported their symptoms eased by 50 percent in the first three months—but so did 42 percent of study volunteers who got placebos. Studies of Requip also showed a benefit of both the drug and a placebo.

These widely advertised drugs can have strange side effects, including gambling, intense sexual urges, and binge eating. For one in four people, long-term use of Mirapex may worsen RLS symptoms. Side effects in the first month of use include nausea, dizziness, fatigue, and insomnia. ■

Snoring

In a quiet lab equipped with microphones, University of Minnesota scientists learned that men really are the loudest snorers—sometimes at a decibel level that exceeds federal noise regulations. Everything from blocked nasal passages to a deviated septum to congestion from a cold can cause nighttime snuffling and snurfling. But if your snoring is a sign of sleep apnea, when tissue in the back of your mouth or throat blocks your air passages over and over again while you sleep, you're at risk for a host of serious health problems, so don't ignore it.

WORKS

✔ **Weight loss** When University of Wisconsin Medical School researchers tracked 690 Wisconsin residents for four years, they found that whenever weight increased by 10 percent, sleep apnea got 32 percent worse. A 10 percent weight loss lessened apnea by 26 percent. Extremely overweight people who underwent surgical weight-loss procedures to drop 25 to 50 percent of their body weight saw a 70 to 98 percent drop in sleep apnea in one study.

Experts say weight loss can quiet garden-variety snoring as well because it shrinks flabby tissue in the throat.

✔ **Sleeping on your side or stomach** Having a silent night may be as simple as rolling onto your side or tummy. When you lie on your back, your tongue partially blocks your breathing and makes tissue in your throat vibrate. A change of position can also help about 50 percent of people with mild sleep apnea, say Israeli researchers. If you're a back sleeper, sew a pocket onto the back of your pajama top or a big T-shirt and put a tennis ball in it before you hit the sack.

✔ **Continuous positive airway pressure (CPAP)** The gold standard treatment for obstructive sleep apnea, CPAP uses a small air compressor to push air through a mask over the sleeper's nose. The pressure keeps airways open so you breathe normally all night. When researchers analyzed 36 CPAP studies involving people with sleep apnea, they found that those who used this system decreased daytime sleepiness by nearly 50 percent, cut sleep interruptions by eight per hour, and boosted the amount of oxygen in their blood significantly. Their blood pressure dropped to healthier levels, too. In a study at the National Jewish Medical and Research Center in Denver, people with sleep apnea who had memory problems saw memory improvement with CPAP. If you have diabetes and sleep apnea, CPAP could even improve your blood sugar control.

✔ **Oral appliances** Fitted by a specially trained dentist, these snore stoppers look like a cross between a plastic sports mouth guard and a kid's metal braces. They work by keeping your throat open at night, often by gently repositioning your lower jaw. While these appliances aren't quite as effective as CPAP, many people prefer them because they're less cumbersome. In a University of Toronto review of 115 studies of various types of "mouth hardware," researchers found that snoring was reduced by 45 percent.

Oral appliances are best for mild to moderate apnea and for loud snorers who don't have apnea, according to a review conducted by the American Academy of Sleep Medicine.

WORKS FOR SOME

● **Surgery** If CPAP and oral appliances don't work for your apnea, surgical removal of excess tissue from your nose or throat might. This tissue sags when you lie down and is responsible for the noise of snoring and the blockage of air passages. The most widely used technique, uvulopalatopharyngoplasty (UPPP), trims tissue from the rear of your mouth and top of your throat; tonsils and adenoids are usually whisked out at the same time. The catch: It doesn't help everyone. UPPP improves apnea for just 40 to 60 percent of those who have the procedure, say Israeli researchers who reviewed dozens of apnea studies—and it's impossible to predict who the lucky ones will be.

For extreme snoring caused by a deviated septum, two procedures, called submucous resection (SMR) and septoplasty, can help. Both involve removing some cartilage from this bony divider between your left and right nasal cavities. In one study from Thailand, septum surgery significantly quieted snoring for 28 out of 30 study participants.

● **Singing or playing a wind instrument**
When 20 chronic snorers performed 30 minutes a day of singing techniques that shaped up their throat muscles, their snoring quieted, report researchers from England's University of Exeter. Simply belting out show tunes in the shower probably won't do the trick; the exercises (such as energetically singing the sound "ung-gah" to familiar tunes) that seem to work are designed to build strength in muscles that support your soft palate, the tissue at the back of your mouth that vibrates if you snore. You can order the program at www.singingforsnorers.com.

If you're more of a "blowhard" than a singer, get out that old clarinet, flute, or tuba and honk away. When 25 snorers at a Swiss sleep clinic took up the didgeridoo, a breath-powered instrument that looks like a long, hollow tree branch, snoring lessened by about 22 percent.

● **Nose strips** Studies on these adhesive strips designed to open nasal passages have been mixed; one sponsored by the US Air Force concluded that they're ineffective, but a Swiss study found that they quieted snoring after about two weeks of use. If you tend to breathe through your mouth, the strips may work for you. Be ready to wear them at night for at least a week to get used to breathing through your nose. They may also help if you have a slightly deviated septum.

● **Lubricating sprays and snore-squelching pillows**
When 40 snorers tried these popular over-the-counter products, researchers at Wilford Hall USAF Medical Center in San Antonio concluded that neither one worked. But there are plenty of anecdotal reports that they do. Try them to see if they work for you. ■

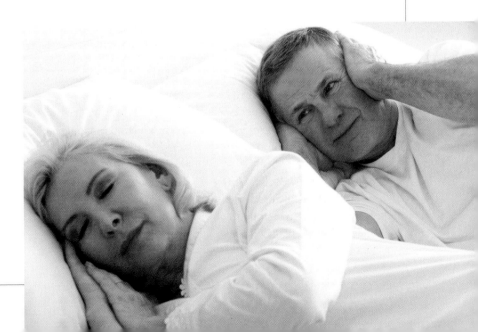

Ulcers

Ulcers and stress used to be as tightly linked as the chains in a friendship bracelet. That was before the discovery that most ulcers are caused by the bacterium *Helicobacter pylori*. That said, stress may make the lining of your gastrointestinal tract more vulnerable. Also, overdoing certain pain relievers certainly increases your risk. Before you start downing antacids like candy, talk to your doctor; you may need help from prescription meds.

WORKS

✔ **Proton-pump inhibitors (PPIs)** Drugs such as omeprazole (Prilosec), lansoprazole (Prevacid), and esomeprazole (Nexium) can heal ulcers and relieve symptoms such as burning and pain. They work by reducing the amount of acid your stomach produces.

One analysis of 32 trials found that these drugs healed all ulcers (stomach and intestinal) in more than 95 percent of patients within four weeks and stomach ulcers in 80 to 90 percent of patients at eight weeks. Another analysis of 24 trials found that they reduced the risk of bleeding after patients had already had a bleeding ulcer by 51 percent and the need for surgery following a bleeding ulcer by 39 percent.

Stick to four weeks of treatment; there's no evidence that using PPIs longer than that makes any difference.

✔ **Triple therapy** If you have an ulcer and are infected with *H. pylori*, you need to not only heal the ulcer but also get rid of the bacteria. That's where triple therapy comes in. Seven to 14 days of treatment with a PPI combined with the antibiotics clarithromycin and amoxicillin or metronidazole typically wipes out the bugs. Eradicating the bacteria slashes your risk of another intestinal ulcer from 67 to 6 percent and of getting another stomach ulcer from 59 to 4 percent.

✔ **H_2 blockers** These drugs, which include cimetidine (Tagamet), famotidine (Pepcid), and ranitidine (Zantac), work by blocking the production of stomach acid—but proton-pump inhibitors work better. H_2 blockers, on the other hand, are cheaper. Since H_2 blockers work differently, doctors sometimes prescribe one of these drugs along with a PPI.

DON'T BOTHER

✖ **Garlic** There is some evidence that garlic supplements can keep *H. pylori* under control, but it won't get rid of the bacteria, according to studies.

✖ **Following a bland diet** Milk and cottage cheese won't do diddly for your ulcer. In fact, milk appears to increase stomach acid. Meanwhile, there's some evidence that spicy ingredients like hot peppers can help eradicate or at least damp down *H. pylori*. (If they irritate your ulcer, of course, avoid them.)

✖ **Probiotics** These "good" bacteria, found in yogurt with active cultures and sold as supplements, won't heal or prevent ulcers, according to an analysis of nine studies. They can, however, reduce the risk of diarrhea associated with the use of antibiotics. ∎

Our BEST ADVICE

Go easy on the aspirin, ibuprofen, and naproxen. Overuse of these drugs, along with *H. pylori* infection, is a leading cause of ulcers. If you must take a painkiller regularly, talk to your doctor about also taking a proton-pump inhibitor, which reduces the risk of ulcers when taking these drugs.

Urinary Tract Infections

Half of all women get at least one urinary tract infection (UTI). Everything from frequent sexual intercourse to declining estrogen levels after age 55 may be factors; some research even suggests that women with the blood types AB and B may be at higher risk. Researchers haven't solved the mystery of why some women never get a UTI and others get many, but they know how to cure a raging UTI—and how to cut your risk of getting another one.

WORKS

✔ **Antibiotics** At the first sign of a UTI, such as a burning sensation during urination and the need to go more often, head to the doctor, who will probably prescribe an antibiotic. Three days of treatment with trimethoprim-sulfamethoxazole (Bactrim or Septra) cures 94 percent of UTIs—and is just as effective as five or more days of treatment, say Israeli researchers. Longer courses of antibiotics doubled the risk of side effects such as yeast infections.

Unfortunately, the bacteria that cause UTIs are becoming resistant to these drugs. If you've been treated for a UTI in the past six months, or you live in an area where drug-resistant UTIs are rampant, your doctor may prescribe a different, possibly stronger, antibiotic. Some strong antibiotics, such as ciprofloxacin (Cipro), are quite effective with just a single dose.

✔ **Cranberry juice** The tart, tangy juice contains compounds that prevent bacteria from attaching to the wall of the bladder or urethra. In one review of cranberry studies, women who drank cranberry juice or took cranberry extract tablets daily for 12 months cut their risk of repeat UTIs by 39 percent. Various studies have used 6 to 25 ounces of juice a day, but in one study, people who drank 10 ounces of cranberry juice cocktail daily for six months cut their risk of infection in half. We recommend unsweetened cranberry juice, though, mixed with seltzer if you can't drink it straight.

✔ **Vitamin C** When pregnant women took daily vitamin supplements either with or without 100 milligrams of ascorbic acid (vitamin C) for three months, those in the ascorbic acid group had half as many UTIs as those in the other group. Ascorbic acid may help by making urine more acidic and less hospitable to bacteria.

✔ **Yogurt with active cultures** Finnish women who ate fermented milk products such as yogurt three or more times a week had an 80 percent lower risk of UTIs than those who ate them less than once a week, reported researchers from Finland's University of Oulu. The beneficial bacteria in yogurt with active cultures may prevent the overgrowth of the "bad" bacteria that cause UTIs.

Not a yogurt fan? Try a probiotic ("good" bacteria) supplement. A Greek review found that the bacterial strains *Lactobacillus rhamnosus* GR-1, *L. reuteri* RC-14, *L. casei shirota*, and *L. crispatus* CTV-05 all seem to help.

Varicose Veins

Inside your leg veins, tiny valves prevent blood from flowing backward. But if you've inherited a tendency for weak valves, are on your feet most of the day, or have had several pregnancies, these little gates can malfunction, allowing blood to pool. The result: Twisted, bulging veins—and tired, achy, itchy, swollen legs. At best, varicose veins are a cosmetic problem. At worst, they can lead to inflammation and even ulcers if the skin near a vein is deprived of blood. If you have a parent with varicose veins, your odds of developing them are five times the average. While you can't trade in your genes, there's plenty else you can do.

WORKS

✔ **Compression stockings plus simple exercises** Elastic compression stockings gently squeeze your legs so blood can't move backward. The result? Less aching and swelling. When Japanese researchers measured the legs of 20 people with varicose veins, they found that all grades of compression stockings (from light to strong pressure) reduced swelling but that medium and strong-grade stockings worked best. These are stockings labeled "22 mmHg" or "30–40 mmHg."

Compression stockings aren't perfect, though. When stocking-clad volunteers in a Hong Kong study changed position—from sitting to standing to rising on their toes—pressure at various points along their legs rose and fell. Often the scientists found a serious design flaw: Pressure at the calves was higher than at the ankles, even though the opposite should be true to encourage blood to move toward the heart.

Their conclusion: Compression stockings are worth wearing if you're on your feet for hours every day, but don't forget to do simple lower-leg exercises designed to help pump blood through these thin veins. These include rising on your toes several times an hour, shifting your weight from one foot to the other, bending your legs, flexing your ankles, and walking in place.

✔ **Horse chestnut seed extract** When Harvard Medical School doctors reviewed 16 well-designed studies of 11,776 people with chronic venous insufficiency—the "weak veins" that lead to varicose veins—they found that those who took this herbal extract had four times less pain than those who took placebos. Half saw a decrease in swelling, and 70 percent had less itching. They also reported improvement in feelings of fatigue and heaviness in their legs. Meanwhile, British researchers who reviewed seven horse chestnut studies concluded that this botanical might be as effective as compression stockings.

Horse chestnut seeds contain the compound escin, which is said to strengthen capillary walls. In lab studies, it has improved pressure and blood flow in veins. A typical dose is one 300-milligram tablet twice a day.

✔ **Flavonoids** These antioxidant compounds derived from fruits, vegetables, and seeds have been shown to reduce the swelling associated with varicose veins. Flavonoids come in a variety of types with curious names like rutin, hesperidin, diosmin, and oligomeric proanthocyanidin complexes (OPCs). In one German study of 133 women with chronic venous insufficiency, those who took a form of rutin called oxerutin had twice the reduction in leg swelling compared to those who took a placebo. Benefits continued for six weeks after treatment ended.

✔ A daily glass of wine

Spanish researchers who analyzed the health records of 1,778 people found that those who enjoyed a glass of wine a day had a 50 percent lower risk of varicose veins than those who drank less—or more. Other research suggests that flavonoids and saponins in wine can help keep blood vessels flexible and healthy.

✔ Getting off your feet

When researchers at Finland's Tampere University Hospital asked thousands of people with varicose veins about their daily lives, they found that having a job that keeps you on your feet for long periods of time increased the risk of bulging veins by 60 percent. If you have a stand-up occupation, such as teaching or retail sales, sit down when you can take a break and be sure to elevate your feet.

✔ Surgery

The most common varicose vein surgery is called ligation and stripping—tying off a big vein and then pulling it out. In one study of 100 people, published in the *Annals of the Royal College of Surgeons of England*, 90 percent said their legs were "much better" or "cured" a few months after the surgery. Ten years later, 60 percent said their legs still felt or looked better. But surgery is no cure-all. When

Our BEST ADVICE

Guys: Stop straining in the loo. University of Edinburgh researchers found that straining to have a bowel movement raises the risk of vein problems by 94 percent for men (but not for women). Straining puts pressure on veins in the lower legs. Eat enough fiber and drink enough fluids, and you should have less of a challenge.

Italian researchers followed varicose vein surgery patients for 10 years, 30 percent said their vein problems returned within 5 years, and 40 percent saw a recurrence within a decade. There are risks, too: The odds of nerve damage can be as high as 1 in 10.

WORKS FOR SOME

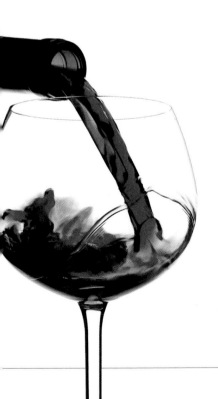

● Sclerotherapy for small and medium-size veins

Injections of saline or a newer foaming agent irritate the lining of the vein, eventually creating scars that close off veins. Experts at the Cleveland Clinic report that the procedure works about 90 percent of the time, but studies from England and Italy suggest that varicose veins can return up to 50 percent of the time. The procedure seems to work best for small to medium-size veins. Spider veins may fade in three to six weeks, and bigger veins within four months.

● Radiofrequency and laser surgery

In these procedures, performed under local anesthesia, strong pulses of light or radio waves (delivered through a catheter inserted through tiny incisions) make the vein fade and disappear. The downside? You may need repeat therapies to keep varicose veins at bay. Like foam sclerotherapy, these high-tech surgeries haven't yet been analyzed in long-term studies. ■

Warts

No, you can't catch a wart from a toad. The unsightly growths, caused by the human papillomavirus, appear mysteriously—and disappear just as mysteriously, often regardless of what you've used to treat them. In fact, warts are notoriously susceptible to the placebo effect; if you believe a treatment may rid you of a wart, there's a decent chance it will. Otherwise, treatments can be maddeningly hit or miss. And all too often, warts reappear, even if you've had them treated in the doctor's office—so take our "Works" recommendations with a grain of salt.

WORKS

✔ **Salicylic acid** The active ingredient in over-the-counter wart remedies and patches, salicylic acid works by peeling off infected skin. It causes mild irritation that may also help by mobilizing your immune system to fight off viral invaders in the area. In one review of 13 well-designed studies, salicylic acid cured 75 percent of warts. But be patient—it may take weeks or months to banish a wart (by which time the wart may have actually healed itself). And be sure to follow the directions. For best results, soak your wart in warm water first, then rub away dead skin with an emery board before applying the remedy each time.

✔ **Freezing (cryotherapy or liquid nitrogen therapy)** You'll need to see a doctor for these therapies. Liquid nitrogen destroys a wart by prompting a blister to form around it. After about a week, the whole thing sloughs off. But you may need multiple treatments to see results. In one study of 225 people, it took 12 treatments to get a "cure rate" of just 45 percent. Other studies suggest that salicylic acid is just as effective as standard cryotherapy. Freezing is painful and isn't recommended for kids.

✔ **Garlic extract** Compounds in garlic have been shown in lab studies to fight viruses and stop them from replicating inside infected cells. Could this kitchen herb knock out warts? In one placebo-controlled trial, garlic extract dabbed daily on warts "cured" them in three to four months.

✔ **Duct tape** In 2002, a headline-grabbing study found that duct tape knocked out more warts than cryotherapy. Volunteers in the duct tape group stuck wart-size pieces of the tape over their warts and left them in place for six days, then removed them, soaked the warts, and scrubbed off the dead skin with an emery board or pumice stone. The warts were left uncovered overnight, then the cycle was repeated. After repeating these steps for two months, warts were gone for 85 percent of the duct tape group compared to 60 percent of the cryotherapy group.

A more recent study, however, found much less benefit from "duct tape therapy," though it could be because the researchers used clear duct tape, not the standard gray type. The gray kind contains rubber, while the clear kind doesn't.

DON'T BOTHER

✖ **Curretage and cautery** Surgically removing warts, then burning the skin, has a 65 to 85 percent success rate, but it's painful and causes scars. On top of that, 30 percent of warts return anyway. ∎

Yeast Infections

At the first telltale signs of a yeast infection, you know what's coming—and you want relief fast. Don't bother heading to the drugstore unless you're *certain* it's a yeast infection. Instead, head to your doctor for a diagnosis and a prescription. If you get frequent yeast infections, look to the root causes, which include taking antibiotics (these kill the beneficial bacteria in the vagina, allowing fungi to get a foothold), corticosteroids, and birth control pills; using spermicidal creams; and oral sex.

Our BEST ADVICE

Think you have a yeast infection? Don't be so sure. Other common triggers of vaginal itching and discharge are bacterial infection and trichomoniasis (caused by a parasite). Each requires different treatment. Self-treatment without an accurate diagnosis could be a waste of time and money.

If you do self-treat with an over-the-counter antifungal, see your doctor if your symptoms don't improve with one course of treatment.

WORKS

✔ **Antifungals** Most antifungals come as creams or inserts sold over the counter, but the one that works best for yeast infections is a prescription pill that you swallow. A single dose of fluconazole (Diflucan) works as well as a vaginal cream or insert used for one to three days, improving symptoms and wiping out the fungi in 80 to 90 percent of women.

If you get four or more infections a year, using the antifungal for six months after the initial infection can help prevent additional infections. One major study found that women who took a weekly dose of fluconazole for six months after treating their initial infections with three oral doses of fluconazole, 72 hours apart, were half as likely to have recurrences in the year following the initial infection as women who didn't take the maintenance therapy. It took an average of 10 months before they had another yeast infection compared to 4 months in the control group.

If you get frequent yeast infections, ask your doctor whether you should take a prescription antifungal to prevent an infection when you have to take an antibiotic.

WORKS FOR SOME

● **Probiotics** Taking these "good" bacteria (also found in yogurt with active cultures) helps restore healthy levels in the vagina and may help prevent recurrent yeast infections. Some women use these supplements whenever they're taking an antibiotic. But studies are mixed on their benefits, and most are poorly designed. Still, there's enough evidence that they may help—with few if any side effects—to make them worth a try. Not any probiotic will do (there are thousands). For yeast infections, stick with *Lactobacillus rhamnosus* GR-1, *L. acidophilus*, or *L. fermentum* RC-14.

DON'T BOTHER

✘ **Cutting out sugar** Many women believe this will help prevent yeast infections. While cutting down on sugar is a good idea for many reasons, there's no good evidence that diet contributes to yeast infections. ■

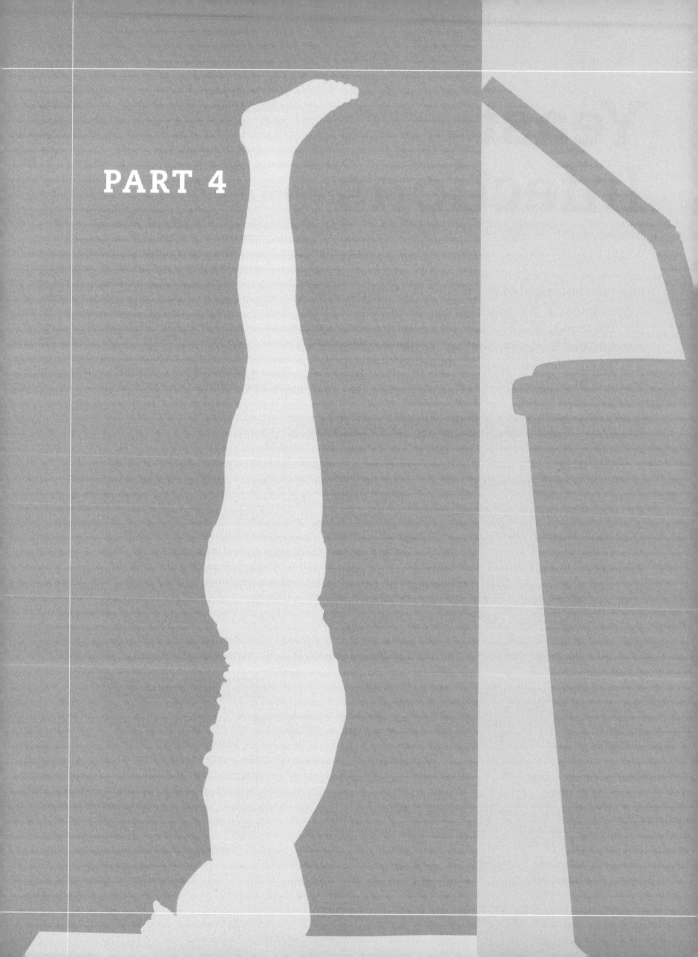

PART 4

is it safe

or dangerous?

ACUPUNCTURE

Acupuncture

Doctors have been debating for years whether acupuncture really works. But you may have a far more immediate concern: Is it safe to let someone stick needles in my flesh? Acupuncture needles are hair-thin, far finer than the hypodermic needles doctors prick you with. Still, they may plunge a few centimeters beneath the skin into nerves, muscle, and other sensitive tissue. That's cause for a few "pointed" questions about acupuncture.

Can acupuncture hurt?

YES You may barely notice the needles being inserted, but some patients say the procedure leaves them in pain later on.

Acupuncturists say that patients usually feel nothing more than mild pinpricks, if anything, as needles are inserted. Since the needles can stimulate nerves, the patient may also feel a dull ache. Otherwise, the procedure is relatively painless, acupuncturists insist. In one survey, practitioners of this ancient art reported just three instances out of nearly 32,000 consultations in which needle sticks caused lingering pain.

Patients tell another story. A second survey by the same researchers found that about one of nine acupuncture patients said they felt pain at the site of a needle insertion during or after the procedure, though the discomfort

eventually faded. It's important to note, however, that an even greater number of patients said they felt "energized" or "relaxed" after their acupuncture sessions, and most said they would return for further treatments.

Aside from pain, is acupuncture risky?

NO Like virtually any other medical treatment, acupuncture can have side effects, but serious complications are rare.

Researchers polled nearly 2,000 acupuncturists about more than 34,000 acupuncture treatments they performed over a one-month period and turned up no reports of major problems. Infections from poorly sanitized needles, once a concern, have become uncommon thanks to the widespread use of disposable needles. Even minor complaints tend to be rare. Less than 1 percent of patients

bleed or become nauseated during treatments, for example. One study found that nearly one in four patients felt drowsy or tired afterward, though, so it may be wise to have a friend drive you home, at least until you find out how acupuncture affects you.

One extremely rare but serious complication is a form of collapsed lung called pneumothorax, which can happen if needles are inserted in certain parts of the chest. A collapsed lung causes shortness of breath and chest pain and can be fatal in very rare cases. One review found just nine cases of pneuomothorax caused by acupuncture reported over a 20-year period. ■

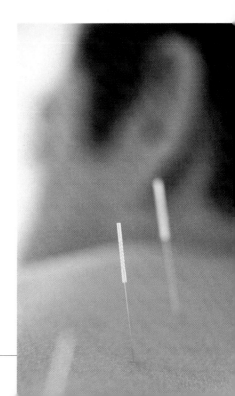

Anesthesia

Anesthesia has come a long way since the days when surgery patients were given a swig of whiskey and a bullet to bite. But the drugs used today to induce the deep sleep of general anesthesia also alter your breathing, blood pressure, and other body functions, so it's no surprise that they can cause side effects. What's more, anesthesiologists may provide the wrong dose or fail to take necessary actions when a patient has a bad reaction.

Can anesthesia make me sick—or worse?

YES The drugs used to induce unconsciousness and relax muscles for surgery may cause side effects, though they are usually minor.

A Canadian study of nearly 113,000 surgery patients found that about 1 in 10 experienced aftereffects from anesthesia. The most common problems were nausea, vomiting, and sore throat. Only a tiny portion of those complaints—less than half of 1 percent—were serious. Surgery patients do die from anesthesia, but that probably occurs in fewer than 1 in 10,000 operations.

Is it possible to "wake up" in the middle of surgery?

YES One or two patients regain consciousness during surgery per 1,000 surgeries.

It has become fodder for Hollywood filmmakers and talk show hosts: A patient wakes up during surgery but is unable to speak or let anyone know that the anesthesia has failed. About half the time, these patients later report that they could hear sounds during the surgery, such as doctors and nurses talking. One of four "anesthesia awareness" patients feel the pain of scalpels cutting their flesh or tubes being inserted down their throats, according to a study by Emory University anesthesiologist Peter S. Sebel, MD, and his colleagues.

It's important to note that anesthesia awareness is rare. Dr. Sebel estimates that about 26,000 patients in the United States experience the phenomenon, but more than *20 million* people undergo general anesthesia. The problem usually arises when a patient receives too little anesthesia, due to an error by the anesthesiologist or equipment failure. Patients are more likely to become aware during certain procedures, including cardiac surgery, that

may require lower doses of anesthesia or while being treated for trauma, since it's harder to deliver the right dose of anesthetic during emergency surgery.

While only a minority of patients who experience anesthesia awareness feel physical pain, the memory of being awake during surgery can leave emotional scars. Two years later, about half of patients have symptoms of post-traumatic stress disorder, which can include flashbacks and recurring nightmares. ∎

ANTIBIOTICS

Antibiotics

Once upon a time, a simple infection could rob you of life or limb. Today doctors can turn to more than 100 antibiotics that are capable of quashing bacteria of all sorts. Unfortunately, we've used these drugs so much that the germs are adapting; some are now "immune" to the drugs' effects. Meanwhile, taking antibiotics may not always be the smartest course of action for you.

Should you take antibiotics for colds or flu?

NO It won't help, could make you sicker, and contributes to a public health crisis.

The common cold and the flu are caused by viruses. Antibiotics kill bacteria; they are useless against viruses. Taking antibiotics will not relieve cold or flu symptoms nor will it shorten the time you spend feeling sick.

In fact, taking antibiotics may make you feel sicker. A review of six studies compared cold sufferers who took antibiotics with others who did not. Not only did the review show that taking antibiotics was no help, but adults who took the drugs were two to three times more likely to have upset stomachs and diarrhea than those who didn't.

Worse, the overuse of antibiotics adds to the growing problem of antibiotic resistance, in which germs develop ways to escape the effects of the drugs. Studies have shown, for instance, that children in communities where doctors prescribe the most antibiotics are most likely to test positive for pneumonia germs that are resistant to penicillin.

Can antibiotics cause yeast infections?

YES These germ killers may wipe out "good" bacteria, making women more vulnerable to uncomfortable infections.

Taking antibiotics clears up infections, but the cure may come at a cost. These infection fighters seek and destroy bacteria, but they don't discriminate. Unfortunately, antibiotics can kill beneficial bacteria, like those in the vagina that normally control the population of *Candida albicans*, a fungus that causes yeast infections.

Many other factors may promote an overgrowth of yeast in the vagina, such as douching, birth control pills,

diabetes, pregnancy, and even stress. However, doctors have known since the 1950s that women who take antibiotics are at risk for yeast infections, which can lead to burning, itching, pain during intercourse, and a white discharge. The magnitude of the risk was unknown until recently.

In a 2006 Australian study, researchers studied 233 women who had received prescriptions for antibiotics. At the outset, 21 percent tested positive for *Candida*. After each woman completed the course of antibiotics, that number jumped to 37 percent. This study's authors suggest that women who are prone to yeast infections and have to take antibiotics may avoid this uncomfortable condition by taking an antifungal medication at the same time. ■

Antidepressants

The story of antidepressant medications begins in the 1950s, when doctors noticed that the moods of patients undergoing treatment with experimental tuberculosis drugs seemed to brighten. Inspired by this discovery, scientists developed drugs that helped relieve depression but had a long list of unpleasant side effects. The introduction of Prozac and other newer antidepressants reduced the problem of side effects, but controversy has nonetheless haunted this new generation of mood enhancers.

Do antidepressants *cause* more suicides than they prevent?

NO Despite the scary headlines, many experts believe that the benefits of antidepressants far outweigh the risks.

It seems like the cruelest of ironies: Some research suggests that medications meant to lift mood and erase despair may make people *more* likely to commit the ultimate act of hopelessness. Concerns that antidepressants make people suicidal emerged in the 1980s, when Prozac (fluoxetine) and other similar drugs first became available. The threat appeared to be greatest among children and teens taking the drugs.

At first, the concerns were based largely on anecdotal reports, including several high-profile incidents in which youths for whom the drugs were prescribed began acting strangely before taking their own lives. Then, in 2004, the FDA looked at 25 studies and determined that antidepressants double the risk of suicidal thinking in children under 18 who suffer from depression.

Skeptics have pointed out that the FDA focused largely on suicidal *thoughts*, which are common among teens (about one in five think about suicide in a given year). In fact, none of the young people studied actually killed themselves. Few even attempted suicide.

Other research contradicts the theory that antidepressants make people suicidal. For instance, a 2007 review of 27 studies found no significant increased risk of suicide among young people taking antidepressants. On the contrary, University of Illinois biostatistician Robert D. Gibbons, PhD, and his colleagues have shown that the suicide rate dropped 13 percent in the United States during the 1980s and 1990s as the number of people taking antidepressants increased fourfold. When concerns about young people harming themselves led doctors in the Netherlands to cut back on prescribing Prozac and similar antidepressants by 22 percent, the suicide rate among youths *rose* by nearly 50 percent. These studies suggest that far from causing people to harm themselves, antidepressants help to prevent the leading cause of suicide: untreated depression. ∎

Far from causing people to harm themselves, antidepressants help to prevent untreated depression—the leading cause of suicide.

Artificial Sweeteners

If you're watching your weight, you can potentially slash hundreds of calories a day just by switching from regular soda to diet. But is it a devil's bargain? Saccharin (better known as Sweet'n Low) was the first artificial sweetener on the market, invented back in 1879. Later it gained notoriety for reportedly causing cancer in lab animals. Today the reputation of artificial sweeteners has been rehabilitated—mostly.

Does saccharin cause cancer?

NO There is little solid evidence that artificially sweetened foods and beverages increase the risk of cancer in humans.

If you hesitate before sipping a diet soft drink or downing a container of calorie-free yogurt, relax: Most research suggests there's no harm in eating artificially sweetened foods in moderation. Not that anyone would blame you for worrying.

Way back in 1911, a board of US scientists declared the sugar stand-in to be an "adulterant" that should be banned from foods. Later, studies in the early 1970s showed that laboratory rats fed saccharin developed bladder cancer. Canada banned saccharin, while the United States and other countries required warning labels on products containing it.

Experts immediately spotted problems with the scary studies, however. Not only were the rats fed ultra-high doses of saccharin, but scientists pointed out that rodents process the sweetener in a unique way that makes their urine contain cancer-causing chemicals. The same process does *not* occur in humans. What's more, rates of bladder cancer did not rise during or after World War II, when saccharin was widely used. Nor was there any evidence that bladder cancer was more common among people with diabetes, who presumably consumed more of the sweetener. The United States no longer requires warning labels on products that contain saccharin.

Does aspartame cause brain cancer?

NO These concerns have been dismissed.

Just when it seemed safe to slurp diet soda again, questions arose about an artificial sweetener introduced in 1981, aspartame (sold as NutraSweet and Equal). In 1996, a group of scientists published a controversial paper showing that the rate of brain cancer had risen in the United States and several other industrialized countries since 1980,

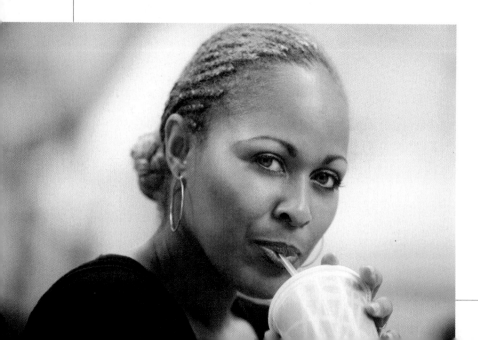

suggesting that the growing use of aspartame in foods and beverages might be to blame.

However, critics pointed out, by the same logic, you could also blame the rising tide of brain cancer on personal computers, VCRs, rap music, and just about any other phenomenon that flourished during the 1980s and 1990s. Several studies, including one by the US National Cancer Institute involving nearly a half million men and women, found no connection between aspartame and brain cancer. The validity of studies linking aspartame to leukemia and lymphoma in rats has been contradicted by other research, too.

Don't take this news as an excuse to guzzle diet soda all day, though. Studies suggest that consuming very large amounts of artificial sweeteners—the equivalent of 9 or 10 cans of aspartame-sweetened soda per day—may modestly increase the risk of cancer. Several newer artificial sweeteners have been introduced in recent years, including sucralose (Splenda), acesulfame-K, and neotame. Studies in animals and humans haven't linked these products to cancer, though longer-term studies in large groups of people are needed to know for sure.

Are sugar substitutes completely safe?

NO Some people should avoid foods that contain aspartame, while overindulging in certain sugar replacements may disrupt your digestion.

People with a rare condition called phenylketonuria (PKU) should avoid aspartame, since it raises levels of an amino acid called phenylalanine. People with PKU lack an enzyme needed to break down phenylalanine, so consuming too much aspartame could be toxic.

Other potential health threats are sugar alcohols such as sorbitol, which are used to turn cookies, cakes, and other fattening foods into diet-safe splurges. Sugar alcohols (which are neither sugar nor alcohol) aren't technically artificial sweeteners; they're produced by tinkering with the chemical structure of starch and other carbohydrates. Consuming too much sugar alcohol—especially mannitol and sorbitol—can send your tummy for a tumble, causing bloating and diarrhea. Doctors have reported cases of people who chew sorbitol-sweetened gum all day and develop chronic diarrhea and lose up to 20 percent of their body weight. (The problems clear up when patients stop chewing the gum.)

Another reason to go easy: Unlike artificial sweeteners, sugar alcohols are not entirely calorie-free; they provide about two calories per gram, so overindulging can pad your hips.

Do artificial sweeteners make you fat?

NO According to one theory, sugar substitutes cause you to overeat. However, studies in humans show that weight loss is more likely.

Based on research in lab animals, scientists theorized that artificially sweetened foods fail to damp the appetite; in fact, they "train" the brain to perceive all sweet-tasting foods and drinks as calorie-free, leading you to overindulge. No one knows if it's true in humans—and maybe it doesn't matter, because studies show that people who replace sugary foods and beverages with artificially sweetened products lose weight.

Don't expect to shrink from a size 10 to a 2 by sipping diet cola, however. A 2006 review of 24 studies estimated that replacing sugary foods with similar products sweetened with aspartame would result in a loss of slightly less than a half pound per week—still nothing to sneeze at.

Other studies show that choosing artificially sweetened foods over a long period may help stave off the return of lost pounds. Over a three-year period, one trial showed that dieters who ate and drank products sweetened with aspartame regained less than half as much weight as a similar group who avoided the fake stuff. ■

Barbecued Meat

Scientists really know how to chill the thrill of the grill. The biggest concern about barbecuing used to be that your crazy uncle Eddie would get careless with the lighter fluid and set his eyebrows on fire. However, recent research has revealed that eating too much meat cooked at high temperatures—even skinless chicken breasts or slabs of salmon—may be a recipe for health problems.

Does eating barbecued meat increase the risk of cancer?

YES Eating barbecued steaks, hot dogs, and other meats appears to increase the risk of several cancers.

The bad news for barbecue fans comes from lab and population studies. First, chemists discovered that cooking most types of beef, pork, poultry, and fish at high temperatures—such as when you grill or pan-fry—produces compounds called heterocyclic amines (HCAs) and polycyclic aromatic hydrocarbons (PAHs). Both cause cancer in lab animals. Grilling or pan-frying meat until it's well done produces large amounts of these compounds; roasting, stewing, braising, and other low-temperature cooking methods produce far smaller amounts. (Unfortunately, gravy made from pan drippings is also high in HCAs.)

The National Cancer Institute found that people who prefer their meat medium-well or well done are three times more likely to develop stomach cancer than those who like their steaks and chops rare or medium-rare. A recent study showed that postmenopausal women who had consumed the most grilled or smoked meat over their lifetimes had a 47 percent increased risk of breast cancer. Other research has linked an appetite for barbecued meat to high risk of colon and pancreatic cancers. ■

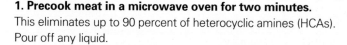

KEEP THE FIRES BURNING

Following a few simple rules can slash your intake of cancer-causing compounds.

1. Precook meat in a microwave oven for two minutes. This eliminates up to 90 percent of heterocyclic amines (HCAs). Pour off any liquid.

2. Prevent flare-ups. Avoid grilling meat directly over hot coals or flames. Form the charcoal in a ring around the edges of the grill and cook the meat in the center. Using a gas grill? Get one with two burners and cook food between them. Trimming excess fat helps, too.

3. Marinate meat before grilling. Marinating meat for a few hours can cut HCAs by up to 90 percent. Use a marinade that contains an acidic ingredient, such as vinegar or citrus juice.

4. Eat your meat rare or medium-rare. Longer cooking times produce more cancer-causing compounds.

5. Get out the skewers. Small cuts of beef, such as those used for kebabs, require brief cooking times.

6. Flip burgers frequently. This seems to prevent the formation of HCAs.

Blood Transfusions

If you are in a serious accident or require major surgery, there is a good chance you will need a blood transfusion. Donor blood saves lives, but receiving a transfusion carries risks. Patients may have reactions, ranging from itching and fever to hives and nausea, to blood that's not their own. But the most worrisome threat may be what's in the blood that shouldn't be.

Is there a significant risk of getting infected?

NO Thanks to improvements in methods for screening donors and blood, the risk of infection from transfusions is tiny.

News reports of people who developed exotic and terrifying conditions such as West Nile and mad cow disease after receiving transfusions have called attention to the problem of tainted blood. It will never be possible to safeguard the blood supply against all infectious diseases that emerge, but there's comfort in knowing that scientists are able to respond to new threats rapidly by developing effective screening tests.

For example, scientists discovered in 2002 that West Nile virus can be transmitted through blood transfusions. (The disease may cause a range of symptoms, from headaches and fatigue to high fever and convulsions.) That year, at least 23 people in the United States developed West Nile disease after receiving transfusions of infected blood. Within a year, blood centers were able to test for the virus, and the reported number of people infected through transfusions dropped to 6. By 2005, there were none.

What's more, rigorous screening of donors and superior testing methods have dramatically reduced the threat to the blood supply from more common infectious diseases over the past two decades. For instance, the risk of receiving blood infected with human immunodeficiency virus (HIV) or hepatitis C is roughly 1 in 2,000,000. (The odds of being struck by lightning in a given year are about 1 in 700,000.)

There's also little danger of acquiring cancer from donated blood. A 2007 study by Swedish researchers showed about 3 percent of blood donations come from people who have undetected cancer. However, recipients of their blood do not have an increased risk for any form of the disease. ∎

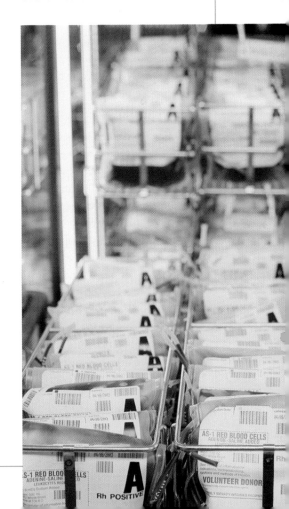

BREAST IMPLANTS

Breast Implants

Women have been going under the knife to get bigger breasts for over a century. The surgery has always carried the risk of complications, but in the 1990s, concerns arose that the implants themselves were making women sick. The ensuing controversy caused fear, confusion, and heated debate. In the end, plenty of women proceeded with breast augmentation, which remains one of the most common forms of cosmetic surgery.

Do breast implants cause any disease or illness?

NO The courts may have found breast implants guilty, but there is practically no evidence that they pose a health threat.

The purported hazards of silicone breast implants were one of the hottest medical news stories of the 1990s. Alarming headlines told of women who believed that their ruptured implants had caused silicone to spill into their bodies and make them sick. Women complained of many different illnesses, but the most common conditions attributed to leaky implants were connective tissue diseases such as rheumatoid arthritis, lupus, and scleroderma.

No one ever doubted that these women were ill, but overwhelming evidence shows that implants were not to blame.

First, what's not in dispute: Breast implants rupture. After five years, up to 10 percent of them spring a leak, and the risk continues to rise over time. Escaped silicone can cause the implant to lose shape and may form lumps or knots around the breast or in the armpit. In some cases, the leak may cause tingling or burning. Nor is there any question that breast implants carry risks. Scar tissue can form around the implant, which can cause the breast to become hard, deformed, and even painful. Some women lose sensation in the nipples.

There is no evidence, however, that breast implants cause connective tissue diseases or any other major disease. In a study published in the *New England Journal of Medicine*, doctors from the Mayo Clinic in Rochester, Minnesota, found that women with implants had about the same risk as other women of developing rheumatoid arthritis, lupus, and a long list of other autoimmune diseases. In fact, there have been at least 17 studies showing that women with breast implants do not have an increased risk of connective tissue diseases, according to a 2000 report by the Institute of Medicine. The same report determined that breast implants do not cause any form of cancer.

Can breast implants interfere with mammograms?

YES But women with breast implants aren't more likely to end up with advanced breast cancer, though no one is sure why.

A breast implant shows up as a solid white mass on a mammogram, so it may block the view of up to half of the breast tissue, depending on where it's positioned. (Implants placed in

There is no evidence that breast implants cause any major disease.

front of the chest muscle block more of a mammogram than implants placed beneath the muscle.) Both silicone and saline breast implants pose this problem. A study published in the *Journal of the American Medical Association* by researchers in Seattle found that mammograms missed 55 percent of breast tumors in women with implants, compared to 33 percent in women without them.

As a result, you might expect breast cancer to be more advanced when it's finally discovered in women with implants. Yet the Seattle study found that was not the case. Their tumors were no more dangerous than those in women without implants.

There are several possible explanations. It may be that women with implants have less of their own breast tissue to check during self-exams, so they check more thoroughly, or that the implant acts as a firm surface to press against, making it easier to feel anything unusual. Also, doctors instruct women to check their implants frequently, so they may be more likely to find lumps. Whatever the case, all women with implants should follow standard recommendations for undergoing mammograms. Try to find a clinic where the technicians and radiologists have experience producing and evaluating mammograms of women who have implants. ∎

Bug Spray

To DEET or not to DEET? That's the question facing gardeners, hikers, and anyone else wanting protection from mosquitoes, some of which carry disease. There's little question that this chemical is more effective than any other form of insect repellent, but some people avoid it as if it were Agent Orange, convinced that it's toxic to humans.

Is DEET a health threat?

NO When used properly, this popular insect repellent is safe and effective.

Mosquitoes and other bugs track down humans through their antennae, but scientists believe DEET jams the signal. It's no wonder that short of holing up indoors, the best defense against bugs is to wear the right clothes (such as long-sleeved shirts and long pants) and apply an insect repellent that contains the chemical.

Concerns about DEET surfaced in 1989, when public health officials in New York reported that four children and an adult had seizures after using insect repellent containing it, though all five recovered. Other research has suggested that exposure to the chemical lowers sperm count. Some studies have shown that laboratory rats exposed to it suffer brain damage.

Many people today refuse to use DEET on themselves or their children, but fear of this

Our BEST ADVICE

Beware of "natural" insect repellents, which may wear off long before you're done enjoying the outdoors. A study published in the *New England Journal of Medicine* found that most bug sprays containing botanical ingredients such as citronella, lemongrass oil, peppermint oil, and others protected against mosquito bites for only about 20 minutes. One product, made with soybean oil, repelled bugs for about 90 minutes. However, that paled in comparison to a DEET-based spray, Deep Woods Off, which lasted for five hours. (A caveat: Wristbands containing DEET were worthless.)

Bug Spray
(continued)

bug beater appears to be misguided. University of Toronto researchers combed the medical literature for reports of children who had seizures after having DEET-based insect repellent applied to their skin. They found just 10 cases over a 50-year period, and none after 1992. However, millions of children are slathered with insect repellent each summer. What's more, seizures are relatively common in kids; 3 to 5 percent experience one each year. In other words, if a child has a seizure after having bug spray applied, it could be a coincidence.

The same study determined that DEET poses no threat to pregnant or nursing women. Several other groups of researchers have found that the repellent carries a low risk of causing other health problems (including low sperm count). However, these studies emphasize that DEET is safe when users follow label instructions. Most critical: Keep DEET away from the eyes and especially the mouth; there's no question that *ingesting* large amounts can cause seizures and may be fatal. ■

Cell Phones

Cancer scares come and go, but this one seemed to ring true. After all, who was surprised to hear that placing a radiation-emitting device next to your noggin several times a day might cause brain tumors? While scientists have debated the purported link between cell phones and disease, lawmakers in some countries have taken steps to keep one particular group—motorists—from talking themselves into trouble.

Is it likely that cell phones cause cancer?

NO Most studies suggest that cell phones don't cause brain cancer or any other type. But stay on the line; the signals about long-term use are fuzzy.

Worries that talking on a cell phone increases the risk of brain cancer emerged in the early 1990s when several high-profile lawsuits claimed these wireless wonders caused the disease. A decade later, several studies by Swedish researchers suggested that using cell phones more than doubled the risk.

The radio waves generated by cell phones and other electronic devices are a low-energy form of radiation known as non-ionizing radiation. While some forms of radiation can cause cancer, it's not clear whether non-ionizing radiation has any negative health effects. Some lab studies have failed to show that radio waves comparable to those delivered by cell phones can cause brain tumors.

Furthermore, in the years since the alarming Swedish study, a number of other studies have failed to indict cell phones. A 2006 study of more than 420,000 cell phone users in Denmark showed no increased risk of brain cancer. Likewise, a 2007 review of nine studies published in the *Journal of Neurooncology* found that overall, cell phone users were no more or less likely to develop brain tumors.

The same study leaves open the possibility that long-term use of a cell phone—10 years or more—could pose a cancer

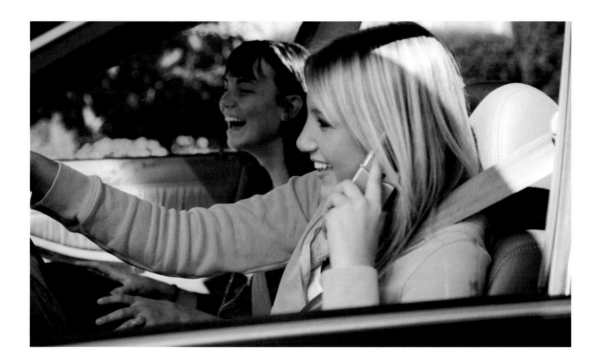

risk. However, long-time users are also more likely to have owned old-style analog cell phones, which some experts say may be the culprits. (Most cell phones sold today use digital technology.)

Does talking while driving make you more likely to crash?

YES The science is as powerful as an eight-cylinder engine: Yakking on a cell phone behind the wheel makes you a much worse driver.

It's illegal to use a cell phone while driving in many parts of the world for a good reason. One study by a team at the University of Utah found that talking on cell phones—either handheld or "hands-free" models—slowed reaction time by 18 percent and resulted in twice as many rear-end collisions.

Thankfully, that study occurred in a lab, with volunteers using a driving simulator. In the real world, however, other studies have found that distracted cell phone users are far more likely to miss traffic lights and stop signs, with predictable consequences. In a study published in the *British Medical Journal*, Australian researchers analyzed the cell phone records of 456 people who crashed their automobiles. Using accident reports to estimate the time of the incidents, they determined that gabbing while driving increases the risk of a crash *fourfold*. ■

Our BEST ADVICE

Until researchers clear up the static over cell phones and cancer, you can limit exposure to radio waves by keeping your cell phone's antenna as far as possible from your head. The best way to do that is to attach a headset to the phone instead of pressing the device to your ear.

Chiropractic

Chiropractors are truly hands-on healthcare professionals. They believe that many of the body's aches, pains, and other ills can be traced to nerve problems created by misaligned vertebrae in the spine. Spinal manipulation—physically realigning vertebrae with pressure applied by hand—is the chiropractor's basic tool, though these healers may use similar techniques on muscles and joints. Once-skeptical physicians now refer patients with lower-back pain and other conditions to chiropractors. However, some say the risks of treatment are understated.

Can a neck adjustment cause a stroke?

MAYBE Chiropractors say the risk is minuscule, but some doctors worry that neck adjustments may damage arteries in the neck.

Even if you've never had a neck adjustment, you've probably seen one in a movie or TV show, often for comic effect. The chiropractor places his hands on the sides of the patient's head, then abruptly rotates it to one side (cue crackling sound effects and a laugh track). However, some doctors insist there is nothing funny about neck adjustments. They claim that rotating the neck with force stretches arteries there, which could cause one to tear and result in a stroke.

Chiropractors use neck adjustments to treat neck pain, some types of headaches, and other conditions, claiming that they restore mobility and prevent muscle spasms. The American Chiropractic Association calls neck manipulation "remarkably safe," citing statistics showing that only about one in six million patients who have the procedure suffer strokes.

But skeptics say the number of people who have strokes is unknown and could be higher. A 2007 review in the *Journal of the Royal Society of Medicine* identified 200 cases of patients who experienced serious "adverse events" after undergoing spinal manipulation between 2001 and 2006. The most common complication was a torn vertebral artery. Several of the patients died or had long-term effects, such as paralysis (though most others made full recoveries). Critics say that many strokes and other injuries caused by neck adjustments probably go unreported.

The true risk of injury from a neck adjustment will probably never be known. Even critics acknowledge that it happens infrequently, making it difficult to study. Another 2007 study of more than 50,000 neck adjustments turned up no reports of strokes or any other serious aftereffects.

Can a session with a chiropractor leave me feeling *worse*?

YES Up to half of patients report soreness and other symptoms after a session, though the discomfort is usually brief.

In an ideal spinal manipulation session, the chiropractor straightens out your off-kilter backbone and presto, you're pain-free. While some patients do walk out of a single session feeling like new, studies show that others feel worse before they get better. In a survey published in the journal *Spine*, researchers interviewed 280 patients with neck pain after their first trips to a chiropractor. About 30 percent complained of pain, stiffness, headaches, and other side effects after the session, though the problems usually cleared up within a day or two. Other studies have found the rate of minor complaints among chiropractic patients to be as high as 50 percent.

What's going on? Chiropractors say that an adjustment loosens stiff joints that are "locked" in place, allowing them to move freely. As part of this process, muscles and ligaments may feel sore as they realign. However, they say, the aches are no worse than what you might feel after a hard workout and disappear just as quickly. ∎

Commuting

The typical employed American spends more time each year driving to and from work—about 100 hours—than on vacation. Although roads are getting increasingly clogged, congestion is not new: Traffic tie-ups were so bad in Rome during the first century B.C. that Julius Caesar banned the use of delivery carts during the daytime. But scientists know today that people who log lots of miles and frequently find themselves stuck in traffic may be taking the short route to some serious health problems.

Can driving to and from work make you sick?

YES If your commute drives you crazy, chronic stress could be making you vulnerable to minor and major health threats.

Many of us just can't leave our tension behind after a stressful commute. University of California psychologist Ray Novaco, PhD, and his colleagues showed that people who consistently feel the most harried as they drive home from work also report feeling the most irritable, impatient, tired, and sad in the evening. Dr. Novaco found that women find long commutes and heavy traffic more stressful than men do, probably because they are most often the parents who must get home in time to pick up the kids at soccer practice and put dinner on the table.

Since stress weakens the immune system, it's not surprising that the research team found a direct link between the amount of traffic a commuter must fight each day and how often he or she got sick. The research also showed that people with the longest commutes tend to have the highest blood pressure. Beware if you routinely blow your stack when traffic backs up: A study published in the *Journal of the American Medical Association* found that people with "Type A" personalities who are impatient and often feel rushed have a 50 percent increased risk of developing high blood pressure.

Getting plenty of physical activity each day is essential to staying healthy, of course, and people who drive to work may shortchange themselves. Just 14 percent of people who commute by car take at least 10,000 steps per day as

COMMUTING

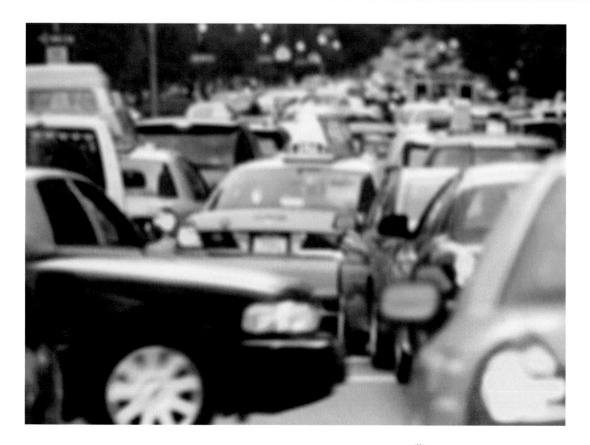

recommended by the US Centers for Disease Control and Prevention. One study found that about 40 percent of train riders attained this goal, probably because twice a day they had to walk from their cars to the platform and from the platform to their workplaces.

Is a long daily commute bad for your back?

YES Sitting behind the wheel for too many hours seems to be even more damaging than sitting at a desk.

That's probably due to stress on spinal disks from vibration and swaying back and forth as you take turns, speed up, or slow down. Furthermore, using your feet to operate the accelerator, brake, and clutch (if your car has manual transmission) means they are not available to support your back, which increases strain.

A number of studies suggest that the more you drive, the more likely you are to develop some form of back injury. British scientists reported that people who drove 20 hours or more a week as part of their jobs missed six times more work days due to back pain than people who drove 10 hours or less. ■

Our BEST ADVICE

Take public transportation to work if possible. A recent study that followed two groups of commuters for three years found that people who traveled by train from New Jersey to their jobs in New York City every day reported feeling significantly less stress than a similar group of commuters who drove to work.

Cookware

What's worse for you: a fat, juicy steak loaded with saturated fat and cholesterol or the skillet you fry it in? Simmering concerns about safety have long plagued aluminum and nonstick cookware. Purists who cook with only cast-iron or copper pots and pans can skip this section, but most home chefs favor budget-friendly, easy-to-clean cookware. Do low cost and convenience come at a price?

Does eating food cooked in aluminum pots and pans cause Alzheimer's disease?

NO Suspicions that aluminum cookware causes dementia once reached a boil, but later studies have turned down the heat on this controversy.

Worries about aluminum pots and pans have been around for at least a generation. In 1965, a study showed that injecting aluminum into the brains of rabbits caused damage resembling the changes that occur in humans with Alzheimer's disease. Later studies revealed that people who have Alzheimer's often have large deposits of the metal in their brains. Before long, home chefs around the world began replacing their aluminum cookware. To this day, some won't even heat up leftovers wrapped in aluminum foil. But these measures probably aren't necessary.

When you cook with an aluminum pot or pan, the metal can leach into food, but it's only a tiny amount, and your body is exposed to other sources of aluminum all day. It's in the air and drinking water as well as soft drink cans, cosmetics, and some antacids.

If you have sworn off aluminum cookware, you should toss out your tea bags, too—the hot brew is a rich source of the metal. Yet Alzheimer's disease is not rampant in countries where tea is popular. Likewise, studies do not consistently show that people who work in aluminum factories have high rates of dementia. And the early research indicating that Alzheimer's patients have high levels of aluminum in their brains has

been challenged by more recent studies suggesting that's not the case. Scientists say that more research is needed to know if exposure to aluminum increases Alzheimer's risk, though most agree that at worst, it poses a minor threat.

Can fumes given off by nonstick cookware make you sick?

YES When the pans are heated to very high temperatures, they can give off fumes that cause flu-like symptoms.

First, the bad news for parakeets and cockatiels: When heated to high temperatures, the coating on nonstick cookware can break down and send particles into the air, producing fumes that are toxic—often fatal—to a winged one's lungs. Remember that small birds have sensitive respiratory systems, which is why miners took canaries into coalmines to help detect noxious gases.

Of course, you and your family inhale the same fumes, which can cause symptoms such as a cough, headache, and chills that may last a few days and are often mistaken

If you have sworn off aluminum cookware, you should **toss out your tea bags, too.**

Cookware
(continued)

for the flu. Doctors have known about "polymer-fume fever" since at least the early 1950s. You can avoid getting sick and protect your pet bird, if you have one, by not over-heating nonstick pots and pans. DuPont, the maker of Teflon, says that its nonstick coating may begin to deteriorate at 500°F. The company recommends using low to medium heat when cooking with nonstick pots and pans. (The consumer watchdog Environmental Working Group recommends getting rid of nonstick cookware altogether, especially if you own birds.)

Scientists are currently studying whether chemicals used to make nonstick cookware cause more serious health concerns for humans. Perfluorooctanoate (PFOA) causes cancer in lab rats, and some research shows that babies born to women with high levels of the chemical in their blood tend to be small. Yet most people have PFOA in their blood—not surprising, since the chemical is used in making many products, such as carpets, furniture, and clothing. The EPA says there is no reason to stop using nonstick cookware. ∎

Dental Fillings

"Silver" dental fillings aren't made exclusively from that precious metal. Instead, they are formed from a powder consisting of silver, tin, copper, and other metals, which is combined with liquid mercury. Dentists have been using these "amalgam" fillings to repair teeth for nearly two centuries. Although other types of fillings are available, amalgam is strong and budget friendly. But is it safe?

Does the mercury in amalgam fillings cause health problems?

NO Studies have failed to show consistently that people with amalgam fillings experience any related health problems.

Dentists used to insist that the mercury in amalgam fillings remained safely in the teeth. It's now clear, however, that fillings give off mercury vapor, especially when you chew. It's also long been known that chronic exposure to large amounts of mercury can harm the kidneys and cause tremors, depression, irritability, memory loss, and other neurological problems. (Mercury was once used to make felt for hats, which spawned the phrase "mad as a hatter.")

Worries about mercury-based fillings date back to at least the mid-19th century. Skeptics have claimed that mercury leaching from fillings causes a variety of conditions, particularly diseases of the central nervous system. But there is no clear proof that these fillings cause brain damage or any other health woe, even if you have a mouth full of them.

University of California epidemiologist Michael N. Bates, PhD, surveyed the medical literature in 2006 and found no scientific evidence that people who have amalgam fillings have an increased risk of chronic fatigue syndrome or kidney disease. What about Alzheimer's disease? Past research raised concerns that exposure to mercury increased the risk of neurological conditions such as Alzheimer's and

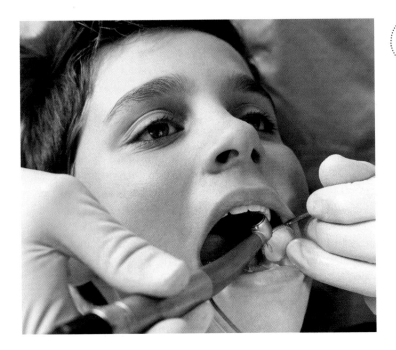

If you are concerned about having mercury in your mouth, talk to your dentist about composite fillings the next time you have a cavity. These tooth-colored alternatives to amalgam are made of glass or quartz combined with resin. Not only do they look more natural, but they also require the removal of less of an existing tooth, so they're usually smaller, too. Composites may cost up to twice as much as amalgam fillings, however, and typically need to be replaced within 5 to 10 years. (Amalgam fillings last 15 years or longer, on average.) Some studies show that amalgam fillings may be the longest-lasting choice for repairing bicuspids and molars, the large teeth in the back of the mouth that do the most chewing.

Parkinson's disease. But those studies looked only at occupational exposure to mercury and never linked amalgam fillings to neurological diseases. A few studies suggest that mercury from fillings may cause multiple sclerosis, but that research is inconclusive.

Several recent studies appear to rule out claims that children with amalgam fillings are at risk for learning disabilities. One study found that kids have normal memory, concentration, motor skills, and other neurological measurements seven years after receiving amalgam fillings.

The FDA says there is no evidence that mercury-based fillings are harmful, though Dr. Bates and other scientists say that more studies are needed.

Is there a good reason to have silver fillings removed?

NO There is no evidence that removing amalgam fillings cures or relieves the symptoms of any disease.

"Holistic" or "biological" dentists often claim that removing mercury-based fillings will relieve pain and symptoms of chronic disease. In many of the studies that appear to support this theory, researchers typically asked patients to describe their symptoms before and after removal of their amalgam fillings. These studies may be greatly influenced by the placebo effect, which casts doubt on their results. That is, people may feel better because they believed strongly that their fillings were toxic.

In one experiment, researchers in Norway found that patients with various chronic disorders who had their amalgam fillings removed rated their symptoms as improved seven years later. However, their symptom ratings matched those of a group of similar patients who did not have their fillings removed. ∎

DEODORANT

Deodorant

You may recall a time when the only worry you had about deodorant (other than whether it would keep working) was that spraying aerosol under your arms was destroying the ozone layer. Switching to roll-on took care of that concern, but then another one arose: Instead of making the planet sick, could deodorant be harming *you*?

Does deodorant cause breast cancer?

NO Despite what you may have read on the Internet or heard from your neighbor, there is no solid evidence to back up this rumor.

This stubborn rumor wasn't started by a prankster. On the contrary, several scientists have raised the possibility that using deodorant and other cosmetics may expose women to cancer-causing chemicals. One study found that women with breast cancer who used deodorant and shaved their underarms most often tended to be diagnosed at a younger age, especially if they began these habits before age 16. In theory, nicks from shaving might allow dangerous compounds in deodorant to enter the bloodstream. Parabens, which are preservatives commonly used in deodorant, are one suspect, since they mimic the activity of estrogen, which is known to promote breast tumors. Other scientists have suggested that aluminum, an ingredient in antiperspirant formulas, causes cancer to arise in breast cells.

However, these theories are contradicted by the only study ever to examine the link between breast cancer and deodorant. Scientists at the Fred Hutchinson Cancer Research Center in Seattle interviewed 813 women with breast cancer and a similar group of healthy women. They found no difference in how often the women applied deodorant or antiperspirant. Nor was there a difference in how often the women shaved their underarms. While more studies would help resolve the matter once and for all, most scientists agree that there's no reason to fear using deodorant. ■

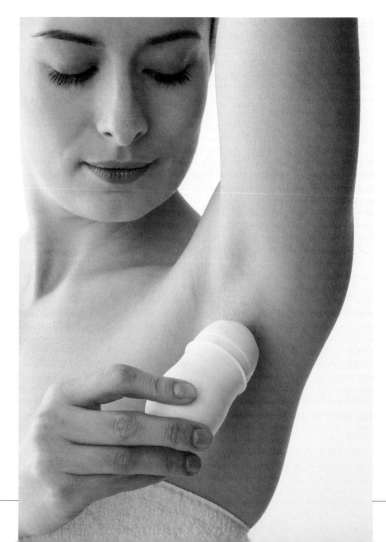

Flu Shots

A flu shot can spare you from aches, fever, and chills and could even save your life. So why don't more people get them? Anyone can benefit from being vaccinated (and some people can opt for nasal spray instead of the needle), though small children, the elderly, pregnant women, and people with chronic illnesses need it most. Yet many people shun this annual ritual, fearing it poses a serious health threat.

Can flu shots *cause* the flu?

NO Yet surveys show that many people don't get vaccinated due to this mistaken belief.

Yes, a flu shot contains the flu virus. Each year, scientists identify the flu strains they believe are most likely to cause widespread illness. These strains are included in the vaccine, which is reformulated annually. But the viruses are inactivated—that is, dead (or weakened, in the case of nasal spray vaccine). In other words, they can't cause the flu. Yet they coax your immune system into producing germ-killing proteins called antibodies, which learn how to recognize and destroy the flu virus should you encounter it.

Another source of confusion: Sometimes people are vaccinated and then come down with the flu a few days later. The flu vaccine is up to 90 percent effective in healthy young people but offers less protection to others who are older or sicker. In other words, you can still get the flu after getting a flu shot. If you catch the bug right away, you may think that the jab in the arm made you ill. But the flu shot didn't make you sick—the timing was coincidental.

Also, don't be surprised if you feel a little under the weather immediately after a flu shot. It's perfectly normal to develop a low-grade fever or feel achy for a day or two.

Should I ask for mercury-free flu shots for my child or if I'm pregnant?

MAYBE There is little evidence that vaccines containing mercury are unsafe for humans. Nevertheless, concerns about exposure to this metal—especially in children and pregnant women—are mounting.

Most flu shots contain a preservative called thimerosal,

Our BEST ADVICE

Getting a flu shot in October or November is an annual ritual for many. But what if December or January rolls around and you still haven't gotten vaccinated? Get the shot anyway. The vaccine takes about two weeks to become effective, so that still gives your immune system time to rally its defenses for the height of influenza season in January and February.

which is made with mercury. Early research suggested that vaccines containing mercury caused neurological problems in children, such as attention deficit disorder and delayed speech. Now, however, most scientists say those studies were flawed. A number of later studies failed to show a clear, consistent link between a child's exposure to thimerosal and developmental problems, including autism. Major public health groups insist that thimerosal is safe.

Even so, if you have banned swordfish and other mercury-rich fish from your dinner table, you may wonder, Why should I let a doctor inject mercury into my child? A dose of thimerosal-containing flu vaccine for an infant has 12.5 micrograms of mercury; a can of tuna has about 11 micrograms, while a serving of salmon has far less. It's known

FOOD COLORINGS

Flu Shots
(continued)

that high doses of mercury can cause brain damage. A few studies suggest (but don't prove) that boys who receive vaccines containing thimerosal are somewhat more likely to develop tics and twitches.

It's possible, says Columbia University researcher Mady Hornig, MD, that some people are born with genes that make them more sensitive to mercury. Dr. Hornig's research shows that lab mice whose immune systems are sensitive to mercury develop enlarged brains and behavioral problems when exposed to vaccine-like doses of thimerosal.

Drug makers now offer the option of flu vaccines that are mercury-free or contain only traces of the preservative. However, manufacturers make a limited supply, so it's not always easy to find a clinic that offers mercury-free flu shots. Another way to guard against the flu and avoid mercury is to opt for the nasal vaccine LAIV—better known as FluMist—though it has not been approved for children under age 2. FluMist is available for people ages 2 to 49 who are healthy and not pregnant. Further studies are needed to determine whether FluMist is safe for people 50 and older. ■

Food Colorings

Your taste buds help you decide if a food tastes good, but your eyes help you decide whether to eat it in the first place. Food manufacturers make their wares more appetizing by adding food coloring, often relying on synthetic dyes to do the job. Over the years, critics have charged that artificial colorings cause health problems, especially behavior disorders in children.

Hasn't the theory about food coloring and ADHD been debunked?

NO In fact, recent research refreshes concerns that artificial dyes added to foods and drinks may cause or worsen hyperactivity.

In the 1970s, pediatrician Benjamin Feingold, MD, introduced a theory that gave hope to parents of hyperactive children: Eliminating certain food ingredients and additives, including artificial colorings, from their kids' diets, could reduce unruly behavior and improve concentration. Most mainstream physicians rejected Dr. Feingold's theory, arguing that diet does not influence the condition now known as attention deficit hyperactivity disorder (ADHD).

However, recent research suggests that cutting back on artificial colorings just may make kids less restless and more focused after all. Doctors at Columbia University analyzed 15 studies in which parents and teachers rated children's behavior before and after the youngsters consumed artificially colored drinks and foods. They estimated that eliminating these products

Cutting back on artificial colorings may make kids **less restless and more focused.**

improved conduct and concentration about one-third to one-half as effectively as ADHD medications. More study is needed, but feeding kids fewer foods with added coloring can't hurt and may help keep order in the house and classroom.

Are natural food colorings necessarily safe?

NO Some natural dyes come from surprising sources that may, in rare cases, cause allergic reactions.

It may bug you to learn that your raspberry yogurt or pink lemonade could contain a dye made from insects—beetles, to be precise. A variety of foods and beverages get their brilliant colors from red dyes called carmine and cochineal, which are made from ground-up cochineal beetles.

Vegetarians and people who follow a kosher diet often react with anger upon learning that they have unwittingly consumed insect parts. But at least they don't break out in hives or struggle to breathe, which is what happens to a small number of people who are allergic to these dyes. Some develop full-blown anaphylactic shock. The Center for Science in the Public Interest, a watchdog group, estimates that about 400 people in the United States experience bad reactions to these bug dyes each year, many serious enough to require a trip to the emergency room or hospitalization.

Many people don't discover that they are allergic to carmine and cochineal colorings until they have a bad reaction. Unfortunately, these dyes aren't always clearly identified on product ingredient lists. However, a growing number of manufacturers list carmine and cochineal by name, while others have stopped using them altogether. ■

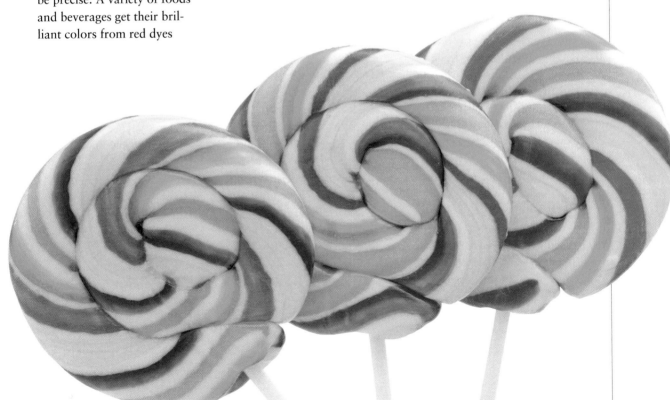

GENERIC DRUGS

Generic Drugs

Generic drugs offer high-end medical therapy at Wal-Mart prices. Or do they? By law, generic drugs are supposed to provide the same dose of medicine that you would get from more expensive brand-name medications. Insurers save billions by refusing to pay for brand-name drugs when a generic becomes available. However, studies show that some generic drugs may not deliver as promised.

Should you think twice before agreeing to take a generic drug?

YES Generic drugs are supposed to be just as effective as their brand-name counterparts, but in some cases they aren't.

You've probably heard the speech about generic drugs from your doctor or pharmacist: They are just as potent as brand-name drugs. They are held to the same quality standards. They work the same.

But that's a tough pill to swallow if you've ever felt your condition worsen or become plagued by new side effects after switching to a generic drug. This may happen more often than makers of generics would have us believe. For example, a 2007 study reported that 20 patients being treated successfully for anxiety with Celexa had their symptoms return within a month, on average, when they were switched to generic citalopram. It wasn't a matter of the patients convincing themselves that the generic drug wouldn't work, since their doctors never told them about the swap. After they were able to take Celexa again, their anxiety eased.

There have also been reports of patients whose depression returned after switching to paroxetine, the generic version of Paxil. Studies have also shown that the generic version of the anti-anxiety drug Valium (diazepam) is less potent and takes longer to start working and that many epilepsy patients are no longer able to control their seizures after switching from brand-name drugs to generic.

What's going on? Generic drugs are not necessarily identical to their brand-name counterparts. Makers of generics are allowed to copy a brand-name drug's formula but can't always duplicate its "delivery system," or method of releasing medicine into the blood, which may be protected by a patent or be a trade secret. As a result, generics may dissolve and enter the bloodstream at a different speed.

ConsumerLab.com, a watchdog Web site, compared the dissolution speed of the antidepressant Wellbutrin XL with the generic version, bupropion. Two hours after the test started, four times more of the generic had dissolved. In a patient, that means a dose of Wellbutrin XL, which is supposed to last all day, could wear off too soon. In fact, many Wellbutrin XL users whose insurers forced them to switch to the generic complained that their depression recurred, and they developed headaches, insomnia, and other symptoms. ∎

High-Fructose Corn Syrup

"Franken-syrup." "A coronary on the cob." Those are a few of the damning nicknames that critics have pinned on high-fructose corn syrup. It's probably no surprise that this commercial sweetener is ubiquitous in soft drinks. But did you know that it's also added to ketchup, salad dressing, canned soup, bread, and a long list of other foods? And now that you do, should you swear off the stuff?

Does consuming too much high-fructose corn syrup make you fat?

YES But no more than eating too much sugar does.

Ironically, one of the main faults of high-fructose corn syrup (HFCS) is that it's so darn cheap to produce (thanks to government subsidies of corn crops). That's the principal reason soft drinks have grown exponentially in size but not in price. And yes, Americans' addiction to giant soft drinks is probably part of the reason behind our expanding … behinds.

HFCS and table sugar are chemical twins—not identical, but they look very much alike under a microscope. Corn refiners make HFCS by converting some of the glucose in corn syrup to fructose, the main sugar in fruits (which doesn't make it any healthier). Despite its name, HFCS is only "high" in fructose compared to pure corn syrup, which is all glucose, the most common sugar in all of nature.

Can you guess which other widely used sweetener is also half fructose and half glucose? That's right, table sugar. HFCS is really just table sugar in liquid form. Some "foodies" claim they can tell it apart from sugar, but your hips and waist don't know the difference: Both have four calories per gram. Apart from the fact that HFCS has allowed beverage makers in particular to sell larger products and reap bigger profits, there is no solid scientific evidence that consuming HFCS makes you any

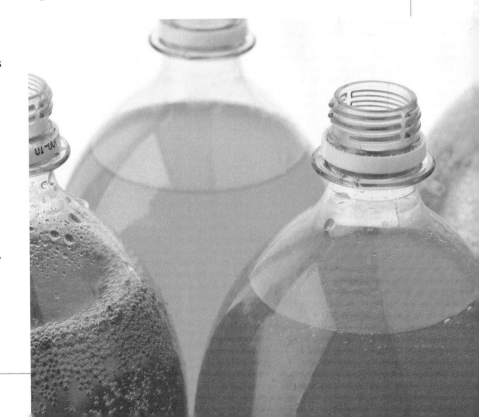

HIGH-FRUCTOSE CORN SYRUP

fatter than eating an equal amount of sugar.

Does consuming too much HFCS increase the risk of heart disease and diabetes?

YES Again, eating too much sugar is bad for you, too. But some evidence suggests that HFCS may be even worse for your body.

When you think of "heart attack" foods, you probably imagine fat steaks and cream sauces, not soft drinks and other sweets. But they can tax your ticker, too. For instance, studies show that a diet rich in fructose—whether from HFCS or table sugar—causes the liver to produce large amounts of artery-clogging fats called triglycerides. One study at the University of Minnesota found that triglyceride levels soared 32 percent in young men fed a high-fructose diet for six weeks.

And that's not the only bad news for your heart when you chronically overdose on foods sweetened with HFCS or table sugar. Studies show that people who consume a lot of either have low levels of HDL ("good") cholesterol, the stuff that helps keep arteries free of gunk. What's more, animals fed high-sugar diets develop high blood pressure, and studies suggest the same may be true of humans.

As we pointed out in Part 2, women who consume one or more nondiet soft drinks per day increase their risk of type 2 diabetes by 83 percent. That doesn't mean that a bottle of "natural" soda sweetened with pure cane sugar is a health tonic, of course. But some research suggests that soda made with HFCS poses a greater diabetes threat. For example, researchers at Rutgers University have shown that carbonated soft drinks sweetened with HFCS—but not table sugar—contain exceptionally high levels of compounds called reactive carbonyls, which damage human tissue. Chalk up the carbonyls in HFCS to the fact that in this liquid form of sugar, the glucose and fructose aren't bound together as they are in table sugar. Recent research has linked unbound glucose and fructose to carbonyls. People with diabetes have high levels of reactive carbonyls in their blood. ■

A diet rich in fructose causes the liver to produce **large amounts of artery-clogging triglycerides.**

Hormone Replacement Therapy

Menopause means more than coping with hot flashes, vaginal dryness, and other unwelcome symptoms. At midlife, a woman's risk of heart attacks, brittle bones, and other major health problems soars. Estrogen plummets during menopause, so doctors once believed that restoring this hormone to youthful levels would guard against these threats. However, hormone replacement therapy (HRT) may cause more problems than it solves.

Does taking HRT increase the risk of heart attacks and breast cancer?

YES Contrary to early claims, HRT actually increases the threat of heart attacks as well as raising the risk of breast cancer and other conditions.

What does it take to make sales of one of the most widely used drugs in the world to nosedive overnight? How about word that the medication increases the threat of heart attacks, breast cancer, ovarian cancer, and other diseases? That's what happened on July 17, 2002, when the *Journal of the American Medical Association* published two large studies showing that women who use HRT may be putting themselves at risk for serious health problems.

One of the studies involved women over 50 who took estrogen and progestin (the latter is included with estrogen therapy to lower the risk of uterine cancer). Compared to other participants who took placebos, women on combination HRT were 26 percent more likely to develop breast cancer, 29 percent more likely to have heart attacks, and 41 percent more likely to have strokes. Their risk of developing blood clots in their legs or lungs doubled.

The second study found that postmenopausal women who used estrogen-only therapy (prescribed to women who have had their uteruses removed) are 60 percent more likely to develop ovarian cancer. A later study of women on estrogen-only HRT showed an increased risk of strokes and blood clots in the leg.

Reduced use of these drugs may be paying off. For example, in the three years after legions of women in the United States gave up HRT, the breast cancer rate fell 8.6 percent, according to a 2007 study reported in the *New England Journal of Medicine*. A second study, of women in the Pacific Northwest, showed an even greater decrease—18 percent. Other factors undoubtedly contributed to this trend, but estrogen does fuel the growth of breast cancer.

Does this mean a woman is crazy to use HRT?

NO Doctors say that women who are struggling with menopause symptoms can safely use HRT for a limited time.

You drank soy milk until you couldn't stand another sip. You took black cohosh, red clover, and every other herbal remedy you could find. You wore sleeveless blouses when everyone else was bundled up. Yet you still couldn't cope with the relentless hot flashes and other unpleasant menopause symptoms.

That doesn't mean you have to sweat them out. Doctors say

Hormone Replacement Therapy

(continued)

that short-term use of HRT remains a reasonable option for women whose lives are disrupted by menopause symptoms, provided they understand the risks associated with treatment.

It's important to put those risks in perspective. For instance, the 26 percent increase in breast cancer sounds scary, but in the real world it means that an additional 8 women will develop breast cancer each year for every 10,000 who use combination HRT. The actual risk of heart attacks and strokes is similar. (Blood clots are a greater concern but still pose a small absolute risk.) Consider, too, that the alarming HRT studies found no difference in death rates between women using the drugs and those taking placebos.

The news about HRT isn't all bad, by the way. Studies show that it lowers the risk of osteoporosis and colon cancer. Doctors generally prescribe the lowest dose that works and advise women to use the medication for no more than a year or two. If a woman's prime complaint is vaginal dryness, vaginal creams and rings may be preferable to oral HRT, since they provide smaller doses of estrogen than pills. ■

Hospitals

Not so long ago, most hospital patients figured the greatest threats to their well-being were bad food and chatterbox roommates. But a 1999 report by the Institute of Medicine shone a light on an age-old problem: Sometimes patients get sicker or even die due to mistakes by doctors, nurses, and other staffers. The report pegged the number of deaths from medical errors at 98,000 per year, most of them in hospitals and other healthcare facilities. Cries for reform followed, but has anyone listened?

Is patient safety still a major problem in hospitals?

YES Some medical centers have instituted changes to make patients safer, but a lot of problems remain.

Where would you rather be if your heart started beating erratically—in a hospital or a casino? Put your money on the casino. Most are equipped with defibrillators, and the odds are better than 50-50 you'll survive cardiac arrhythmia if you keel over on the craps table. By comparison, just one-third of arrhythmia patients in hospitals survive. Granted, people in hospitals are much sicker to begin with, but a 2008 study showed that 30 percent of patients who need defibrillator "shocks" fail to get them within the recommended two minutes.

Wait—weren't hospitals supposed to shape up after the headline-grabbing Institute of Medicine report we mentioned above? The authors called for a 50 percent reduction in deaths from medical errors, but five years after the report was published, an editorial in the *New England Journal of Medicine* complained that not much had changed.

Some doctors say the alarming statistics about medical errors are overblown. Nonetheless, hospitals will soon feel pressure to do more to protect patient safety. A growing number of insurers, including the US Medicare plan, have announced they will no longer pay for treatment related to "never events"— incidents that should never happen to a hospital patient. Some states now require hospitals to report never events, which helps to show how much work remains. For example, in just one year, hospitals in Minnesota reported that 26 surgery patients had

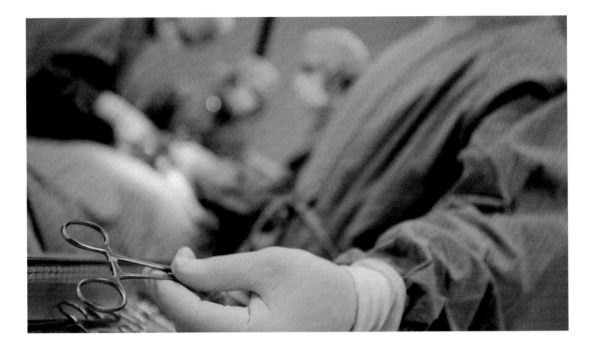

foreign objects (such as sponges or instruments) left in their bodies after operations, 16 had the wrong body parts operated on, 8 had the wrong operations, and 2 were mixed up with other patients. Another 31 patients developed severe bedsores, and 7 died or became disabled because of medication errors.

Are hospitals germ factories?

YES The threat of infections doubles the risk that you will become even sicker or die if you are admitted to a hospital.

If you need to be hospitalized, the complication you're most apt to develop is an infection, which happens to as many as 1 out of 10 patients. Hospitals are full of sick people, many with depressed immune sys-

tems. That means some infections are probably inevitable— but many others are not.

For instance, the most common infection a patient may pick up is a urinary tract infection (UTI). Up to one in four patients must have a catheter, or tube, inserted into the urethra to remove urine from the bladder. Bacteria on the catheter can cause a UTI, so keeping these tubes clean and removing them when no longer needed should be major priorities. Yet a University of Michigan study found that three-quarters of hospitals in the United States have no system for tracking how long a patient has had a catheter or whether it has been removed.

While antibiotics can usually take care of a UTI, other common infections are more serious. Skin incisions may

become infected after surgery, a problem that can be reduced by giving antibiotics before an operation. But a study in New York State found that hospital staff failed to give antibiotics properly before surgery 27 to 54 percent of the time. More serious still, patients who need ventilators or feeding tubes are at risk for lung infections that cause pneumonia, the leading cause of infection in intensive care units.

Microbes that are resistant to one or more antibiotics cause nearly 70 percent of hospital-acquired infections. You may have heard about the most notorious super-bug of all—methicillin-resistant *Staphylococcus aureus,* or MRSA. "Staph" infections picked up in the hospital used to be easy to treat with antibiotics, but MRSA is staph on

HOSPITALS

steroids. It often requires several courses of powerful antibiotics and can be deadly. In 1974, MRSA caused 2 percent of staph infections in hospitals. Today, it accounts for 63 percent of all staph infections. Unfortunately, MRSA infections have become more common outside hospitals, too.

Are sleepy medical staff members a danger to patients?

YES Sleep deprivation makes people foggy-brained. You probably don't want a drowsy doctor taking your medical history, much less taking out your appendix.

Medical interns routinely work shifts that last 24 hours or longer. Research shows that the cognitive and behavioral effect of going without sleep for a day or more is similar to that of getting drunk. Not surprisingly, a 2006 survey found that sleep-deprived doctors in training said they had fallen asleep during lectures, while examining patients, and even in the middle of surgery.

Laws now limit the number of hours medical interns can work, but they still log plenty of long shifts. A 2004 study found that medical interns working shifts of 24 hours or longer made 36 percent more serious errors than other interns who worked shorter hours. Errors included misdiagnosing a patient's condition and giving the wrong medication. Some mistakes were recognized in time, but others were not.

Interns aren't the only staffers at your local hospital downing espresso to stay awake. With nurses in short supply, these caregivers often work long hours, too. One study found that nurses are twice as likely to make errors when they work 12.5 consecutive hours or longer. The same study found that 20 percent of nurses said they had fallen asleep during a shift, and sleepiness was a problem during both the day and night shifts. ■

STAYING SAFE WHEN YOU NEED SURGERY

In Part 1, we offered some tips on avoiding infection during a hospital stay ("Don't Touch That Remote!" on page 32). If you need surgery, you should take these further precautions to keep the bugs at bay.

• **Ask your doctor if you should be tested for methicillin-resistant *Staphylococcus aureus* (MRSA).** You'd need the test a week before you enter the hospital. If it's positive, the staff can take extra steps to keep the bacteria on your skin or in your nose from being transmitted into your body.

• **Scrub up before your operation.** Some authorities recommend showering or bathing with chlorhexidine soap for three to five days in advance. However, recent studies suggest that using special soap isn't necessary—any kind will do as long as you bathe thoroughly.

• **Ask your doctor to use clippers or depilatory cream if you need hair removed from the incision site.** Studies show that shaving with a razor increases the risk of post-surgery skin infections.

• **Remind your doctor or nurse that you need an antibiotic one hour before surgery.** Surgical wounds are another major source of infections, yet patients often fail to receive protective antibiotics prior to an operation.

• **If you're told you need a urinary tract catheter, ask if it's really necessary.** Urinary tract infections are the most common type you can pick up in a hospital. If you do need a catheter, ask to have it removed as soon as possible.

• **If a wound dressing becomes loose or wet, tell a nurse.** The dressing is there, in large part, to prevent bacteria from entering the wound.

Hot Tubs

Whether you're lucky enough to take that stress-busting, muscle-relaxing soak in a spa, a luxury hotel, or your own backyard, 10 minutes in a hot tub can be divine indeed. Surely such a blissful, soothing experience couldn't pose any dangers (besides getting addicted)? Actually it can, though a hot, bubbly soak can still be safe as long as you know the water's clean, and you take some smart precautions.

Can a hot tub make me sick?

YES Germs can breed if the frothy warm water remains unchanged for too long—or stews too many bodies between changes. Both are common problems.

While it may be the epitome of relaxation, a dip in a hot tub or Jacuzzi can pose several health threats. To start, if the heated water isn't kept clean and frequently treated with a disinfectant such as chlorine, it can harbor bacteria that may cause skin rashes and infections—or worse.

The most common culprit is the *Pseudomonas* bacterium, a bug that can cause folliculitis, or red, itchy bumps around hair follicles. "Dead skin and skin oils become food for the bacteria, so you'll basically be sitting in a bacteria soup if you don't watch it," says microbiologist Charles Gerba, PhD, a germ expert at the University of Arizona in Tucson.

"Women are at greater risk for *Pseudomonas* infection because their tight bathing suits hold the bacteria closer to the skin."

The more people who use a hot tub, the faster the disinfectant is depleted, and the likelier it is to contain dangerous levels of bacteria. "If I saw a hot tub filled with people, I wouldn't go in," says Dr. Gerba.

The *Pseudomonas* bacterium is the most common germ to lurk in hot tubs, but more dangerous villains such as *Mycobacterium* (which causes lung infections) and *Legionella* (which causes Legionnaire's disease, a form of pneumonia) have been known to visit them, too. In the United States, there are an estimated 8,000 to 18,000 cases of Legionnaire's disease each year (many aren't diagnosed correctly), and studies have suggested that dirty hot tubs are among the most common routes of transmission.

Our BEST ADVICE

If you have a hot tub at home, follow the maintenance directions religiously. Make sure you add disinfectant regularly (usually every three days) and change the water at least every two months. Before sitting in a hotel, gym, or spa hot tub, give it the nose-and-eye test, advises Charles Gerba, PhD. First, take a sniff while standing near the tub; you should smell chlorine. Second, dip a clear plastic cup into the water and hold it up to the light. The water should be clear. "If the water is cloudy, don't go in," warns Dr. Gerba.

Can hot tubs harm kids?

YES In the United States alone, about 33 children drown in hot tubs each year, and there are many close calls.

While bacteria exposure from dirty water is the number one risk hot tubs carry, it's not the only one. Unsupervised children can become trapped in the powerful suction of a drain.

"Many parents leave their children unsupervised around hot tubs because they think that they're too shallow to be dangerous," says Ed Kang, spokesperson for the US Consumer Product Safety

HOT TUBS

Commission in Bethesda, Maryland. "They don't realize that hot tubs are just as dangerous to children as swimming pools."

Before using a hot tub—with or without a child—make sure the drain cover is intact, and replace a drain cover that's more than 20 years old.

Burns and scalds are another risk, especially when broken temperature regulators or thermometers or other faulty parts allow the water temperature to exceed 104°F. "Always dip a toe in a hot tub first to test the temperature of the water," says Andrew Harris, vice president of Robert's Hot Tubs in Richmond, California, who has served as an expert witness in lawsuits involving hot tub injuries.

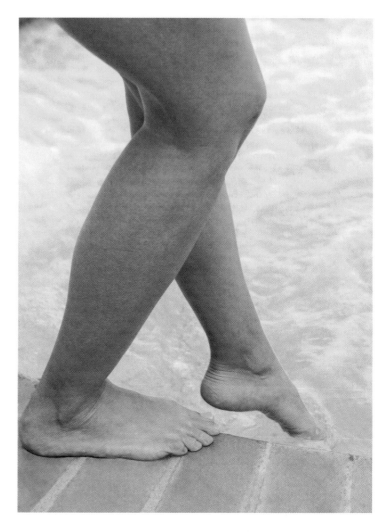

Should I worry about a soak if I have a health problem?

MAYBE Sitting in hot water raises your body temperature, and that can be risky for pregnant women and people with diabetes or high or low blood pressure.

Since the water in hot tubs is normally hotter than 100°F, soaking for prolonged periods (say, longer than 10 minutes) can be dangerous for people with certain health conditions, such as diabetes, heart disease, or high or low blood pressure; they should get clearance from

a doctor first. Doctors also advise pregnant women to avoid hot tubs, as the prolonged heat may harm an unborn baby. A study of 1,060 pregnant women conducted by the Kaiser Foundation Research Institute in Oakland, California, found that those who used hot tubs two or more times a week were twice as likely to have miscarriages as women who never used hot tubs.

Finally, while they may be romantic, hot tubs are not the

perfect aphrodisiac for couples looking to conceive. Fertility doctors have speculated for years that the heat from hot tubs can lower sperm count in men, though no studies have proven this absolutely. One small Brazilian study showed that 11 men with fertility problems had a rise in their sperm counts when they stopped using hot tubs regularly—as long as they were nonsmokers. ■

Household Cleaners

Many of the cleaning products in your under-sink cabinet contain a witches' brew of chemicals that can be lethal if misused. No surprise there, right? But if you don't do anything stupid, such as pour the bleach into your iced tea or hand your baby the drain declogger, do you still have to worry?

If you use common sense, can household cleaners still harm you?

YES There are many combinations of cleaning products that could produce toxic fumes or caustic liquids and irritate your eyes and lungs.

Hopefully, most of humankind knows to never, ever mix ammonia and chlorine bleach. The combo can produce highly irritating chlorine gas, which can cause nausea, eye tearing, headaches, and severe coughing—and send offenders to the emergency department if they're exposed too long in an unventilated room.

While this evil mixture is infamous, there are several other potentially nasty combinations that are less well known. It's one reason that cleaning products caused nearly 10 percent of the more than two million cases of poisoning reported in the United States in 2005. Bleach, which is poisonous as well as a skin and eye irritant on its own, can react with many common acidic cleaners in addition to ammonia, such as those containing hydrochloric acid, sulfuric acid, muriatic acid, or lye.

Never mix products that contain bleach with toilet cleaners, vinegar, drain cleaners, oven cleaners, floor and glass cleaners (which often contain ammonia), shower tile cleaners, and mildew-fighting cleaners. On purpose or even by accident, it's easy to use a chlorine-bleach cleanser and a mildew remover back to back on a bathtub, or an oven cleaner followed by all-purpose cleaning spray that contains bleach—but don't do

CLEANING PRODUCTS AND AIR PURIFIERS DON'T MIX

A study at the University of California, Berkeley, found that many common ingredients in cleaning products become toxic when they mix with ozone. That's not usually a problem—unless you live in a smog-filled city, you're surrounded by large office equipment (such as photocopiers that release ozone), or you use an ionizing air purifier that pumps out ozone. The latter have become quite common.

The researchers found that ozone is especially dangerous when mixed with terpenes, chemicals found in products with a lemon, orange, or pine scent. The combination can produce small amounts of carcinogens as well as formaldehyde, which can irritate your eyes, nose, and throat and worsen asthma symptoms. Some air fresheners may also react with ozone to produce these agents. Occasional mild exposure isn't likely to cause problems, but frequent exposure in a room without good ventilation could be dangerous. So click off that ionizing air purifier and open a window.

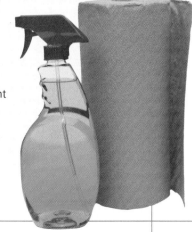

HUMIDIFIERS

Household Cleaners

(continued)

it. Accidentally making bad combinations is even more likely now that so many cleansers are "Now with Bleach!"

Exposure to cleaning products can hurt you in sneaky, indirect ways, too: A 2007 study of 3,503 Europeans found that those who were exposed to cleaning sprays (especially glass and furniture cleaners and air-freshening sprays) were more than 50 percent more likely to develop adult-onset asthma.

Our advice: Don't mix any cleaning products, even if they're the same type of cleaner (but a different brand) or intended for the same use. ■

Humidifiers

Some folks like breathing in dewy air reminiscent of the rainforest, and thanks to humidifiers, even people in the driest climates can. A humidifier can combat a dry heating system to keep your home pleasantly moist in winter. Sadly, moist air isn't all you'll breathe in if you don't keep that machine whistle-clean.

Can a humidifier make you sick?

YES A dirty machine can spew bacteria and mold into the air that can cause flu-like symptoms, or worse.

Have you ever heard of "humidifier lung"? It's an inflammation of the lungs (also known as hypersensitivity pneumonitis) caused by breathing fungus-laden air. It'll saddle you with coughing, fever, chills—the works.

If you don't change the reservoir water, empty the drip pan daily, and clean the inside of the water tank frequently, fungi and bacteria will start to grow—as evidenced by those little black dots and the faint layer of scum you see floating in humidifier water that's been neglected too long. Those bugs can hide in internal parts, too, so cleaning them out and disinfecting your humidifier may not be an easy task. If you get lazy, the fine mist emanating from your humidifier will carry those little stinkers throughout your room and into your lungs, where they

can irritate your respiratory system, worsen asthma, cause an allergic reaction, or chronically build up into the dreaded humidifier lung.

To keep your humidifier clean, follow this advice.

• Every three days, unplug the machine, empty the tank, and use a brush or scrubber along with a 3 percent hydrogen peroxide solution to remove any film or scaly deposits. Wipe all surfaces dry. Perform any other steps according to the manufacturer's directions.

• Clean or replace the unit's filter at intervals specified in the directions.

• Refill with distilled water rather than tap water. Tap water often contains minerals that can clog filters, encourage bacteria growth, and end up as a fine white powder on your furniture.

• By a hygrometer at a hardware store to measure the humidity in your home and don't let it exceed 50 percent—above that level of humidity, mold can grow quickly in your walls and elsewhere. ■

Mail-Order Drugs

With prescription drug prices in the stratosphere, saving money is a real concern. Enter mail-order pharmacies, which ship drugs to your door at lower prices than community pharmacies charge. It sounds perfect—and it just may be. Mail-order pharmacies can be convenient money savers that spare you from hearing another pharmacist say, "Come back in about 20 minutes." But they can have shortcomings, too.

Are mail-order pharmacies appropriate for everyone?

NO They're best for people with stable chronic conditions who don't forgo doctor visits.

The savings you get with mail-order pharmacies are real: Insurance copayments for drugs can be 50 percent cheaper than those charged at drugstores. And many mail-order pharmacies allow you to order a three-month supply of some drugs, yielding even more dramatic savings. You may not even have a choice in the matter, since some health insurance providers insist you use these pharmacies for certain drugs.

"For certain patients in certain circumstances, mail-order pharmacies can be a great option," says Ian Blumer, MD, a physician in the Toronto area and author of *Understanding Prescription Drugs for Canadians for Dummies*. What kinds of patients? Those who are successfully managing a *stable* chronic condition (such as treated high blood pressure), need the same medication in the same dosage at regular intervals, and keep in regular touch with their doctors.

The last point is critical, says Dr. Blumer. "Some patients stop seeing their doctor when they begin using a mail-order pharmacy because they no longer need to see him for refills," he explains. "That's dangerous because the doctor can't monitor the patient's condition without those visits."

Is a mail-order pharmacy just as safe and reliable as your corner pharmacy?

NO Mail-order pharmacies make fewer mistakes, but in some cases the drugs you get may not be exactly what the doctor ordered.

As far as mistakes go, studies have found that highly automated mail-order pharmacies

MAIL-ORDER DRUGS

that fill more than 10,000 prescriptions per month had significantly lower error rates than brick-and-mortar pharmacies that fill prescriptions by hand. But at your corner drugstore, the service can obviously be more personal, and a pharmacist can potentially catch an error during small talk by noticing, for example, that a teenager probably shouldn't be taking a drug for, say, Parkinson's disease.

What about the drugs themselves? According to Dr. Blumer, some mail-order pharmacies achieve their savings by filling prescriptions in foreign countries, even though their contact address and phone number may be domestic.

"Some drugs have completely different names in different countries, and it's not uncommon for a patient to get the wrong drug," he says. In 2003, the FDA found that Americans were ordering medications from Canadian mail-order pharmacies that filled prescriptions in Canada and used versions of drugs that weren't approved in the United States, including a version of the common anti-clotting drug warfarin that was a different formulation and potency than the US-approved pill.

Finally, the perils of "shipping and handling" can play havoc with certain drugs. They

ONLINE PHARMACIES: FRIEND OR FAUX?

"VIAGRA—PENNIES A PILL!"

You've never received an e-mail with that subject line? You're fortunate. Pill sellers—legit, criminal, and everything in between—have infested the World Wide Web with their services, and their number continues to grow. In 2007, a US Senate investigation found 394 Web sites selling prescription drugs online, up from 168 sites in 2006. All promise anyone with a computer that they're just a click and a day away from cheap prescription drugs.

Do you sense a catch?

"Disreputable online pharmacies are notorious for doing three things," says Toronto physician Ian Blumer, MD. "They either never send you the drugs, give you counterfeit drugs, or give you drugs that lack the active ingredient you need."

Many of these "pharmacies" are nothing but shams. The 2007 Senate investigation found that 84 percent of the online pill shops didn't require a prescription at all. The other 16 percent? Half of those required only a faxed prescription, which can be easily forged (or sent to 50 such pharmacies simultaneously). That left a scant few that operated like professionals.

Online pharmacies have all the same perks and drawbacks as all mail-order pharmacies, and applying the same proving standards can help you make sure you're dealing with a legal, trustworthy operation. One big key is to find the VIPPS seal on their Web site. That's the Verified Internet Pharmacy Practice Sites seal, indicating that the site has been checked out and approved by the National Association of Boards of Pharmacy.

can lose potency if they bake in your mailbox (or a delivery truck) on a hot day, whereas the shipments sent directly to pharmacies are handled with particular care. A 2004 study conducted by researchers in Phoenix (where the summer heat sizzles) found that the inhaled asthma drug for- moterol lost half its potency after baking at 150°F—which simulates the inside of a metal mailbox or sealed car roasting in the sun—for four hours. Ask your doctor if the drug you're taking is particularly sensitive to extreme heat or cold, and try not to let drugs sit in a very hot or cold mailbox. ■

Manicures

Many women—and even some men—simply feel more attractive and better groomed with manicured hands (and in summer, pedicured feet). Just be smart when you visit a nail salon, or you may take home more than beautiful nails.

Can I get an infection from a manicure?

YES But if you take some precautions, you can greatly reduce your risk.

In most clean nail salons staffed by conscientious workers, you won't have to worry about contracting a serious disease from a manicure or a pedicure; such cases are rare. A study reported in the *Journal of Viral Hepatology* did find a small statistical connection between hepatitis C and manicures, however; if contaminated instruments nick your cuticles or the skin under your nails, there's a small but real chance that the hepatitis virus can enter your bloodstream. But there are far more frequent problems that plague manicure lovers.

One of the most common is paronychia, says D'anne M. Kleinsmith, MD, a dermatologist in West Bloomfield, Missouri. "It's an infection around the base of the nail as a result of having the cuticles cut or pushed back," she explains. That's why you should never let a manicurist do this (or do it yourself); your cuticles protect your nails from infection. The bugs at work can be *Candida albicans* (a type of yeast), *Staphylococcus* bacteria, or others.

To stay safe, whether you're having a manicure or pedicure, use these tips.

• Make sure both the salon and the workers are licensed.

• Bring your own manicure tools, such as nail clippers and emery boards.

• Ask how tools are sterilized; the salon should use an autoclave or soak tools in a disinfectant solution for at least 10 minutes.

• Don't patronize a salon that smells of fumes; it's a sign of dirtiness and poor ventilation.

• Notice whether the nail technician washes her hands before working on a client. If she doesn't, the hygiene standards are too low. Go elsewhere.

• Wash your own hands thoroughly with an antibacterial soap before the manicure.

• Don't trim or push back your cuticles, and don't allow the manicurist to do so.

• Don't let the technician clean under nails with an instrument; it's not necessary. "This will frequently break the seal that keeps the skin attached to the underside of the nail plate," says Dr. Kleinsmith. The nail then lifts, inviting yeast, bacteria, or fungi to breed underneath it.

• Get a "polish change" instead of a full manicure. It can yield similar results if your nails are in good shape.

• Don't shave your legs before having a footbath; this will help prevent an infection (from the common *Mycobacterium*) that causes boils and may require antibiotics to treat.

Are glue-on nails risky?

YES Make sure the nail technician is highly experienced in applying artificial nails; a shoddy job can allow bacteria can grow between the real and artificial nails. Also, "since the acrylic nails are so tough, the nail will frequently be lifted off the underlying skin, again leading to various infections," says Dr. Kleinsmith. If you still want glue-on nails, don't wear them for longer than a month. ■

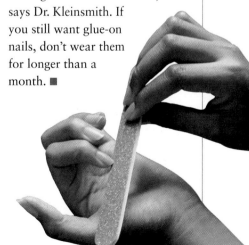

MICROWAVE OVENS

Microwave Ovens

The wondrous technology that boils water in a minute and cooks a hot dog in 55 seconds doesn't carry any particularly scary health concerns—as long as you use the right materials and respect the power of the phenomenon called superheated liquid. And get comfortable with the idea of eating a little plastic now and then.

Are microwave ovens dangerous sources of radiation?

NO Years of studies have found that microwave ovens leak too little radiation to be a health hazard. Just be sure that your microwave never operates while the door is open. If it does, its safety switch is broken and needs repair. Fun fact: The cooking power of microwaves was discovered while the, uh, door was open. In 1940, a British engineer trying to improve radar technology accidentally exposed himself to microwaves leaking from his equipment. A chocolate bar in his pocket melted, and that lit a lightbulb above his head.

Is it safe to use plastic wrap in a microwave oven?

YES But the FDA cautions that you shouldn't let plastic wrap touch the food, since it can melt or allow chemicals to leach into the food.

The bad news: Several terrible-sounding substances can seep from plastic wrap into your food during microwaving—or while stored in the refrigerator, for that matter. One is diethylhexyl adipate, or DEHA, which is used to make plastic wrap flexible and clingy.

Others include polyvinyl chloride and polyethylene. The less-bad news: Animal studies have found that the tiny amounts of these substances that you ingest from microwaved foods are well below toxic levels and probably harmless. At least that's the official verdict as of 2008, and these food wraps have been around for decades. To be safe, follow the FDA's advice and keep plastic wrap from touching the food (give it a one-inch clearance). If you're still worried, use glass or china in the microwave instead of plastic.

What about other sources of plastic, like Tupperware containers? Use only containers clearly marked as "microwave safe," since you can be sure they've been tested. Many plastic containers that are labeled as safe still allow

AVOID GETTING BURNED

We mean that literally. Have you ever heated water for tea in the microwave and had it boil over in a furious froth when you added a tea bag or sugar? That's thanks to a phenomenon called superheated water, or water that's heated past the boiling point. Oddly enough, the water remains eerily still while in the microwave. It's a function of physics, partly due to the smooth container remaining cooler than the water (as microwave ovens heat only the water, while kettles and pots on a flame heat the container as well). To lessen the odds of creating superheated water, put a wooden coffee stirrer or a spoonful of sugar or salt in the cup before microwaving.

Another potential burn hazard: Ready-to-microwave soups. A study at the University of California, Davis, found that these were frequent causes of burns, mostly from spills due to the awkward shape of the containers. Many are tall and narrow, allowing them to tip easily—and spill their hot cargo on you.

minuscule amounts of the aforementioned chemicals to seep into food during microwaving, but again, the white-coats say this is not dangerous to your health.

Never use old yogurt, margarine, or other packaged food containers in the microwave, since they can allow larger amounts of chemicals to seep into your food. And don't use frozen-food trays as microwave dishes more than once. Keep grocery store plastic bags out, too. And while it seems all too natural to throw Chinese takeout containers into the microwave, the sparking metal handles and possible resultant fire will quickly remind you that it's a bad move.

Can I pop microwave popcorn kernels in a brown paper bag?

NO Brown bags (as well as newspaper) are definite microwave no-nos; they can contain contaminants and tiny metal shards that can ignite.

Is it safe to use small amounts of aluminum foil in a microwave?

YES Microwaves can't penetrate aluminum foil, so some advanced chefs use foil to shield certain parts of food that may cook too quickly

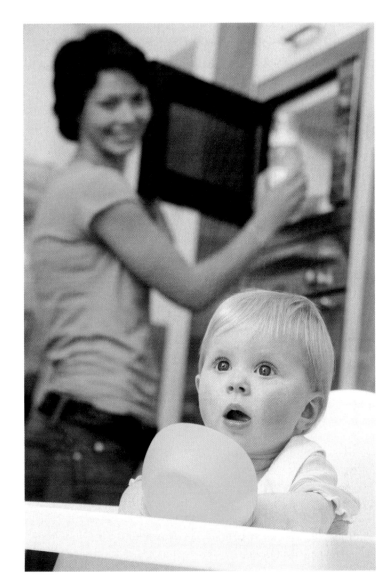

(such as the wings on a Cornish game hen). According to the FDA, if you use new, smooth foil (creases can promote sparking), keep the amount small (no more than a hand's width), and place the foil at least two inches away from the wall of the microwave to prevent burning, all should go well.

Are microwave ovens still a danger to pacemakers?

NO If you had your pacemaker installed more than 20 years ago, ask your doctor if it's safeguarded against microwaves. Otherwise, if it's a current model, passing by or hovering near the oven while it operates poses no threat. ■

Monosodium Glutamate (MSG)

"You will soon develop a headache, flushing, and a general miserable feeling." You probably haven't cracked open a fortune cookie and found those words. But many people who dine on Chinese food say they meet that fate about an hour after they set their chopsticks down—or just about when they're hungry again, according to another scrap of popular wisdom. And MSG gets all the blame.

Is the MSG in Chinese food likely to give you a headache?

NO The best studies to date have shown no link between MSG and headaches or the mysterious "Chinese food syndrome."

In the late 1960s, doctors finally gave a name to the headaches, nausea, and malaise that some patients claimed to experience after visiting their local house of lo mein: They called it Chinese food syndrome. Most researchers pinned the blame on the flavor enhancer MSG, which is made from the crystallized powder of glutamic acid, a naturally occurring amino acid. It has been added to foods for at least 60 years to enhance a meaty, "savory" flavor.

Small, poorly controlled studies in the late 1960s and 1970s seemed to show a link between MSG and Chinese food syndrome. But from the 1980s onward, follow-up studies failed show any strong connection. More definitively, a recent analysis reviewed over 40 years' worth of clinical research and found that those studies "have failed to identify a consistent relationship between the consumption of MSG and the constellation of symptoms that comprise the syndrome." The study also found no evidence linking MSG to migraine headaches or asthma attacks.

So why do we love to vilify it? According to study author Matthew Freeman, CNP, MPH, compared to natural-sounding ingredients like sugar or salt, "monosodium glutamate has a processed, artificial, scientific sound to it," even though it occurs naturally in many foods.

The most telling evidence that MSG doesn't cause headaches is that many people eat MSG every day without visiting Chinese restaurants. Milk, broccoli, peas, grapefruit juice, walnuts, packaged sauces, soy sauce, condensed soup, and Roquefort and Parmesan cheeses are rich sources of MSG—"but nobody has ever complained of a 'Parmesan cheese headache,'" Freeman comments.

Am I just imagining that headache after eating a Chinese meal?

MAYBE Although studies haven't found strong evidence to support this theory, a very small number (less than 2 percent, researchers estimate) of people may indeed have an unusual sensitivity or allergy to MSG—which you could quickly determine by eating the common foods mentioned above. For everyone else, any postmeal suffering could be due to overdosing on salt and fat. Or it could be the placebo effect: If you believe that Kung Pao chicken will make your head throb, it just might. ∎

Salad Bars

There, spread before you, is a cornucopia of nature's fresh bounty, from crisp salad greens to glistening olives to brightly colored vegetables. But "fresh" is relative—and who's to say the person before you didn't sneeze on the food while filling a plate? If you do manage to avoid germs—and if the food's been kept at the proper temperature—can you manage to enjoy a healthy lunch at a salad bar? That depends on what you serve yourself (go easy on the cheese, croutons, and creamy dressings).

Do salad bars pose health risks?

YES Even if the food's been washed properly, it can spoil if not kept at the proper temperature. And customers may introduce germs.

In theory, salad bars seem like a perfect idea. There's no waiting for your food. You can choose from dozens of items and take only those you like. You want exactly 22 bacon bits? Done. Russian dressing only on every third cucumber slice? You have the power—and the stainless steel tongs.

In practice, though, salad bars pose some dangers, mainly due to two unpleasant realities: (1) you aren't the only person enjoying the cornucopia, and (2) the employees caring for the salad bar may be doing a crummy job. Yes, of course, you're always gambling a little whenever you eat a restaurant meal, but salad bars carry extra risks.

First, they're usually stocked with prepackaged raw foods that may not have been washed properly. Second, the foods tend to sit out, exposed to the air, for hours on end. Third, many of the foods need to be kept either very cold (such as salad dressings) or very hot (such as soups) so that bacteria don't breed.

Some foods also need to be tossed frequently. Fourth and maybe most important, the food is constantly fondled, poked, and pawed by that notoriously filthy and careless destroyer of food safety named John Q. Public. That's you and me, with unwashed hands. And our kids, with dirty hands *and* runny noses.

A survey conducted at the University of California found that restaurant salad bar patrons committed all sorts of sins, including handling food with their fingers, ducking their heads under the plastic sneeze guard to reach distant foods, and—no kidding—even dipping their fingers into the salad dressings to get a taste.

Then you helped yourself—and *Salmonella*, *Escherichia coli*, and *Norovirus* may have been waiting for you.

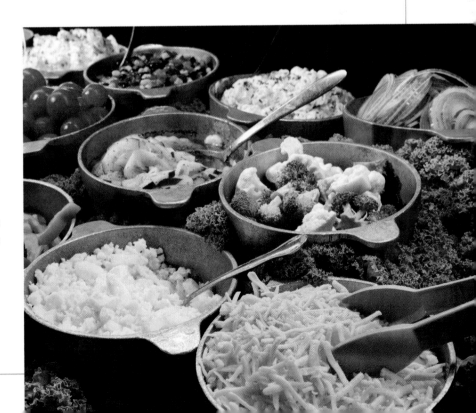

SALAD BARS

Are you likely to get sick?

NO If you use good judgment, the chances that you'll get sick are relatively small.

It's a wonder that more food poisoning outbreaks aren't blamed on salad bars. Exact figures are hard to pin down since many cases of food poisoning go unreported. Of the 1,247 food-borne disease outbreaks reported to the US Centers for Disease Control and Prevention in 2006, which sickened a total of 25,659 people, only 4 were traced back to salad *bars*. Yet nearly 100 were traced to salads of various types and their accoutrements, almost all of which were eaten away from home.

That said, many salad bars offer the healthiest fare that restaurants serve. And if you decide to take your chances, the odds are with you. Even if we triple or quadruple the food poisoning statistics given above to account for unreported cases, your odds of getting sick from a salad bar are still relatively low. In one encouraging study from the United Kingdom, analysis of 2,950 self-service salad bars found that only 3 percent of the vegetables tested had dangerous amounts of bacteria such as *E. coli*. ∎

EATING SAFELY AT SALAD BARS

To reduce your odds of suffering tummy troubles at the hand of a salad bar, do some detective work before filling your plate, advises Joan Salge Blake, MS, RD, LDN, clinical assistant professor of nutrition at Boston University.

• **Look for a sneeze guard** that's difficult for an average-size person to duck under. If there isn't one or it's dirty, off you go.

• **Eyeball the lettuce.** Is some of it brown and slimy? If so, the staff lets the food stay out too long or keeps it too warm.

• **Check for cleanliness.** Are there spills on the salad bar? Are tongs and other utensils in the wrong bins or sitting inside food containers? These are signs of a breeding ground for food-borne bacteria.

• **Look for a supply of clean plates next to the salad bar.** If there are none, and diners refill their own plates, that means salad bar utensils touch dirty plates.

• **Quiz the manager.** Ask at what temperatures he keeps the food in the salad bar. By law, hot food should be kept at 140°F or higher and cold food at 41°F or lower. If the manager can't recite these specific temps to you instantly, take a walk. And don't accept vague nonanswers such as "We keep everything on ice" or "It's electronically controlled."

• **Ask a staffer,** "Do the salad bar vegetables come prewashed, or do you wash them before putting them out?" It's a trick question. "They're prewashed" means "We just rip open the bags and fill the bins," in which case you should leave and find a restaurant with a staff that at least *tells you* they wash the food.

• **Watch how meticulously the staff cares for the salad bar.** Do they change foods frequently and whisk away empty bins quickly? Do they wear gloves when touching the food?

• **Choose plain oil-and-vinegar dressing.** Vinegar isn't a friendly host for bacteria.

• **Forgo the raw sprouts unless you really trust the restaurant.** They're prone to bacteria. "Just rinsing them is not okay. They need to be cleaned properly [and need] safer handling and storage," says Blake.

Sleeping Pills

Swallow a pill, succumb to sleep. If you're a chronic or occasional insomniac, it sounds too good to be true—and it usually is. While sleeping pills do help many occasional users get a little extra shuteye (the operative word is *little*), others find their side effects worse than losing sleep.

Can sleeping pills be dangerous?

YES But most side effects are more annoying than risky.

From the looks of sleeping pill sales, more people are popping pills than counting sheep. But apart from the real question of whether or not the pills work (see page 303), there is the issue of safety.

The bottom line: Generally speaking, sleeping pills are indeed safe. "The most common risks are daytime sedation or hangover effects," says Karl Doghramji, MD, director of the Jefferson Sleep Disorders Center at Thomas Jefferson University Hospital in Philadelphia. "The morning after taking them, people may have sleepiness, fogginess, imbalance, dizziness, wooziness, forgetfulness, and sometimes some depression." In other words, you may feel like half of your brain is still asleep—and the other half is not happy about being awake.

Drugs with short half-lives (which means they exit your system faster) are less likely to give you a medication hangover the next morning. They also help you fall asleep faster. Popular pills with short half-lives (under three hours) include zolpidem (Ambien), ramelteon (Rozerem), and zaleplon (Sonata). These are best for people who have trouble falling asleep but no problem staying asleep. Sonata has the shortest half-life.

Other than feeling groggy the next morning, some people may experience other side effects, such as an allergic reaction, dry mouth, or headache, but these are uncommon.

Also uncommon are the kinds of truly bizarre side effects that have grabbed headlines. Some Ambien users reportedly had sleepwalking incidents in which they stuffed themselves full of food or drove their cars—and remembered nothing of it the next morning. Others complained of hallucinations. Soon similar reports involving triazalam (Halcion), Sonata, and other pills surfaced. However, the number of sleeping-pill takers who experience such odd side effects is very low (less than 1 percent).

There's one big caveat with both prescription medications and over-the-counter sleep aids: There are no reliable long-term studies showing that *prolonged* use of sleeping pills is safe, as studies generally lasted only weeks or months. These pills aren't intended to be taken for long periods.

Are they addictive?

YES But only psychologically, not physically.

Clinical studies—many of which are admittedly short, lasting only several months at the longest—show that sleeping pills are generally not *physically* addictive. Your body doesn't crave them the way a junkie craves the next fix. Most doctors' experiences with the drugs show this as well. Sleeping pills can, however, be very *psychologically* additive, says Dr. Doghramji.

"All of these sleeping medications can cause rebound insomnia," he explains. In other words, if you take the drug for too many days in a row, it may be even harder to fall asleep when you stop.

STYROFOAM CUPS

Sleeping Pills
(continued)

Rebound insomnia can lead people to continually experiment with new drugs and dosages as their insomnia persists. Interestingly, the condition is more likely in people who take sleeping pills with short half-lives.

Are sleeping pills less safe for elderly people?

YES And for those who are seriously ill. It's rare, but sleeping pills can put these vulnerable folks into a *deep* sleep—permanently.

"Most sleeping pills have the possibility of causing respiratory suppression," explains Dr. Doghramji. In plain English, enough of the drug will cause you to stop breathing. Many varieties of sleeping pills contain a benzodiazepine, a drug that depresses your central nervous system. Frail people who aren't in good health can be especially susceptible to the drug's sedating effects, and their central nervous systems may shut down. As long as a person doesn't overdose on sleeping pills, the risk of respiratory suppression is usually a worry only for elderly or extremely sick people who are already in a weakened state. They should take sleep aids only under a doctor's strict supervision. ■

Styrofoam Cups

On the one hand, you have to appreciate Styrofoam: It keeps drinks hot or cold and prevents blistered fingers when your coffee is steaming. But aside from its impact on the environment, it also seems like a great candidate to be one of those substances that, one day, we'll find out was killing us slowly.

Do Styrofoam cups leach chemicals into hot liquids?

YES But the amounts are tiny and not harmful, according to the latest science (though not everyone agrees).

In the past three decades, several studies have found that small amounts of Styrofoam (or, to use its chemical name, polystyrene) can indeed "migrate" into foods from containers. Foods or liquids that are hot (like soup) or rich in fat (like ice cream, yogurt, and butter) pull more polystyrene from the cup or bowl— and trace amounts of the substance have even been found in human cells. But the FDA and EPA say that consuming these trifling amounts poses no real health threat. Still, if it buys you peace of mind, it can't hurt you (or the environment) to switch to reusable mugs. ■

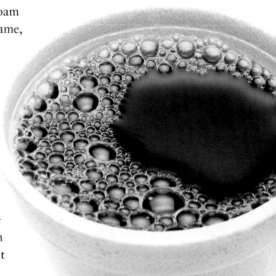

Sushi

Once popular only in Asia, sushi is now a favorite across the world. Even people who once turned their noses up at the idea of eating raw fish are giving it a try. After all, fish is healthful! Or is it? Fears and rumors about sushi abound: Dining on tuna rolls will inject you with toxic mercury, parasites, mercury-contaminated parasites ... What's fact and what's paranoid hype?

Should I worry about the mercury in sushi?

MAYBE If you eat sushi no more than once a week, you should be fine, especially if you avoid bluefin tuna.

Worried about the mercury in your seafood? Overall, experts say the benefits of eating fish far outweigh the risks (except for pregnant women and young children) *if* you avoid the fish highest in contaminants. The trouble is, many of the prized cuts used in sushi come from long-living, larger fish that are ocean predators, such as tuna, king mackerel, swordfish, tilefish, and shark—exactly the fish that tend to contain the most contaminants.

Food safety officials as well as sushi chefs often have little clue how much mercury is in the fish on your plate, as levels can vary greatly even among identical fish in the same catch. One thing is clear, however: Research has shown that a great deal of sushi contains more mercury than experts previously thought—and more than is allowed by law.

In 2007, Oceana, a marine conservation organization based in Washington, DC, tested sushi samples from 23 cities in the United States. They found that a third of all tuna samples had higher mercury levels than the FDA allows, and half of the samples were pretty close to the bar. Soon after the survey surfaced, the *New York Times* had labs test sushi samples from 20 restaurants and stores in Manhattan. They found that 5 of the establishments—or 25 percent—were selling fish that had unacceptably high mercury levels, with bluefin tuna topping the mercury charts. That's no doubt why some environmental groups advise that no one eat bluefin tuna.

Eating just six pieces per week of the sushi the *Times* tested would put a diner's mercury intake over the FDA's safe threshold. Yet experts noted that these levels would probably cause problems only after months of regular consumption.

Yellowfin tuna is a bit lower in mercury than bluefin, according to the Oceana test findings, and will usually be your most prudent tuna option at the sushi bar—but it still contains far more mercury than freshwater fish such as salmon. Of all fish, according to Oceana's report, your lowest-mercury choices include salmon, shrimp, cod, pollock, tilapia, scallops, and mackerel (but not *king* mackerel).

Can you pick up a parasite from eating sushi?

YES But it's, uh, rare. You can get worms from eating raw freshwater fish, such as salmon and herring, but some precautions should ward off all stowaways.

Mercury, worms—you're about ready to bid your local sushi chef a fond farewell, aren't you? Don't. Millions of people on Earth eat sushi regularly and outlive those that don't. Still, that doesn't change an off-putting fact: Sushi eaters have been known to pick up little friends who take up residence in their guts.

The flesh of raw or under-cooked freshwater fish such as mackerel, herring, cod, trout, striped bass, carp, pike, and freshwater eel can have worms that can survive in your gastrointestinal tract—if they

SUSHI

manage to get there alive. (Saltwater fish are less likely to carry parasites, although saltwater salmon can be iffy since it spawns in fresh water. Never order your salmon fillet "rare" at a restaurant.)

In the United States, the Centers for Disease Control and Prevention estimates that there are perhaps a few hundred cases of parasite infection due to consuming raw fish each year. Relatively few are confirmed, because cases are either unreported or undiagnosed (after a few days of nasty stomach pains, some people will vomit or pass the worms, recover, and never know they had visitors).

While they're nauseating to contemplate, the parasites that people tend to get from eating contaminated sushi rarely cause fatal conditions. All the same, take this advice to enjoy sushi without getting an unwanted bonus.

Eat only at *busy* sushi restaurants. "You should patronize reputable seafood stores and restaurants that turn over seafood stock frequently," says Keri M. Gans, RD, MS, spokesperson for the American Dietetic Association in New York City.

Ask the sushi chef how long the fish has been frozen. In the United States and Europe, by law, all fish destined for sushi must be frozen for at least 72 hours (at a temperature between –4° and –31°F) to kill parasites. If the chef boasts, "The fish was never frozen, it's all fresh," mosey on to a better joint.

Ask the chef if he's skilled at "candling." This is a method of detecting worms by holding fish up to a candle. If he seems befuddled, out you go.

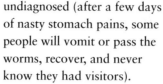
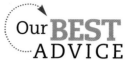

Our BEST ADVICE

If you like sushi, keep eating it. It's packed with protein and healthful omega-3 fatty acids. But to be safe, eat sushi no more than once a week (tests have shown sushi to contain mercury levels that could *potentially* harm even healthy adults if they eat it more often) and avoid bluefin tuna. Women who are pregnant, trying to conceive, or breastfeeding; children under age 5; and people older than 75 or who have an immune system disorder should avoid fish high in mercury, whether it's sushi or cooked seafood.

Notice whether the chef is using gloves to handle the rice and fish. The careful ones do.

Make sure the fish looks fresh. It should be bright and colorful, with deep purples and reds. "The deeper the color, the better," says Gans.

Use wasabi and add vinegar to your rice. Studies have found that this can kill any bacteria on sushi, further lowering the odds of food poisoning.

If you get severe stomach pains or persistent diarrhea in the days after eating sushi, see a doctor. ∎

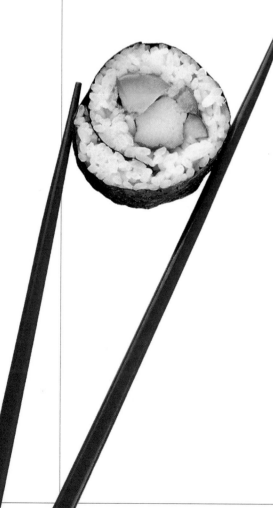

Tanning Salons

Why do many people still use tanning beds? That's a good question. Why do people still smoke? Or drive without wearing seatbelts? The world may never know. But there are no mysteries surrounding the dangers of tanning beds.

Our BEST ADVICE

Instead of a tanning salon, turn to a drugstore bronzer or sunless tanning lotion for a natural-looking tan without the risks—and for less money.

Is it safe to occasionally use tanning salons?

NO They ravage your skin with ultraviolet radiation in far higher doses than you'd get during the same amount of time in the sun. If wrinkles don't scare you, skin cancer should.

The lure of tanning salons is unmistakable: Enter one, and after 20 minutes or so, you can emerge with a tan that may have taken you several hours on the beach to achieve. But there's a serious health tradeoff.

You tan fast in a salon because the tanning bed bombards your skin with a far more powerful dose of ultraviolet radiation than you'd get from natural sunlight in the same time period. This can cause cellular damage, premature aging, and skin cancer—not to mention a scaly sunburn if you stay in too long or temporary blindness because you neglected to wear eye shields. Studies have even found that some people become addicted to using tanning beds, continuing to use them several times a week as they watch their skin suffer irreparable damage.

The dangers are clear. A study conducted at Dartmouth University Medical School found that adults who had ever used tanning beds were 1.5 to 2.5 times more likely to develop basal or squamous cell carcinomas, respectively, which are the most common skin cancers. Another study of more than 100,000 women in Norway and Sweden found that those who used tanning beds once or twice a month were 55 percent more likely to develop melanoma, the deadliest form of skin cancer.

Bottom line: Just like cigarette packs, all tanning beds should carry a large-print warning that reads, "The US National Institutes of Health (NIH) has determined that exposure to sunbeds and sun-lamps is known to be a human carcinogen based on sufficient evidence of carcinogenicity from studies in humans, which indicates a causal relationship between exposure to sunbeds and sunlamps and cancer."

But isn't using a tanning bed a good way to boost vitamin D levels?

NO Proponents of tanning beds (usually tanning bed manufacturers and salon owners) point out that our bodies need exposure to ultraviolet radiation to produce vitamin D. But merely exposing your hands and face to sunlight for a few minutes a day—say, during a walk outside—will allow your body to make adequate levels of D without the hazards of tanning. If your doctor determines that you need more vitamin D than you can produce naturally through normal daily sun exposure, taking a supplement can do the job more safely than using a tanning bed or sunbathing. ■

Tattoos

Today it seems like every other person you meet has a little design somewhere on his or her body. Tattoos are more popular than ever, but they're not without risks—even if you factor out future remorse (more than one in three people eventually regret getting tattoos).

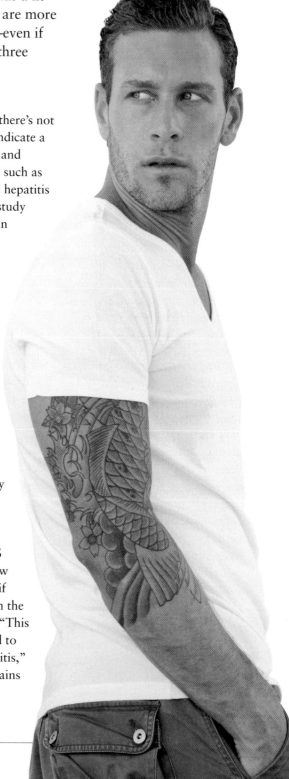

Can I catch a disease from getting a tattoo?

YES It's possible, but not likely, especially if you choose a reputable tattoo parlor.

Dare we say, tattoos are so common they've lost their daring. A whopping 49 percent of Americans ages 18 to 29 claim to have one or more tattoos, as do 28 percent of those ages 30 to 39. In Great Britain, 21 and 35 percent of people in these respective age groups claim to sport at least one tattoo. That's an ocean of ink!

If we can trust the statistics, getting a tattoo from a legitimate artist in a clean parlor is fairly safe. In a Northwestern University study of 500 random tattoo wearers ages 18 to 50 across the United States, few reported any serious or long-term medical problems stemming from their tattoos.

That said, many doctors and health organizations believe that tattoos present a risk for transmitting blood-borne diseases, and they suggest erring on the side of caution. The US Centers for Disease Control and Prevention says there's not enough research to indicate a link between tattoos and blood-borne diseases such as HIV, hepatitis B, and hepatitis C. It cites a 20-year study showing that less than 1 percent of people newly diagnosed with hepatitis C had ever been tattooed. On the flipside, however, a study at the University of Texas Southwestern Medical Center in Dallas found that people who received tattoos in a commercial tattoo parlor were nine times more likely to have hepatitis C than those without tattoos.

Incidentally, the US Red Cross won't allow you to donate blood if you've had a tattoo in the previous 12 months. "This requirement is related to concerns about hepatitis," the organization explains in its blood donation guidelines. It says the waiting period isn't necessary if the tattoo was applied by a state-regulated entity using sterile needles and ink that is not reused, but only a few states currently regulate tattoo facilities, so most donors with tattoos must wait 12 months after tattoo application before donating blood.

Are there other potential dangers?

YES Though unlikely, these range from infection to scarring. Choosing a licensed tattoo artist who uses sterile tools lowers the risks.

While serious diseases and allergic reactions are statistical long shots with tattoos, less serious complications are likelier. A recent study of 824 subjects reported in the *European Journal of Dermatology* found that almost a third of tattoo wearers complained of bleeding or itching as the tattoos healed. Other risks include scarring and bacterial infections (there have even been some cases of antibiotic-resistant infections traced to tattoos). These happen infrequently, but dealing with unlicensed or unclean tattoo artists can increase the odds.

Tattoos have also been known to spread warts, says dermatologist Carolyn Jacob, MD, director of Chicago

Cosmetic Surgery and Dermatology. If the tattoo artist drags a needle through a small wart on the tattoo site, it can spread the human papillomavirus that causes warts to other skin areas. Old tattoos can cause problems with MRI (magnetic resonance imaging) tests due to the magnetic properties of some inks used decades ago.

Is it easy to get a tattoo removed?

NO It may take several painful, costly sessions to remove even a small tattoo, and you could still be left with scarring.

Laser treatments can destroy tattoo pigments and erase tattoos, but they often leave at least some scarring, and certain ink colors are notoriously difficult to remove. Black and dark blue are easy to remove with lasers, while reds, yellows, and greens are more stubborn. "Fluorescent colors, including teal and yellow, are very difficult, if not

Our **BEST** ADVICE

If you want to get a tattoo, stick (sorry!) with a highly reputable artist. Choose a licensed artist who uses disposable needles and clearly shows how the equipment is sterilized. And get a small, dark blue or black tattoo (adding one other color at most) so it can be removed more easily if you decide to do so later.

impossible, to remove," says Dr. Jacobs.

In selecting a doctor to remove a tattoo, insist on a dermatologist who has vast experience in laser tattoo removal, advises Bruce Katz, MD, director of the Juva Skin and Laser Center in New York City. Hint: Pick a specialist who owns (vs. rents) several of the costly lasers used to disintegrate inks. Don't be surprised if that cute $250 tattoo you got in college takes five sessions and $2,500 to erase. ∎

The **US Red Cross won't allow you to donate blood** if you've had a tattoo in the previous 12 months.

TELEVISION

Television

Many of us have a love-hate relationship with the flickering screen we remain glued to for hours a day. No, not the computer—the TV. It was lovingly branded the boob tube back when it fed us four channels and wireless remote controls were still in the realm of science fiction. But is that box your ruin or your reward?

Can watching TV ruin your eyesight?

NO The classic dangers linked to excessive TV watching—mainly by concerned parents, forward-looking social scientists, and assorted curmudgeons—were twofold: Sitting too close to the TV would ruin your eyesight, and watching too much TV would turn your brain to mush. The warnings were often tailored based on the habits of the child being lectured.

Sixty years of ignoring the warnings have proven the eyesight dangers to be a myth, as any ophthalmologist will confirm. As far as the "mush" claim goes, no autopsy has ever revealed the presence of actual mush in a chronic TV watcher's brain, though we do know that stimulating the brain through more challenging pursuits, such as learning to play an instrument or doing crossword puzzles, may help maintain cognitive function.

Then is watching TV totally harmless?

NO While it won't destroy your brain, or your rods and cones, it can do a job on your waist and thighs.

An expanding waistline is the worst danger yet confirmed to come from excessive TV watching. A recent study found that adults who watched more than two hours of TV a day were about 27 percent more likely to be obese than those who watched less than one hour a day. Not surprisingly, the most avid TV watchers were also more likely to have diabetes and high blood pressure, too.

Perhaps more shocking, a study of more than 50,000 women found that each two hours a day spent watching TV raised the women's risk of obesity by 23 percent and their risk of diabetes by 14 percent—even if they exercised as much as women who watched less TV. Why? It isn't completely understood, but one factor is clear: Watching TV spurs snacking. ∎

Our BEST ADVICE

1. Try to watch an average of less than 30 minutes of TV a day. If you have a few days of heavy viewing, get some TV-free days.

2. Make TV time exercise time. Or chore time. Watch TV while you're walking on a treadmill or ironing clothes.

3. Keep your home free of snacks that beg to be eaten mindlessly while you're engrossed in a show.

4. When a fast-food commercial comes on, change the channel.

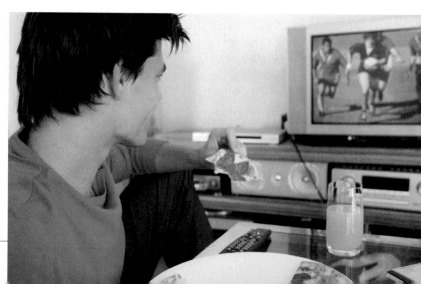

Vaccinations

Vaccinations are undoubtedly one of the most important health achievements of the human race, just about eradicating terrifying diseases like smallpox and polio, once common in our own backyard. When was the last time you heard of someone dying of lockjaw? It probably was not in a developed country or in the past few decades. As wondrous as the benefits of vaccinations are, however, they're not perfect, and we do know they carry some risks. Thankfully, most are minor.

Are vaccinations dangerous?

NO While they may cause unpleasant side effects—or worse problems in a very few people—the known risks just don't warrant fear or serious concern. Being *unvaccinated*, however, can be downright treacherous.

The most common reactions to vaccines are minor muscle soreness or redness at the injection site or a low-grade fever, says vaccination expert Robert H. Hopkins, MD, an associate professor of internal medicine and pediatrics at the University of Arkansas for Medical Sciences in Little Rock. That said, in a small number of people, there are rare problems caused by "live-virus" vaccines such as the measles, mumps, and rubella (MMR) vaccine; the chickenpox (varicella) vaccine; the shingles (zoster) vaccine; and the nasally administered flu vaccine. All of these vaccines use live but weakened viruses to provoke an immune system response, and they're very safe unless given to the wrong people.

"We don't want to give those vaccines to people who have impaired immune systems," says Dr. Hopkins. These include people with HIV, those receiving chemotherapy, or weak and ill elderly people. "The risk is that their immune system may not be able to fight off the weakened virus," he explains. They may develop a "vaccine-associated illness," a condition very similar to the disease the vaccine was intended to prevent. Because doctors are more prudent about to whom they give live-virus vaccines now, this outcome is rare.

Some people have allergic reactions to vaccines, but that's also very rare. Rumors have linked multiple sclerosis and SIDS (sudden infant death syndrome) to vaccinations, but studies have shown them to be unfounded.

Vaccinations decidedly offer more benefits than risks. However, if you believe you or your child has experienced a negative reaction to a vaccination, tell your doctor and then report it to the Vaccine Adverse Event Reporting System at (800) 822-7967 or www.vaers.hhs.gov/reportable.htm.

Has research linked vaccinations to autism?

NO The most exhaustive research to date hasn't found a connection. Further, autism rates are still rising even though thimerosal (one suspected culprit) was removed from vaccines.

In the past decade, there have been persistent rumors that vaccines, specifically the MMR vaccine, may cause some babies to develop autism, a developmental disorder typically diagnosed in the first three years of life. It was fueled by a controversial 1998 study published in the medical journal *Lancet* that suggested there might be a link between autism and the vaccine. But subsequent studies failed to show any connection, and 10 of the 13 authors of the *Lancet* study changed their position.

VACCINATIONS

In a 2004 report on the issue published by the US Centers for Disease Control and Prevention (CDC), the authors concluded that it was time to put the matter to rest, noting that a large review of studies conducted in 2001 by the US Institute of Medicine failed to find any link, as did follow-up studies. "The evidence now is convincing that the measles-mumps-rubella vaccine does not cause autism or any particular subtypes of autistic spectrum disorder," the CDC authors wrote.

But not everyone was convinced. Specifically, some parents believed that thimerosal, a preservative used in the vaccine, gave their kids autism. Thimerosal contains a small amount of mercury, and it's known that mercury toxicity can affect the neurological development of babies and children.

As with the MMR vaccine itself, studies have found no link between thimerosal and autism. In response to the fear and outcry over the use of the preservative, vaccine makers stopped using it in 2001—yet rates of autism continue to rise. Some neurological researchers believe that this increase is due to more liberal and expansive diagnostic criteria for autism that are leading to more children being diagnosed with the disorder, rather than to a medical or environmental pollutant. ∎

BEFORE YOU GET NEEDLED: SOME TIPS

Keep yourself and any young ones in your care up to date on all needed vaccinations. To minimize the already small risks—and to take full advantage of the best that modern vaccination science has to offer—use these tips from Robert Hopkins, MD, of the University of Arkansas for Medical Sciences.

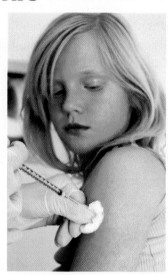

• Schedule a vaccination for when you're feeling well—not when you're saddled with a cold or feeling run down.

• For children who are getting their booster shots, taking an acetaminophen tablet (not aspirin!) beforehand can ease the needle soreness.

• In the days after your child has received a vaccination, don't let him have contact with people who could have impaired immune systems, such as sick or elderly people or those receiving chemotherapy. There's a chance that he could transmit the live virus in a vaccine to the vulnerable person.

• Teens and anyone heading off to college should ask their doctors about getting a meningitis vaccination.

• If it's been 10 years since your last tetanus shot, you probably need another dose.

• Females from adolescence to their midtwenties should ask their doctors about getting an HPV (human papillomavirus) vaccination to lower their risk of cervical cancer.

• On the off chance that you're an adult who's never had chickenpox or been vaccinated for it (the vaccinations started in 1990), ask your doctor if you should be vaccinated. It can be serious in adults.

Video Games

They're addictive, graphic, and much maligned, but video games may not be as evil as some people fear. Will they make your child violent or shorten his attention span? More research will shed new light, but meanwhile, there's at least one known *benefit* of playing the games.

Does playing video games promote violent behavior?

MAYBE Researchers are still arguing the question. Most research suggests that video games may encourage violent behavior only in people who already have violent tendencies.

If you've ever played (or watched someone play) a popular home video game such as, say, Duke Nukem or Mortal Kombat, you know that "violent" is a politely understated description of the virtual adventure. Bodies explode on the screen as you blast away, pumping buckets of bullets into adversaries. You may wonder, How could these games *not* make a person more bloodthirsty in the real world?

Several researchers across the world have investigated the issue, and the answer is somewhat reassuring. While many studies did in fact find that study participants showed greater degrees of aggressive behavior and hostility after playing violent video games, most of the studies suffered from bias—in other words, the research was in some ways designed to come to this conclusion. In a recent analysis of 17 studies, Texas A&M University researchers, correcting for any slanting, concluded that the "studies of video game violence provided no support for the hypothesis that violent video game playing is associated with higher aggression." Playing video games did seem to produce better hand-eye coordination in the study subjects, though.

Other recent research has suggested that if there is a significant or long-lasting link between violent video games and aggression, it's likely only in children and adolescents already prone to violent behavior. Interestingly, while the popularity of graphic shoot-and-kill video games skyrocketed in the United States between 1993 and 2005, violent crimes committed by juveniles *plummeted* by 61 percent.

You'll be hearing more about this debate in the coming years as the experts continue to, uh, duke it out.

Can playing video games contribute to ADHD?

MAYBE Thus far, most studies point to no. People with ADHD tend to enjoy video games, but there's scant evidence that the games cause or contribute to the condition.

Video-game haters like to blame many of society's ills on Pong and its spawn. The highly lamented "short attention span" of the MTV and Nintendo generations is a prime example. Do computer

Playing video games did seem to produce **better hand-eye coordination.**

VIDEO GAMES

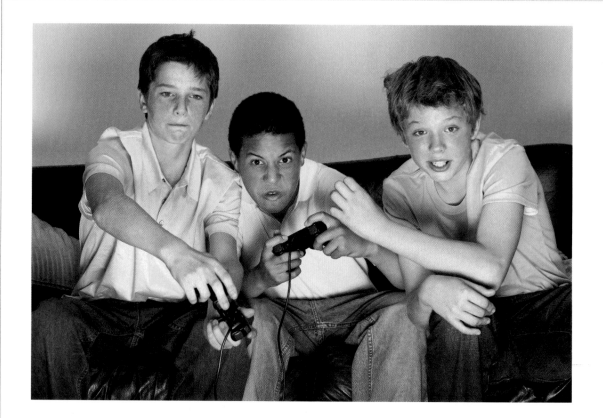

games encourage this phenomenon? More important, can they contribute to attention deficit hyperactivity disorder (ADHD)? It's a good question, and one that hasn't been completely answered.

There have been several small studies investigating the issue, and most haven't found any causal link between video games and ADHD. But there's a definite chicken-and-egg conundrum here. One recent study of 72 high schoolers found that those who played video games for more than one hour a day showed more symptoms of ADHD than those who played for less time. (Only two kids in this study actually had a diagnosis of ADHD.) On the other hand, experts know that children and teens with ADHD (little of this research involves adults) tend to enjoy the rapid stimulation of playing video games, which could explain the connection without implicating the games.

"More severe symptoms of inattention and ADHD behavior were found in students who played video games for more than one hour," the researchers noted, but "it is unclear whether playing video games for more than one hour leads to an increase in ADHD symptoms, or whether adolescents with ADHD symptoms spend more time on video games."

Our BEST ADVICE

Limit your video game time to less than an hour a day, and set similar limits for youngsters. It may help you both in several ways; the heavy gamers in the study of high school students also got worse grades and had poorer social relationships than those who played video games less than an hour a day.

Research has also found that heavy Internet users are more likely to exhibit ADHD symptoms, but again, studies haven't pinned down any causal effect. ∎

Vitamins and Minerals

They're sold over the counter, right next to the toothpaste. Some look like Fred Flintstone. So vitamin and mineral supplements must be perfectly safe, right? Not so fast. Even though smart people you know take them, these supplements can be dangerous in certain dosages and circumstances. Sometimes they can even kill. Even old friends like vitamins C and E can turn on you.

Can taking vitamin and mineral supplements be risky?

YES Though most are dangerous only at high doses.

The government makes sure that the vitamin and mineral pills lining drugstore shelves have been tested for safety and efficacy, right? Wrong.

If you thought that was the case, don't feel bad. A poll found that more than 50 percent of people believe that dietary supplements (from vitamins and herbs to fish-oil capsules) go through the same testing and approval procedures that prescription drugs undergo. That's not the case in the United States and many other countries. The FDA doesn't regulate these products and will typically intervene only if manufacturers start making unsubstantiated claims (such as "Cures Cancer in

7 Days!") or, as happens very rarely, consumers start dropping dead after taking a product.

That means it's up to consumers and their doctors to decide if taking a certain supplement is a good idea. Fortunately, most vitamin and mineral supplements are dangerous only when they contain ultra-high doses of certain nutrients or if you take too many of them. See "How Much Is Too Much?" on page 387 to find out just that.

For more details on common vitamins and minerals, see page 210.

Is it easy to overdose on vitamins and minerals?

YES Sadly, it's all too easy to take "megadoses" of certain vitamins and minerals.

Some supplement manufacturers try to impress consumers with a "more is better" approach. You can easily find multivitamins or single-nutrient supplements that contain doses close to or even above the Tolerable Upper Intake Levels.

In recent years, new data has brought shocking revelations about supplements once considered extremely safe. None was quite as jarring as the 2004 study analysis involving 136,000 subjects conducted by researchers at Johns Hopkins School of Medicine in Baltimore. They found that subjects who took daily supplements of 400 to 800 IU of vitamin E—the amount you find in most over-the-counter formulations—had a higher risk of premature death than those who took placebos. Since vitamin E was the darling supplement of the 1990s, with dozens of small studies suggesting that it offered benefits such as preventing heart disease and dementia, this finding sent shockwaves through the health community.

Not long after this, Danish researchers reported in the *Journal of the American Medical Association* that using

VITAMINS AND MINERALS

antioxidant formulations containing beta-carotene, vitamin A, and vitamin E not only offered study subjects no tangible benefits but also slightly increased their chances of death. (Vitamin C takers also saw no benefits, though they suffered no harm.)

Keep these findings in mind when reading about the potential benefits of the new "hot" vitamin or mineral supplement making headlines. As more research is done, we may again see today's super-nutrient become tomorrow's killer pill.

Do I really need to check with my doctor before taking a supplement?

YES Many common supplements can react dangerously with certain prescription drugs.

Supplements can interfere with or even increase the action of a prescription drug, and the results can be dangerous. For example, folic acid can interact with anticonvulsant medications. And if you're taking a blood thinner such as warfarin (Coumadin) or aspirin, you shouldn't take vitamin E, vitamin K, garlic, fish oil, or ginkgo biloba, all of which also thin the blood. Too much blood thinning could possibly cause bleeding in the brain.

According to the US National Institutes of Health (NIH), if you're taking a cholesterol-lowering statin drug and niacin to reduce your risk of heart disease, avoid antioxidant supplements (which may contain vitamin C, vitamin E, selenium, and beta-carotene). They can reduce the gains in "good" HDL cholesterol produced by the statin drug and niacin.

Finally, smokers should avoid supplements that contain more than 3,000 IU of vitamin A (or beta-carotene),

Our BEST ADVICE

Consumer groups have found that as many as one-third of supplements analyzed contain doses much lower or higher than their labels indicate. If you want to take a supplement, choose a product that bears the United States Pharmacopeia (USP) verification symbol, indicating that the product has met certain quality and consistency standards. Nature Made is one such brand.

which is about the amount you'll find in many multivitamins. Studies have found that taking supplements with high doses of beta-carotene can increase a smoker's risk of contracting lung cancer, though getting beta-carotene from foods such as spinach, kale, squash, and apricots poses no risk. ■

Supplements can interfere with or even increase the action of a prescription drug, and the results can be dangerous.

How Much Is Too Much?

Below are the daily Tolerable Upper Intake Levels (or ULs) of several common nutrients as determined by the US National Academy of Sciences—and what can happen if you exceed those limits for days or weeks at a time. These are *not* the recommended daily doses but the maximums you should never exceed.

NUTRIENT	DAILY UL*	WHAT **MAY** HAPPEN IF YOU EXCEED THE UL
Vitamin A	15,000 IU	Nausea, vomiting, blurred vision, headaches, reduced bone density, birth defects.
Vitamin B_3 (niacin)	35 mg	Flushing, rashes, nausea, liver damage.
Vitamin B_6	100 IU	Numbness in hands and feet, nerve damage.
Vitamin B_9 (folic acid)	1,000 mcg	Could mask a vitamin B_{12} deficiency until irreversible neurological changes occur.
Vitamin C	2,000 mg	Nausea, kidney stones, increased absorption of iron.
Vitamin D	2,000 IU	Nausea, vomiting, constipation, weakness; effects can include heart rhythm abnormalities, mental confusion, and kidney damage.
Vitamin E	1,500 IU	Dizziness, fatigue, headache, weakness, blurred vision. May interfere with absorption of other vitamins; may cause internal bleeding or stroke if mixed with blood-thinning medications. Taking daily doses of vitamin E as low as 400 IU may cause increased risk of premature death.
Calcium	2,500 mg	Decreased absorption of other minerals, kidney stones, impaired kidney function.
Iron	45 mg	Over time, iron can accumulate in the body, possibly causing cirrhosis or cancer of the liver or damage to the heart and pancreas.
Magnesium	350 mg	Nausea, confusion, diarrhea, abdominal cramps, muscle weakness, low blood pressure, irregular heartbeat, kidney damage.
Selenium	400 mcg	Nausea, vomiting, diarrhea, hair loss, nail brittleness, numbness in hands and feet.
Zinc	40 mg	Although usually seen only with consumption of extremely large doses—300 mg to 1 g a day—too much zinc can cause nausea, vomiting, diarrhea, headaches, and impaired immune system function.

*Tolerable Upper Intake Level

X-RAYS

X-rays

The hard truth? Even minuscule doses of x-ray radiation can give you a tiny boost in cancer risk—but refusing to undergo a necessary x-ray is almost certainly more dangerous to your health. Look at it this way: Statistically, your daily commute to work is more dangerous than getting nuked on the x-ray table.

Do x-rays pose a significant cancer risk?

NO If you undergo diagnostic x-rays very infrequently, like most people, the low doses of radiation shouldn't harm you—unless you're a child or a pregnant woman.

When your arm is broken in three places, the last thing you want to think about is getting cancer from the hospital x-ray machine. But it can creep into your mind—especially after you've been zapped 11 times at slightly different angles. And honestly, even "routine" dental x-rays don't feel so routine when the technician drops a lead cloak on you and leaves the room before unleashing the electrons. In either case, is there cause for worry?

That depends on how much you like to worry.

X-rays *do* cause cell mutations and cancer, but the risk is small and difficult to avoid given the benefits (and necessity) of x-ray testing. How small is that small risk? In an analysis spanning 15 countries, British researchers found that the risk of contracting cancer by age 75 specifically due to diagnostic x-rays was about 0.6 percent in the United Kingdom—meaning that about 700 people a year were likely to get cancer from x-ray exposure. In the United States, the rate was 0.9 percent. (Since you asked, the most common malignancies were leukemia and bladder, breast, and colon cancer.) In other words, x-rays are a far less significant cause of cancer than factors such as smoking, poor diet, sun exposure, and genetic vulnerabilities.

Naturally, the risk from x-ray tests depends on how many and which type you get. Some deliver a much bigger dose of radiation than others. For example, a computed axial tomography (CT or CAT) scan of the chest exposes you to 10 millisieverts (mSv), or about as much radiation as you're likely to be exposed to naturally in three years. A mammogram, on the other hand, may expose you to only about 0.7 to 1.0 mSv, or the amount of radiation you'd be exposed to naturally in three months. Dental x-rays expose you to even less—about the amount of radiation you'd get from nine hours of flying at 30,000 feet in a jet. See page 235 for more details.

Can x-rays be harmful to babies and children?

YES Studies have found that pregnant women who undergo x-rays are more likely to have underweight babies or babies with birth defects. A recent study found that Israelis who underwent CT scans as children were slightly more likely to die from cancer in adulthood than those who didn't have pediatric CT scans. The risk was "small but not negligible," according to the researchers. CT scans expose patients to much greater amounts of radiation than traditional x-rays or magnetic resonance imaging (MRI) tests, which may account for the greater cancer risk seen in the study. ■

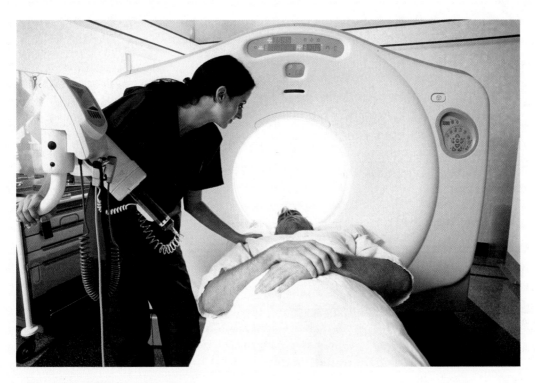

MINIMIZING YOUR RISK

When you need an x-ray, you probably *really* need it—so don't fret too much over radiation risks unless your lifetime tally of x-rays is unusually high, you've had occupational exposure to radiation, or your doctor considers it a worry. But if you want to further minimize the already low risks of x-ray radiation, follow this advice.

• Opt for an MRI over a CT scan when possible.

• Be extremely cautious about exposing unborn babies and children under 10 to x-rays.

• Be judicious (if that's possible, given your circumstances) about undergoing x-rays or CT scans of the chest, cervical spine, pelvis, or hips. They expose more vulnerable organs (such as the breasts and bladder) to radiation and involve higher doses of radiation than other tests.

• Avoid barium enemas.

• If you're a woman, ask your doctor if you should be tested for the BRCA 1 and BRCA 2 genes for breast cancer and how the results may change your mammography options. Evidence suggests that women with these genes are much more vulnerable to mammogram radiation risks and should consider MRI testing as an alternative.

Finally, you may need dental x-rays only every two to three years if you don't have any unusual dental problems, according to the American Dental Association. Your dentist will advise you on the best (and safest) interval to nip any problems in the bud.

YOGA

Yoga

Whether you're into Hatha or Ashtanga, Bikram or Kundalini—or simply trying to keep up with the other 19 people twisting on gym mats at 6:00 a.m.—yoga can pay big dividends. Boosting your balance and flexibility is just the start. Yoga can make you feel stronger, younger, and more energetic. If done carelessly, however, it can also injure you.

Can yoga be risky to your health?

YES Even this relatively safe activity may cause injury by overstretching you or putting pressure on vulnerable parts.

The millions of people who practice yoga know the benefits well. It can help alleviate everything from back pain to migraine headaches, build balance, and offer a haven of serenity in a hectic day. Of course, that doesn't mean it's perfectly safe. Sure, if you're new to yoga, even a session with nothing more difficult than a few downward dog poses may leave you sore the next day; that's normal. Many newbies are surprised to find out just how vigorous certain types of yoga can be.

Most risks from yoga come in the form of sprain and strains. "The most common injuries are overuse or 'pushing too hard' injuries," says Kelly McGonigal, PhD, editor in chief of the *International Journal of Yoga Therapy*. She notes, however, that yoga can also pose specific hazards to people with certain problems like the following.

Osteoporosis: "Some basic yoga moves—such as unsupported forward bending and twisting—will be more risky for this group," says Dr. McGonigal, as weakened bones may break, especially in older participants. "Individuals with osteoporosis will need to find a teacher who knows how to work with the special risks of the condition."

Glaucoma: "Individuals with pressure-related eye disorders should also find a teacher with some knowledge of this condition, as poses that put the head below the heart can be risky," explains Dr. McGonigal. Some research and case reports suggest that inversion moves—such as a headstand or any other pose that puts your head lower than your heart—can increase ocular pressure and make these eye conditions worse.

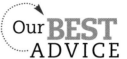

Our BEST ADVICE

Ask your doctor if you have any health problems that could be aggravated by yoga. Take classes with a knowledgeable instructor whose training style makes you comfortable (currently, there is no national yoga certification). Let the instructor know if you have vulnerabilities such as deteriorated knee cartilage, lower-back pain, or a spinal disk problem. Ask the instructor to let you know when to skip or modify a pose to avoid injury. Finally, don't overdo it. It's better to be jealous of more advanced classmates than to be laid up.

What's more, "Everyone should be cautious about breathing exercises that require holding the breath or breathing very rapidly and forcefully," says Dr. McGonigal. There are some reports showing that this can injure your diaphragm and abdominal muscles. "If it feels aggressive, uncomfortable, or forced, it's probably a bad idea," she adds.

Some of yoga's minor but universal risks stem from its popularity. In an overcrowded class, the unsteady person attempting a difficult pose next to you could fall on you. And the mat you're using could be riddled with germs by the third yoga class of the day. ■

Index

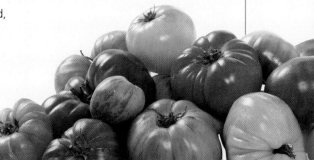

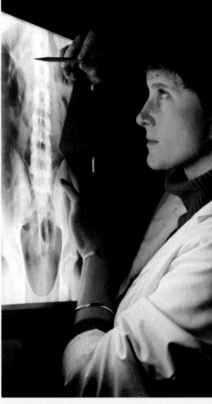

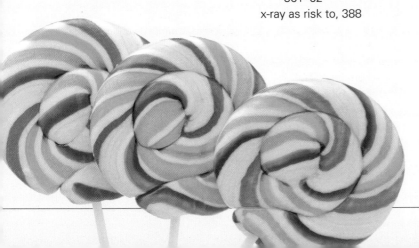

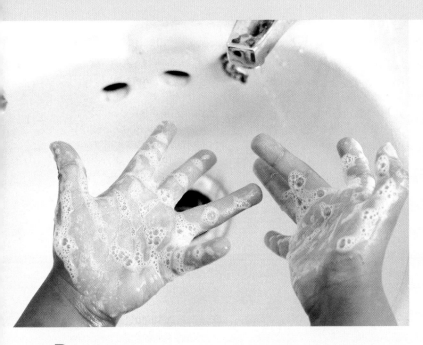

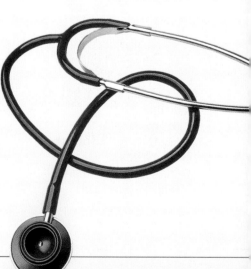

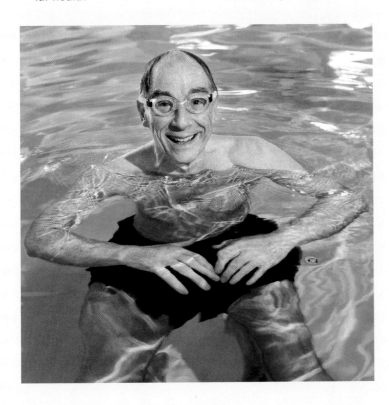

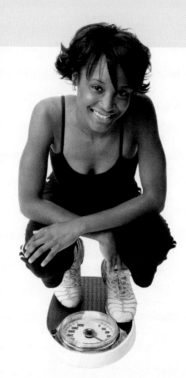

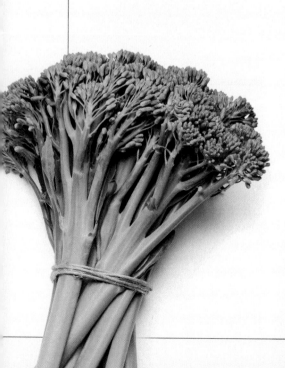

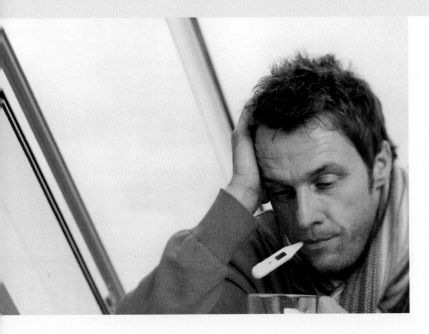

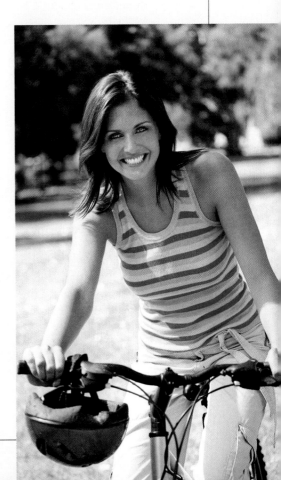

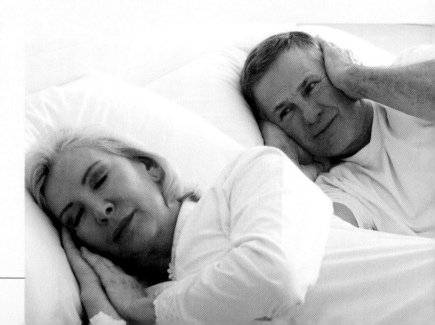

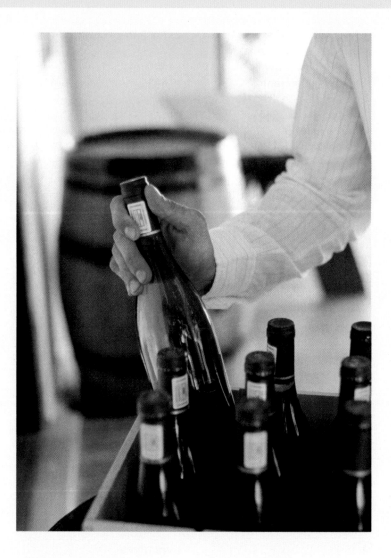

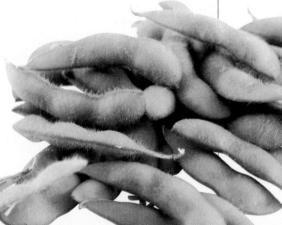

PHOTO CREDITS

Front cover photos courtesy of Getty Images (DAJ, Photodisc, Rubberball, Stockbyte)

Back cover and inside photos courtesy of Jupiter Images (BananaStock, Beauty Archive, Big Cheese Photo, Blend Images, Brand X Pictures, Corbis, Creatas, Dynamic Graphics, FoodPix, i love images, Image100, Image Source Black, Image Source Pink, InsideOutPix, InspireStock, liquidlibrary, MedicalRF.com, Nonstock, PhotoAlto Agency, Photos.com, Pixland, Plainpicture, Polka Dot, Purestock, Rubberball, Somos, Tetra Images, Thinkstock Images, TongRo Image Stock, Workbook Stock)